HIKE LIST

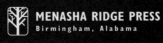

MENASHA RIDGE PRESS
Birmingham, Alabama

60 HIKES WITHIN 60 MILES

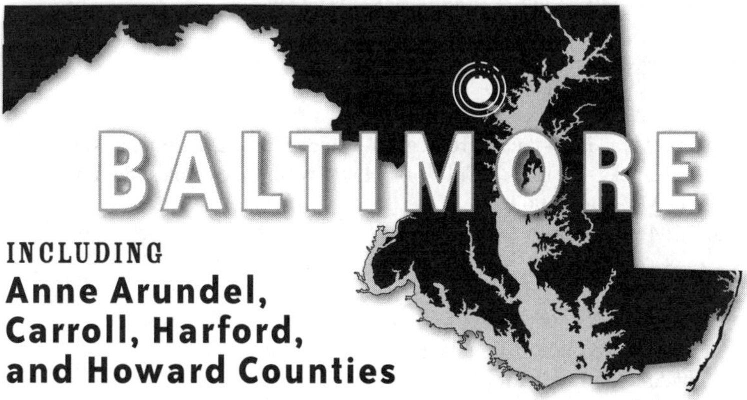

BALTIMORE

INCLUDING
**Anne Arundel,
Carroll, Harford,
and Howard Counties**

SECOND EDITION

EVAN BALKAN

DISCLAIMER
This book is meant only as a guide to select trails in the Baltimore area and does not guarantee hiker safety in any way—you hike at your own risk. Neither Menasha Ridge Press nor Evan Balkan is liable for property loss or damage, personal injury, or death that result in any way from accessing or hiking the trails described in the following pages. Please be aware that hikers have been injured in the Baltimore area. Be especially cautious when walking on or near boulders, steep inclines, and drop-offs, and do not attempt to explore terrain that may be beyond your abilities. To help ensure an uneventful hike, please read carefully the introduction to this book, and perhaps get further safety information and guidance from other sources. Familiarize yourself thoroughly with the areas you intend to visit before venturing out. Ask questions, and prepare for the unforeseen. Familiarize yourself with current weather reports, maps of the area you intend to visit, and any relevant park regulations.

Published by Menasha Ridge Press
Distributed by Publishers Group West
Second edition, fourth printing 2016

Library of Congress Cataloging-in-Publication Data

Balkan, Evan, 1972–
    60 hikes within 60 miles, Baltimore: including Anne Arundel, Carroll, Cecil, Harford, and Howard counties/Evan Balkan. —2nd ed.
      p. cm.
    Includes index.
    ISBN-13: 978-0-89732-692-6
    ISBN-10: 0-89732-692-X
    1. Hiking—Maryland—Baltimore Region—Guidebooks. 2. Baltimore Region (Md.)—Guidebooks. I. Title. II. Title: Sixty hikes within sixty miles, Baltimore.
    GV199.42.M32B342 2009
    917.52'710444—dc22

                    200900362

Cover design by Steveco International and Scott McGrew
Text design by Steveco International
Cover and interior photos by Evan Balkan
Author photo by Shelly Balkan
Cartography and elevation profiles by Evan Balkan, Steve Jones, Scott McGrew, and Jennie Zehmer
Typesetting and composition by Annie Long
Indexing by Jan Mucciarone

Menasha Ridge Press
2204 First Avenue South, Suite 102
Birmingham, AL 35233
www.menasharidge.com

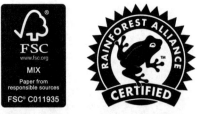

TO AMELIA AND MOLLY—
DON'T LET ANYONE TEACH YOU TO BE AFRAID OF THE WOODS.

—EVAN BALKAN

TABLE OF CONTENTS

ACKNOWLEDGMENTS

I want to thank the many people who create and maintain the trails and areas around them. Their services to the community are invaluable.

I am sorry I did not catch the names of everyone who answered my many questions: the young woman at Irvine Nature Center who identified flowers and birds, another young lady at Hashawha Environmental Appreciation Area who did the same for me there, and the elderly lady cleaning the floors at North Point State Park who told me about her grandchildren. These interactions remain as memories every bit as pleasant as the hikes I did in these places. Of course, these three are by no means an exhaustive list of the many people I came in contact with at the locations in this book. Thanks to all of you.

Special thanks goes to Cheryl Farfaras at the Middle Patuxent Environmental Area. Thanks also to friends Doug Lambdin and Jack Broderick, who accompanied me on some of the hikes. A debt of gratitude goes to Russell Helms at Menasha Ridge, whose exceedingly patient tutorials in the tricky ways of topo software and willingness to make the hard changes in the text that I couldn't bring myself to do were invaluable. A very sincere debt of thanks goes to my wife, Shelly, whose patience and encouragement during this project are extremely appreciated, and also to Amelia, whose smiling face looked out at me from the digital camera I lugged along and often kept me going when my knees began to ache. My family deserves thanks for their general encouragement. I owe my father the biggest debt of gratitude for exposing me to the great outdoors when I was just a boy and for instilling in me a lasting love and awe of the natural world around me. Lastly, I need to acknowledge the best companion a man can ever hope for and who now remains forever in one of our favorite spots—17 years was a good run.

—*Evan Balkan*

FOREWORD

Welcome to Menasha Ridge Press's *60 Hikes within 60 Miles,* a series designed to provide hikers with information needed to find and hike the very best trails surrounding cities usually underserved by good guidebooks.

Our strategy was simple: First, find a hiker who knows the area and loves to hike. Second, ask that person to spend a year researching the most popular and very best trails around. And third, have that person describe each trail in terms of difficulty, scenery, condition, elevation change, and all other categories of information that are important to hikers. "Pretend you've just completed a hike and met up with other hikers at the trailhead," we told each author. "Imagine their questions; be clear in your answers."

An experienced hiker and writer, author Evan Balkan has selected 60 of the best hikes in and around the Baltimore metropolitan area. From urban hikes through the heart of Baltimore to the isolated and rural places of Carroll and Baltimore counties, along beaches, rivers, Chesapeake Bay, piedmont foothills, even a prairie, Evan Balkan provides hikers with a great variety of hikes, and all within 60 miles of Baltimore.

You'll get more out of this book if you take a moment to read the Introduction explaining how to read the trail listings. The "Topographic Maps" section will help you understand how useful topos will be on a hike, and it will also tell you where to get them. And though this is a "where-to," not a "how-to" guide, those of you who have hiked extensively will find the introduction of particular value.

As much for the opportunity to free the spirit as well as to free the body, let these hikes elevate you above the urban hurry.

All the best,
The Editors at Menasha Ridge Press

EVAN BALKAN

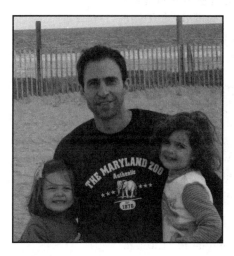

Evan L. Balkan teaches writing and literature at the Community College of Baltimore County. His fiction and nonfiction, mostly in the areas of travel and outdoor recreation, have appeared in numerous publications throughout the United States, as well as in Canada, England, and Australia. He holds degrees from Towson, George Mason, and Johns Hopkins universities, and he lives in Lutherville, Maryland, with wife Shelly and daughters Amelia and Molly.

PREFACE

A good walk is therapy. The fresh air, the sights, sounds, and smells of the natural world: these things can fill a person's senses better than any artificial stimulant. Maryland has long been a leader in programs combating urban sprawl and preserving open spaces. Indeed, what makes Maryland and specifically the Chesapeake watershed the "Land of Pleasant Living" is the wonderful mix of suburban and rural. There is nothing you could want, whether a cultural or historical attraction or a solitary walk in the woods, that you can't find in and around Maryland's largest city.

Maryland is a very varied state topographically, packing extraordinary diversity into a relatively small area. Home to mountains in the west, Atlantic coastline in the east, and the country's largest estuary splitting the state in the middle, everything a nature lover could want is within a few hours' drive. This diversity led Gilbert Grosvenor, the first editor of *National Geographic,* to nickname Maryland "America in Miniature."

This moniker can apply specifically to the Baltimore area. A good-sized city (the country's second largest through the first half of the 19th century), Baltimore is endowed with many fine attractions. But surprisingly to many people—even many who live in the city—Baltimore is also home to an abundance of hiking opportunities. This is a pleasant revelation, coming as it does in an area where millions of people make their homes. Before I began working on the first edition of this book, I thought I was familiar with most, if not all, of these opportunities. I couldn't have been more wrong. It has been an incredible thrill to discover the multitude of places nearby where I can go for a great hike, and in many of these locations I had the place to myself. Amazing to me was the fact that I found even more great places as I began to work on this edition, and I realize now that I haven't even come close to exhausting the options. To that end, I've tried to point out nearby hiking opportunities for many of the hikes in this book.

The basic idea in this book is to catalog 60 hikes within 60 miles. As you'll notice when you look at the locations of these hikes, virtually all of them are within 30 miles of Baltimore. This is intentional. First, you don't need to travel very far from the city center to find great places to hike. Further, as anyone who has sat for hours on I-695 knows, traffic can be tough, and 60 miles often does not equal an hour. Only three of the hikes, Elk Neck State Park, Elk Neck State Forest, and Fair Hill Natural Resource Management Area (all in Cecil County) push the 60-mile limit. But anyone who has hiked in these locations can certainly attest to their deserved inclusion in this book.

It would be an impossible task to include every great hiking destination within 60 miles, and surely at least a few readers will be chagrined to see that their favorite spot was not included. For example, Catoctin Mountain Park and Cunningham Falls State Park, outside Frederick, are within 60 miles of Baltimore and are fantastic places for hiking, but these locations are covered in Paul Elliott's excellent book *60 Hikes within 60 Miles: Washington, D.C.* Because of the thoroughness of that book, I concentrated most of the hikes in this book in the city, north and east of Baltimore, and in the southern and southwestern suburbs. Many hikes in northern Howard and Anne Arundel counties are represented here. In addition, you'll find hikes in Harford, Carroll, and Cecil counties.

My goal in choosing the hikes was to create as much of a spectrum as possible. I chose each hike for its special historical and/or natural interest. The result is 60 hikes that offer a wide array of geographical and topographical diversity.

CHANGES TO THE SECOND EDITION

As a general rule, I've largely eliminated those hikes that could more reasonably be called "walks." Because the average hiker moving on level terrain covers roughly 3 miles per hour, I decided that hikes under 3 miles could be argued as not being hikes at all. (Of course, many of the hikes profiled in this book can be easily shortened if you're short on time.) Accordingly, almost every hike in this book is now 3 miles or more, meaning that hikes could last anywhere from an hour to all day. There are exceptions; notably, Rocks State Park: Falling Branch Area, with Kilgore Falls, which is simply too beautiful to miss.

I've added hikes in Gunpowder Falls State Park (GFSP) and Patapsco Valley State Park (PVSP), as well as a new hike at Loch Raven Reservoir. These are true meccas for Baltimore area hikers, and shouldn't be missed. I've still maintained environmental and geographical diversity, but as these three locations are so fantastic and almost limitless, I felt compelled to add to each. GFSP now has five hikes highlighted here; PVSP now has eight; and Loch Raven has four. In each case, I was careful to make the additional hikes ones that didn't simply repeat what existing hikes in the area offered. Specifically, here are the changes from the first edition of *60 Hikes within 60 Miles: Baltimore.*

• **Anne Arundel County:** I eliminated Kinder Farm Park and replaced it with a wild and scenic hike through the Severn Run Environmental Area. The hike is short, less than 2 miles, but the beautiful nature of the area deserved inclusion.

• **Baltimore City:** I've added Phase I of the new Jones Falls Trail, following the asphalt path from Clipper Mill/Woodberry through Druid Hill Park to Fallsway. I've also added mileage to the Baltimore Waterfront Promenade, the Gwynns Falls Trail, and Herring Run Park. Last, I've reconfigured the hikes at Cylburn Arboretum, as well as the hike along Stoney Run, to include portions of Wyman Park and Johns Hopkins University.

• **Baltimore County:** I've added the following hikes: Loch Raven Reservoir: Northwest Area Trails, Patapsco Valley State Park: Alberton and Daniels Areas, and Robert E. Lee Park: Serpentine / Bare Hills. I've added mileage and/or reconfigured the following hikes: Banneker Historical Park–No. 9 Trolley Line Trail, Loch Raven Reservoir: Deadman's Cove, Patapsco Valley State Park: Glen Artney Area, Patapsco Valley State Park: Hilton Area, Patapsco Valley State Park: Hollofield Area, Robert E. Lee Park: Lake Roland, Torrey Brown–NCRR Trail.

• **Carroll County:** I've reconfigured the hike at Union Mills and eliminated the hike at Gillis Falls.

• **Cecil County:** I've added a wonderful hike at Fair Hill Natural Resource Management Area.

• **Harford County:** I've added Gunpowder Falls State Park: Pleasantville–Bottom Loop (it's a beautiful place, and its absence before was a real omission in the first edition). Likewise, I've made significant changes and additions to Gunpowder Falls State Park: Central Area, which appeared in the first edition as Gunpowder Falls State Park: Lost Pond Trail.

• **Howard County:** I've added Patapsco Valley State Park: Pickall and Hollofield Areas, and made changes to Patapsco Valley State Park: Hollofield Area and Patapsco Valley State Park: Orange Grove and Avalon areas.

Two locations—Susquehanna State Park and Robert E. Lee Park—have two hikes because of the very different nature of their main attractions, and the hikes can be combined in one ambitious and strenuous day. Lastly, I should note that I chose many of the hikes because of their proximity to other attractions, many of which are perfect for family outings. So by all means, grab the kids and go! There are few better ways to spend a day.

A quick note: all of the hike directions begin at Interstate 695 (Baltimore Beltway) or I-83 (Jones Falls Expressway or Harrisburg Expressway, depending on what portion you're driving). Check the directions carefully; depending on where you're coming from, there very well may be quicker and easier routes. If you see any mistakes or omissions—or if you simply have comments for me—please e-mail me at **e.balkan@worldnet.att.net.**

BALTIMORE

Bustling in the 1700s, all but leveled in the Great Fire of 1904, and sunk into economic depression for decades after, Baltimore's rise at the tail end of the 20th century is often cited internationally as a leading example of urban renewal. Sparked by the development of the Inner Harbor, as well as the country's first of the now ubiquitous downtown "old-style" baseball stadiums, many grand old neighborhoods that had fallen into decay have rebounded as well. Not surprisingly, many of these border popular urban green spaces.

Baltimore, which is virtually unmatched in this area, constantly surprises and delights visitors with the large amount of green inside this eastern, industrialized city. This didn't happen by accident. From early on, city leaders recognized the need for and value of open spaces. In 1859, they passed a park tax and raised enough revenue to create and preserve a park system, eventually bringing in famed landscape architect Frederick Law Olmsted to design the city's green spaces. Continued attention to these spaces has resulted in the protection and maintenance of more than 7,000 acres of city parkland, much of it in the adjacent parks at Leakin and Gwynns Falls. These two parks make up part of the largest unbroken urban forest in America, no small feat for a city that is one of the country's oldest.

The abundance of so much green space perfectly complements what makes Baltimore so attractive: this eminently walkable city features a patchwork of unique neighborhoods within easy distance of each other. Beyond the glitz of Harborplace, Baltimore's uniqueness can be found in its diverse neighborhoods: the stateliness of Mount Vernon, the historicity and funkiness of Fells Point and Federal Hill, the grittiness and renewal of Hamden and Canton, the beauty and elegance of Guilford and Homeland, the energy of Charles Village, and the cultural attractions (and restaurants) in Little Italy and Greektown. The list goes on. I've heard many first-time visitors exclaim, "I had no idea how charming Baltimore is!"

All of this charm came somewhat slowly, however. For much of Baltimore's history, the city remained first and foremost a maritime destination. Beginning in the 1600s, its deep and wide natural harbor attracted shippers. This attraction grew as Baltimore did, and its position farther inland than any other major Atlantic port allowed for easier delivery to western locations. Likewise, the system of railways and waterways spreading from the city made its allure as a port almost unparalleled for both cargo and people. Indeed, Baltimore Harbor ranked second only to Ellis Island as a port of entry for New World immigrants.

The city played a well-documented and essential role in the War of 1812. The defeat of the British at Fort McHenry prompted Francis Scott Key to pen the words that served as a rallying point for embattled American militiamen and later became our national anthem. Baltimore's proximity to the Chesapeake Bay made it a logical location for canning factories, which packed and exported the bounty of the bay to other parts of the country. Things waxed and waned in Baltimore for years, but recently another renaissance has begun with major development

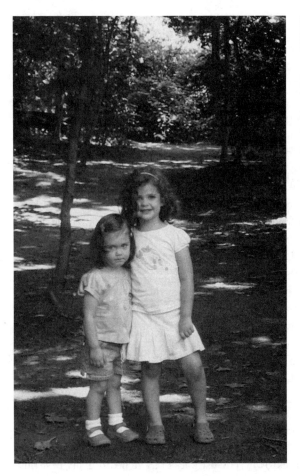

Walking at Robert
E. Lee Park

projects spreading out from the Inner Harbor, which remains the city's major compass point. Major renewals on the west side and Canton waterfront, as well as the addition of a major biopark anchored by Johns Hopkins Hospital, mean that the city continues on its impressive upswing.

Enjoy all the city has to offer, but don't forget about the hiking. The numerous opportunities afforded by our watersheds, rural spaces, and many parks in and around the city help put the charm in Charm City.

THE MECCAS

As I mentioned above, I chose the hikes in this book primarily for their variety in location and topography, but certain locations feature more than one hike, including the state parks at Patapsco Valley and Gunpowder Falls and the reservoir watershed areas of Liberty, Loch Raven, and Prettyboy. These hiking meccas deserve extra attention from the dedicated hiker.

PATAPSCO VALLEY STATE PARK

Patapsco Valley State Park (PVSP) extends along 32 miles of its namesake, the Patapsco River, encompassing more than 14,000 acres in four counties with more than 170 miles of trails, enough to satisfy any hiker. Surprisingly, many of the trails are empty, and you may see 20 times more deer than people. The park has six developed, maintained sections: Hilton, McKeldin, Hollofield, Avalon, Glen Artney, and Orange Grove (the last three share an entrance). Here you will find ball fields, campgrounds, picnic areas, disc golf, playgrounds. A network of maintained trails exists in each of these areas, and I have taken all the separate blazed trails to create long hikes, usually a loop, through each area (a combined hike traverses the Orange

Grove and Avalon areas). I've also included a hike in an unmaintained section of the park, which I've called Granite-Woodstock for its location between those two towns. And, new to this edition, I've added a historic hike through the Alberton and Daniels areas.

GUNPOWDER FALLS STATE PARK

Gunpowder Falls State Park (GFSP) extends almost 18,000 acres along the Big and Little Gunpowder Falls and Gunpowder River. This long, narrow park, which is not always contiguous, envelops a stunning array of topography ranging from tidal marshes and wetlands to steep, rugged slopes. Including the 21-mile Maryland portion of the Torrey Brown–NCRR Trail, which is maintained by Gunpowder Falls State Park but treated separately in this book, GFSP has more than 100 miles of trails. The park also includes three developed areas: Hereford, Central (including Sweet Air, which is popular for equestrian use; Sweathouse Branch Wildlands, popular with bird-watchers and wildflower enthusiasts; and Jerusalem Village, a restored historic town), and Hammerman, plus the NCRR and Dundee Creek Marina. (And for what it's worth, it's now officially my favorite local hiking destination.) With all of these areas to choose from, you can enjoy boat launches, swimming beaches, picnic areas, historic sites, trails galore, and numerous tubing, paddling, and fishing opportunities. You can even stay at the well-appointed Mill Pond Cottage and have park staff arrange itineraries for you. The five GFSP hikes in this book take in the differing areas of the park and, as a result, provide a fantastic mix of scenery.

THE RESERVOIRS: LIBERTY, LOCH RAVEN, AND PRETTYBOY

Loch Raven Reservoir, built in 1881 and holding more than 23 billion gallons, provides the drinking water for most of Baltimore County. Its popularity with joggers, hikers, bicyclists, and fishermen means that parking areas are often at a premium and the chances for solitude are slim. But once you've hiked here, the reasons for its popularity become obvious: it's an absolute gem and a mere 6 miles north of the city line. The four Loch Raven hikes in this book attempt to bring together the best of what the reservoir watershed has to offer.

Every bit as beautiful as Loch Raven, Prettyboy Reservoir in northwestern Baltimore County lies in what is still a relatively rural area and offers the isolation that is sometimes difficult to experience at Loch Raven.

Fishermen routinely catch record-size bass and trout at Liberty Reservoir, which straddles Baltimore and Carroll counties. People also enjoy bird-watching and horseback riding here, as well as hiking, as the two Liberty treks in this book show. Each of these reservoir watershed areas have many more trails and hiking opportunities beyond what this book describes, and I've tried to present the "best of the best." Of course this is a highly subjective choice, and I encourage you to investigate and discover many more of the trails, which are usually marked with orange cables strung between wooden posts, making them easy to spot.

HIKING RECOMMENDATIONS

HIKES LESS THAN 3 MILES IN LENGTH

HIKES 3–6 MILES IN LENGTH

HIKES 6–9 MILES IN LENGTH

HIKES 9-PLUS MILES IN LENGTH

HIKES FEATURING HISTORICAL SITES

HIKES FEATURING HISTORICAL SITES (*continued*)

HIKES FEATURING RIVERS OR LAKES

HIKES FEATURING RESERVOIRS, WATERFALLS, OR CHESAPEAKE BAY

HIKES GOOD FOR CHILDREN

HIKES GOOD FOR CHILDREN (*continued*)

HIKES GOOD FOR SOLITUDE

HIKES GOOD FOR SPOTTING WILDLIFE

HIKES INSIDE THE BELTWAY

HIKES OUTSIDE THE BELTWAY

HIKES OUTSIDE THE BELTWAY (*continued*)

HIKES ACCESSIBLE BY PUBLIC TRANSPORTATION

HIKES GOOD FOR BIRD-WATCHING

60 HIKES
WITHIN 60 MILES

BALTIMORE
INCLUDING

**ANNE ARUNDEL, CARROLL, CECIL, HARFORD,
AND HOWARD COUNTIES**

INTRODUCTION

Welcome to *60 Hikes within 60 Miles: Baltimore.* If you're new to hiking or even if you're a seasoned trail-smith, take a few minutes to read the following introduction. We explain how this book is organized and how to use it.

HIKE DESCRIPTIONS

Each hike contains eight key items: a locator map, an "In Brief" description of the trail, a "Key At-a-Glance Information" box, directions to the trail, a trail map, an elevation profile, a trail description, and a description of any notable nearby activities. Combined, the maps and information provide a clear method to assess each trail from the comfort of your favorite reading chair.

IN BRIEF

A "taste of the trail." Think of this section as a snapshot focused on the historical landmarks, beautiful vistas, and other sights you may encounter on the trail.

KEY AT-A-GLANCE INFORMATION

The information in the Key At-a-Glance boxes gives you a quick idea of the specifics of each hike. The information covers the following basic elements.

LENGTH The length of the trail from start to finish. There may be options to shorten or extend the hikes, but the mileage corresponds to the described hike. Consult the hike description to help you decide how to customize the hike for your ability or time constraints.

CONFIGURATION A description of what the trail might look like from overhead. Trails can be loops, out-and-backs (trails on which you enter and leave along the same path), figure eights, or balloons.

DIFFICULTY The degree of effort an "average" hiker should expect on a given hike. For simplicity, difficulty is described as "easy," "moderate," or "difficult."

SCENERY A rating of the overall environs of the hike and what to expect in terms of plant life, wildlife, streams, and historic buildings.

EXPOSURE A quick check of how much sun you can expect on your shoulders during the hike. Descriptors used include "shady," "exposed," and "sunny."

TRAFFIC Indicators of how busy the trail might be on an average day, and if you might be able to find solitude here. Trail traffic, of course, varies from day to day and season to season.

TRAIL SURFACE A description of the trail surface, be it paved, rocky, dirt, or a mixture of elements.

HIKING TIME The length of time it takes to hike the trail. A slow but steady hiker will average 2 to 3 miles an hour, depending on the terrain. Most of the estimates in this book reflect a speed of about 2.3 miles per hour.

ACCESS A notation of any fees or permits needed to access the trail (if any) and whether pets and other forms of trail use are permitted.

WHEELCHAIR ACCESS Indicates whether all or part of the hike can be enjoyed by persons with disabilities.

FACILITIES What to expect in terms of restrooms, phones, water, and other amenities available at the trailhead or nearby.

MAPS Which maps are the best, or easiest, for this hike, and where to get them.

SPECIAL COMMENTS These comments cover little extra details that don't fit into any of the above categories. Here you'll find information on trail-hiking options and facts, or tips on how to get the most out of your hike.

DIRECTIONS TO THE TRAIL

The detailed directions will lead you to each trailhead. If you use GPS (Global Positioning System) technology, the provided UTM (Universal Transverse Mercator) coordinates allow you to navigate directly to the trailhead.

TRAIL DESCRIPTIONS

The trail description is the heart of each hike. Here, the author provides a summary of the trail's essence and highlights any special traits the hike offers. Ultimately, the hike description will help you choose which hikes are best for you.

NEARBY ACTIVITIES

Look here for information on nearby activities or points of interest.

WEATHER

Hiking can be done pretty much year-round in Baltimore. But as any resident knows, there can be uncomfortable extremes during both summer and winter. While it's not that unusual to get a balmy 60-degree day in December or even January, it's also not unusual to have temperatures with wind-chill readings below zero. A snowfall for an entire winter can sometimes measure a paltry few inches, while several feet of accumulated snow isn't terribly rare either. Likewise, summer days are usually fine for hiking provided you take plenty of water with you. But the sometimes-oppressive humidity that is part of living in the mid-Atlantic region can make some summer days quite unbearable. With the temperature approaching 100° F with 90 percent humidity, it's best to leave the hiking for another day. But generally speaking, these extremes are rare, and you can hike in all seasons. Since the Baltimore area is blessed with pleasant springs and absolutely gorgeous autumns, you may find hiking during these months the most enjoyable, although you may also enjoy the extended light of summer as well as the increased views the leafless winter trees offer.

AVERAGE DAILY TEMPERATURES BY MONTH

	JAN	FEB	MAR	APR	MAY	JUN
HIGH	40°	43°	54°	64°	74°	83°
LOW	23°	25°	34°	42°	52°	61°
	JUL	AUG	SEP	OCT	NOV	DEC
HIGH	87°	85°	78°	67°	56°	45°
LOW	66°	65°	58°	45°	37°	26°

ALLOCATING TIME

I found that the shorter the hike, the more I lingered in one place. Something about staring at the front end of a 10-mile trek naturally pushes you to speed up. That said, take close notice of the elevation maps that accompany each hike. If you see many ups and downs over large altitude changes, you'll obviously need more time. Inevitably you'll finish some of the "hike times" long before or after what I have suggested. Nevertheless, use my suggestions as a guide and leave yourself plenty of time for those moments when you simply feel like stopping and taking it all in.

MAPS

The maps in this book have been produced with great care and, used with the hiking directions, will direct you to the trail and help you stay on course. However, you will find superior detail and valuable information in the United States

Geological Survey's 7.5-minute series topographic maps. Topo maps are available online in many locations. The easiest Web resource is located at **www.terraserver .microsoft.com.** You can view and print topos of the entire United States there and view aerial photographs of the same area. The downside to topos is that most of them are outdated, having been created 20 to 30 years ago, but they still provide excellent topographic detail.

If you're new to hiking, you might be wondering, "What's a topographic map?" In short, a topo indicates not only linear distance but elevation as well, using contour lines. Contour lines spread across the map like dozens of intricate spiderwebs. Each line represents a particular elevation, and at the base of each topo, a contour's interval designation is given. If the contour interval is 200 feet, then the distance between each contour line is 200 feet. Follow five contour lines up on the same map, and the elevation has increased by 1,000 feet.

Let's assume that the 7.5-minute series topo reads "Contour Interval 40 feet," that the short trail we'll be hiking is 2 inches in length on the map, and that it crosses five contour lines from beginning to end. What do we know? Well, because the linear scale of this series is 2,000 feet to the inch (roughly 2-3/4 inches representing 1 mile), we know our trail is approximately four-fifths of a mile long (2 inches represent 2,000 feet), but we also know we'll be climbing or descending 200 vertical feet (five contour lines represent 40 feet each) over that distance. And the elevation designations written on occasional contour lines will tell us if we're heading up or down.

In addition to outdoor shops and bike shops, you'll find topos at major universities and some public libraries, where you might try photocopying the ones you need to avoid the cost of buying them. But if you want your own and can't find them locally, visit the United States Geological Survey (USGS) Web site at **www.topomaps.usgs.gov.** I also recommend **www.topozone.com** as a resource for topographic maps and software.

GPS TRAILHEAD COORDINATES

To collect accurate map data, each trail was hiked with a handheld GPS unit (Garmin Etrex Venture and/or Garmin Etrex Legend). Data collected was then downloaded and plotted onto a digital USGS topo map. In addition to rendering a highly specific trail outline, this book also includes the GPS coordinates for each trailhead. More accurately known as UTM coordinates, the numbers index a specific point using a grid method. The survey datum used to arrive at the coordinates is NAD27. For readers who own a GPS unit, whether handheld or onboard a vehicle, the Universal Transverse Mercator (UTM) coordinates provided on the first page of each hike may be entered into the GPS unit. Just make sure your GPS unit is set to navigate using the UTM system in conjunction with NAD27 datum. Now you can navigate directly to the trailhead.

Most trailheads, which begin in parking areas, can be reached by car, but some hikes still require a short walk to reach the trailhead from a parking area.

In those cases a handheld unit would be necessary to continue the GPS navigation process. That said, however, readers can easily access all trailheads in this book by using the directions given, the overview map, and the trail map, which shows at least one major road leading into the area. But for those who enjoy using the latest GPS technology to navigate, the necessary data has been provided. A brief explanation of the UTM coordinates follows.

UTM COORDINATES—ZONE, EASTING, AND NORTHING

Within the UTM coordinates box on the first page of each hike, there are three numbers labeled zone, easting, and northing. Here is an example from Herring Run–Lake Montebello Park on page 51:

UTM Zone (WSG84) 18S
Easting 363869
Northing 4354855

The zone number (18) refers to one of the 60 longitudinal zones (vertical) of a map using the UTM projection. Each zone is 6° wide. The zone letter (S) refers to one of the 20 latitudinal zones (horizontal) that span from 80° South to 84° North.

The easting number (363869) references in meters how far east the point is from the zero value for eastings, which runs north-south through Greenwich, England. Increasing easting coordinates on a topo map or on your GPS screen indicate you are moving east; decreasing easting coordinates indicate you are moving west. Since lines of longitude converge at the poles, they are not parallel as lines of latitude are. This means that the distance between Full Easting Coordinates is 1,000 meters near the equator but becomes smaller as you travel farther north or south; the difference is small enough to be ignored, but only until you reach the polar regions.

In the Northern Hemisphere, the northing number (4354855) references in meters how far you are from the equator. Above the equator, northing coordinates increase by 1,000 meters between each parallel line of latitude (east-west lines). On a topo map or GPS receiver, increasing northing numbers indicate you are traveling north.

In the Southern Hemisphere, the northing number references how far you are from a latitude line that is 10 million meters south of the equator. Below the equator, northing coordinates decrease by 1,000 meters between each line of latitude. On a topo map, decreasing northing coordinates indicate you are traveling south.

TRAIL ETIQUETTE

Whether you're on a city, county, state, or national-park trail, always remember that great care and resources (from nature as well as from your tax dollars) have gone into creating these trails. Treat the trail, wildlife, and fellow hikers with respect.

1. Hike on open trails only. Respect trail and road closures (ask if you're not sure), avoid possible trespassing on private land, and obtain all permits and authorization as required. Also, leave gates as you found them or as marked.

2. Leave only footprints. Be sensitive to the ground beneath you. This also means staying on the existing trail and not blazing any new trails. Be sure to pack out what you pack in. No one likes to see the trash someone else has left behind.

3. Never spook animals. An unannounced approach, a sudden movement, or a loud noise startles most animals. A surprised snake or skunk can be dangerous for you, for others, and to themselves. Give animals extra room and time to adjust to your presence.

4. Plan ahead. Know your equipment, your ability, and the area in which you are hiking—and prepare accordingly. Be self-sufficient at all times; carry necessary supplies for changes in weather or other conditions. A well-executed trip is a satisfaction to you and others.

5. Be courteous to other hikers, bikers, or equestrians you meet on the trails.

WATER

"How much is enough? One bottle? Two? Three?! But think of all that extra weight!" Well, one simple physiological fact should convince you to err on the side of excess when it comes to deciding how much water to pack: A hiker working hard in 90-degree heat needs approximately ten quarts of fluid every day. That's 2.5 gallons—12 large water bottles or 16 small ones. In other words, pack along one or two bottles even for short hikes.

Serious backpackers hit the trail prepared to purify water found along the route. This method, while less dangerous than drinking it untreated, comes with risks. Purifiers with ceramic filters are the safest but also the most expensive. Many hikers pack along the slightly distasteful tetraglycine-hydroperiodide tablets (sold under the names Potable Aqua, Coughlan's, and others).

Probably the most common waterborne "bug" that hikers face is giardia which may not hit until one to four weeks after ingestion. It will have you passing noxious rotten-egg gas, vomiting, shivering with chills, and living in the bathroom. Other parasites to worry about include *E. coli* and *Cryptosporidium,* both of which are harder to kill than giardia.

For most people, the pleasures of hiking make carrying water a relatively minor price to pay to remain healthy. If you're tempted to drink "found water," do so only if you understand the risks involved. Better yet, hydrate prior to your hike, carry (and drink) six ounces of water for every mile you plan to hike, and hydrate after the hike.

FIRST-AID KIT

A typical first-aid kit may contain more items than you might think necessary. These are just the basics:

- Ace bandages or Spenco joint wraps
- Antibiotic ointment (Neosporin or the generic equivalent)
- Aspirin or acetaminophen
- Band-Aids
- Benadryl or the generic antihistamine equivalent diphenhydramine (in case of allergic reactions)
- Butterfly-closure bandages
- Epinephrine in a prefilled syringe (for people known to have severe allergic reactions to such things as bee stings)
- Gauze (one roll)
- Gauze compress pads (a half dozen 4 x 4-inch pads)
- Hydrogen peroxide or iodine
- Insect repellent
- Matches or pocket lighter
- Moleskin/Spenco "Second Skin"
- Snakebite kit
- Sunscreen
- Water-purification tablets or water filter (for longer hikes)
- Whistle (it's more effective in signaling rescuers than your voice)

SNAKES

Generally speaking, snakes are not a concern in Baltimore, and the prospect of being bitten should never deter a hiker in this area. Maryland has only two native poisonous snakes: northern copperheads, which you may see in Baltimore, and timber rattlers, which live in the western, mountainous part of the state. Although the chances of being bitten by a snake on one of the hikes described in this book are slim to none, take proper caution. If you see a snake and it has an hourglass-shaped head, give it a wide berth.

TICKS

All hikers should be concerned about ticks, especially when hiking along trails that traverse areas of brush and high grass, the insect's favorite hangouts. Your best protection (aside from applying a repellent that contains Deet, which is fairly toxic stuff) is to be vigilant: Check yourself frequently, and look hard. Often the smaller the tick, the greater the chance for subsequent serious health problems. Tiny deer ticks (black-legged ticks), for example, carry Lyme disease; if you find a tick attached to your skin, gently remove it with tweezers, taking care to pull it off gently so the mouth part does not break off and remain attached. Always shower after a hike to wash off any ticks you might not have caught earlier, and check your hair thoroughly with your fingers. (It's a good idea to wear a hat while hiking to prevent ticks from falling from above and burrowing into your scalp.)

In general, ticks pose a major threat only during the warmest months of summer, but an unseasonably mild spring and/or warm autumn can mean a solid six or seven months of "tick season." So do take precautionary measures, but don't let ticks keep you inside. On all of the many hikes and many hours I spent on the trail compiling this book, no tick managed to pierce my skin.

I want to note that Lyme disease tends to be overdiagnosed, but if you see a bull's-eye rash radiating from a tender red spot, see a doctor right away. If you experience flu-like symptoms (intense malaise, fever, chills, and a headache) a day or two after hiking, look very hard for the telltale bull's-eye rash, and see a doctor to alleviate any concerns.

POISON IVY

The old maxim for poison ivy holds true: "Leaves of three, let it be." Poison sumac, however, can contain anywhere from 7 to 13 leaves. Since I am extremely allergic to poison ivy, I always take the following precautions: I do not scratch anything under any circumstances; if poison ivy is sitting on the skin, scratching and then touching skin anywhere else is the surest way of spreading it. Also,

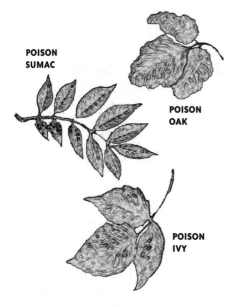

POISON SUMAC

POISON OAK

POISON IVY

Common poisonous plants

in summer I pull up my socks as far as they will go; no, this doesn't look cool, but it's worth it! Third, I always carry alcohol-based moist towelettes, and at the end of the hike, I rub my legs gently with the towelettes to stave off infection until I can get home and shower. (Note: It is very important that these moist towelettes contain alcohol. If they contain just soap, wiping with them will only move the poison ivy oil, urushiol, around, increasing the risk of infection.) Always shower to get rid of any clinging poison ivy oils.

MOSQUITOES

The Asian Tiger mosquito, which spreads the West Nile virus, has been seen in Maryland, especially in places with lots of water, including urban areas. Unfortunately, Baltimore has both (part of its charm, after all).

Protect yourself against mosquito bites by applying an effective repellent. Since many repellents contain toxins, I prefer to use Avon Skin-So-Soft. It has a pleasing smell, and the sweet fragrance repels mosquitoes pretty effectively. Even though West Nile has understandably grabbed headlines in the past few years, your chances of contracting it are extraordinarily slim, and even if you do contract it, a reasonably healthy person who receives medical treatment would be able to stave off the disease's most damaging effects.

HIKING WITH CHILDREN

No one is too young for a hike in the woods or through a city park. Be careful, though. Flat, short trails are best with an infant. Toddlers who have not quite mastered walking can still tag along, riding on an adult's back in a child carrier. Use common sense to judge a child's capacity to hike a particular trail, and always rely on the possibility that the child will tire quickly and need to be carried.

When packing for the hike, remember the child's needs as well as your own. Make sure children are adequately clothed for the weather, have proper shoes, and are protected from the sun with sunscreen. Kids dehydrate quickly, so make sure you have plenty of fluid for everyone.

A list of hikes good for children is provided in the Hiking Recommendations section on page xvi. Finally, when hiking with children, remember that the trip will be a compromise—a child's energy and enthusiasm alternate between bursts of speed and long stops to examine snails, sticks, dirt, and other attractions.

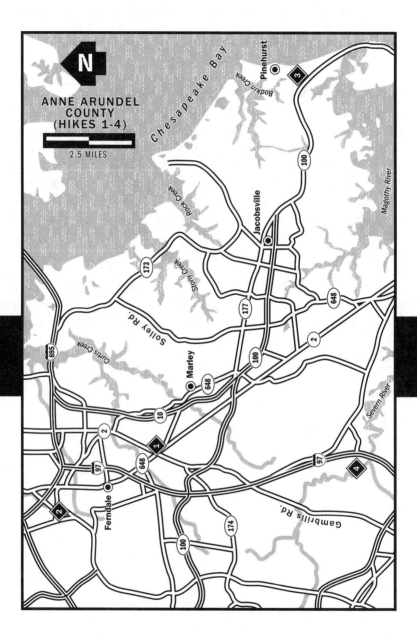

ANNE ARUNDEL COUNTY

01 BALTIMORE & ANNAPOLIS (B&A) TRAIL

KEY AT-A-GLANCE INFORMATION

LENGTH: 12.7 miles (15.5 miles for complete trail)

CONFIGURATION: One-way

DIFFICULTY: Moderate–strenuous

SCENERY: Mixed hardwoods, railroading structures, pocket wetlands

EXPOSURE: Mostly sunny

TRAFFIC: Heavy

TRAIL SURFACE: Asphalt

HIKING TIME: 4–4.5 hours

ACCESS: Sunrise–sunset

MAPS: USGS Relay, Curtis Bay, Round Bay, Gibson Island. A printable map is online at www.aacounty.org/RecParks/parks/aacotrails park/bandamap.cfm.

WHEELCHAIR ACCESS: Yes

FACILITIES: Found all along the trail in nearby businesses

SPECIAL COMMENTS: The hike as described here begins at the Glen Burnie Parking Area and moves south, totaling 12.7 miles. An additional 0.6 miles of trail head north, terminating at Baltimore-Annapolis Boulevard, and a new bike trail adds another 2 miles to Jonas Green Park in the south. Several parking areas along the way make shortening the hike easy.

GPS Trailhead
Coordinates

UTM Zone (WGS84) 18S

Easting 359698

Northing 4336083

Latitude N 39° 9.759471'

Longitude W 76° 37.437007'

IN BRIEF

The B&A Trail is Anne Arundel's linear island in the most congested part of the county. This park is a haven for bikers, strollers, and hikers.

DESCRIPTION

The Baltimore & Annapolis Trail, part of the East Coast Greenway, is a rails-to-trails park that follows the old Baltimore & Annapolis Railroad (1880–1968) from Glen Burnie in the north (not quite Baltimore) to Annapolis in the south. The park itself is 115 acres, running as a 10-foot-wide paved path that follows a more or less straight line along Ritchie Highway and the twistier Baltimore & Annapolis Boulevard to Route 50 heading into Annapolis. It's interesting to note that it was the boulevard and the highway, built to accommodate the increased automobile traffic, that hastened the end of the short line railroad. Nowadays, B&A Boulevard has been increasingly displaced by I-97, the Baltimore–Annapolis Expressway, built to connect Maryland's capital with its largest city. So the railroad corridor, once rendered obsolete, has now become popular again, despite the presence of the boulevard, the highway, and the interstate.

Beginning in the north at Glen Burnie, the trail is fairly urban, with businesses,

-----

Directions ————————————————➤

Take I-695 to I-97 south to exit 15, Aviation Boulevard/Dorsey Road east to Dorsey Road. Take the first right onto MD Route 648, Baltimore-Annapolis Boulevard. Cross Crain Highway and take a right at the "Free Parking" sign in the Glen Burnie Town Center. The trail is just north of the parking garage.

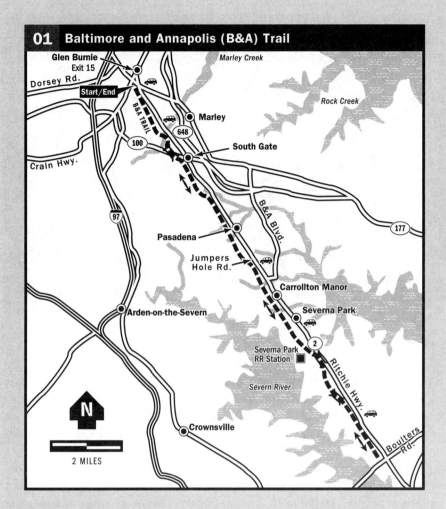

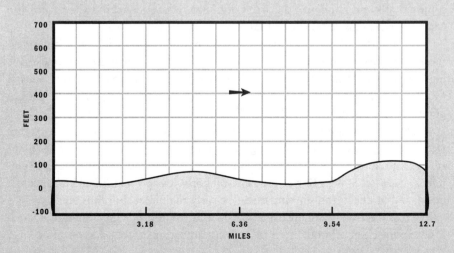

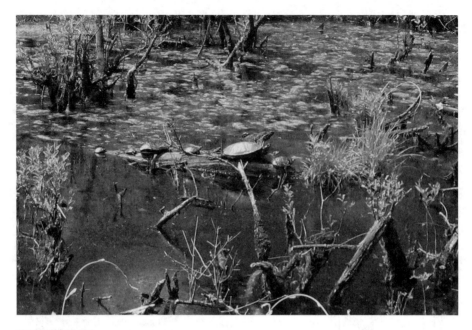

Trailside turtles

residences, roads, and parking lots never too far. From this vantage, it's easy to believe an oft-quoted statistic about the trail: one third of Anne Arundel County's more than 400,000 residents live within a mile of it. The hike begins behind the parking garage at a swing set and benches. There is also a water fountain here.

At 1 mile, you'll see an interesting solar sculpture with some explanatory signs on the sun. There are signs for each of the planets along the trail, spaced out proportionately to follow the pattern from the sun of actual distance in outer space. Beyond the solar sculpture, a wooded buffer turns a bit marshy, with some cattails, a reminder of the area's dominant ecozone: nearby, the Severn and Magothy rivers make their eventual ways to the Chesapeake.

After mile 1.4 is a nice wooded stream valley to the left, full of honeysuckle. The first of several old railroad bridges follows soon after, this one crossing Marley Creek in a forest full of maple, hickory, and oak. Marley Station Mall soon appears on the left. There's abundant parking here, which makes it a popular access point for the B&A. Wildflowers line the edge of the trail.

Cross over Route 100 on a bridge at 2.2 miles. Once beyond, the trail becomes more pleasant and wooded, heading to another parking area at 3 miles on Jumpers Hole Road. There's a gazebo with benches just beyond Jumpers Hole, beginning a nice stretch with flower plantings on both sides of the trail and leading to a marsh full of ducks and sunning turtles, clearly the nicest spot thus far.

Cross East-West Boulevard at 4.2 on a railroad bridge and enter a wooded residential neighborhood. A third parking area can be found soon after, at 5 miles, at Earleigh Heights. This is a good area to rest up; several places to eat are nearby off the trail. A Ranger Station and pond are also just on the other side of Earleigh Heights. There's a trail map there to check your position.

The area feels a bit more aquatic suddenly, and in summer, you'll see dragonflies shuttling back and forth over the trail. Every now and again, you'll cross a tiny one-lane road, but this stretch for the next few miles is nicely wooded and semi-isolated. Pass another series of wildflower plantings—lilies, daffodils, petunias, peonies, coneflowers—at 7 miles. You'll also see the old Severna Park Railroad Station. This is one of the few intact structures left over from the railroad. You will have probably noticed several switch boxes and a power house along the trail as well, but the Severna Park Station (aside from the Ranger Station at Earleigh Heights) is the most stark reminder of this corridor's earlier incarnation. Most "stations" along the route were nothing more than small platforms. These are indicated along the trail by rectangular outlines in stone, along with a little sign telling which station it was.

Cross another wooden railroad bridge at 7.6 miles. A trails maintenance shop follows at 8.4 miles. Just beyond is the only spot along the trail where you can still see railroad tracks—only about 20 feet worth, to the left. By 9 miles, you can hear B&A Boulevard to the left, but a big wooded gulley sits between. To the right is a thickly wooded forest of oak, poplar, and maple. The trail is soon lined with dense stands of bamboo.

At 9.5, as you cross the steel railroad bridge, look to the left for a series of wire-contained rocks, a drainage system. There's a nice rural scene of rolling hills with horses soon to the right, providing a quick view of what the area looked like when the trains still came through. The Arnold Parking Area is at 10.9 miles, followed by a very pleasant couple of miles with nice buffers between the road to the left and neighborhoods to the right. Sometimes, these buffers extend to a couple of hundred feet. The hike ends at Boulters Road. There, a sign points to Route 50 to the left, where you'd find the Annapolis parking area and the bike path extension. (If you've done the trail in reverse, beginning at Annapolis, from the parking area head up Boulters Road east, and you'll very quickly reach the trail.)

NEARBY ACTIVITIES

Because of the B&A's location and configuration, you can choose from a historic capital (Annapolis—just across the bridge on Rt. 50 east), a big city (Baltimore's Inner Harbor is just a few miles north of the trail's end in Glen Burnie), town centers (Glen Burnie, Severna Park, Pasadena, Arnold), more hiking (BWI Trail—see page 16), or shopping (Marley Station Mall, numerous establishments along the trail).

02   BWI TRAIL

KEY AT-A-GLANCE INFORMATION

LENGTH: 11.6 miles

CONFIGURATION: Loop

DIFFICULTY: Moderate

SCENERY: BWI airport, pines, wetlands

EXPOSURE: Mostly sun

TRAFFIC: Moderate–heavy

TRAIL SURFACE: Asphalt, boardwalk

HIKING TIME: 3.5–4 hours

ACCESS: Open

MAPS: USGS Relay; maps online at www.dnr.state.md.us/greenways/bwi trail.html and www.aacounty.org/RecParks/Parks/aacotrails park/bwitrailmap.cfm.

WHEELCHAIR ACCESS: Yes

FACILITIES: None on the trail, but food is available at BWI Plaza and bathrooms and water at various airport and transportation buildings.

SPECIAL COMMENTS: The hike distance and configuration can be altered by taking the light rail. Directions for the hike described here are to the Linthicum Light Rail station. To go to the BWI station, take I-195 toward the airport, exit at Aviation Boulevard (MD 170, Exit 1) east, and follow the signs to Light Rail. Hours: Monday–Saturday, 6 a.m.–11 p.m.; Sundays and holidays, 11 a.m.–7 p.m.

- -

GPS Trailhead Coordinates

UTM Zone (WGS84) 18S

Easting 357028

Northing 4340493

Latitude N 39° 12.116718'

Longitude W 76° 39.346461'

IN BRIEF

Hiking at an airport? It's a lot more pleasant than it sounds. Marvel at the woods and wetlands that still coexist with the airport and be awed by jets flying just above your head.

DESCRIPTION

One caveat: the BWI Trail is an absolute must for aviation aficionados, but it's not for those who crave the solitude of a walk in the woods. Even if you count yourself in that latter group, the BWI Trail is worth a go; it's not hard to find something to like along its well-used route.

Starting across from the Linthicum Light Rail station, take the asphalt path adjacent to the tracks as it parallels a small buffer of woods to the right with a residential neighborhood beyond. You'll quickly come to two small streets: Shipley Road at 900 feet and Music Lane at 0.2 miles. Beyond that the trail is simply the sidewalk that runs along Hammonds Ferry Road. Cross over Andover Road, and pick up the asphalt path on the other side at just under half a mile. Go left and continue to Camp Meade Road. Ignore the signs pointing to the airport to the right, and follow the BIKE ROUTE signs straight ahead over Camp Meade. At just under 0.7 miles, cross over the Light Rail tracks and swing around into a little wooded section. There's a parking area for

- -

Directions

Take I-695 to Exit 6 (Camp Meade Road south); take the second right (Maple Road) and follow Maple to the first light. Turn left onto Hammonds Ferry Road, and then turn left onto Oakdale Road. The trail begins at the end of Oakdale Road across from the Linthicum Light Rail station.

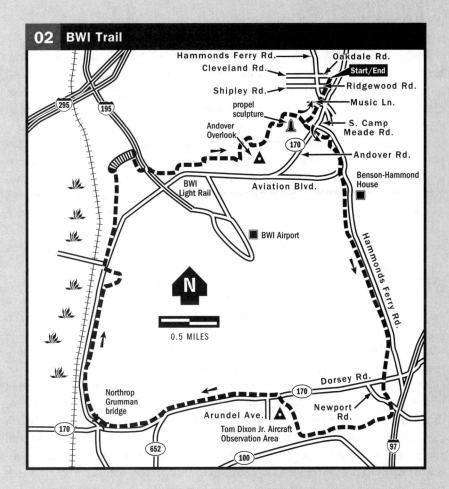

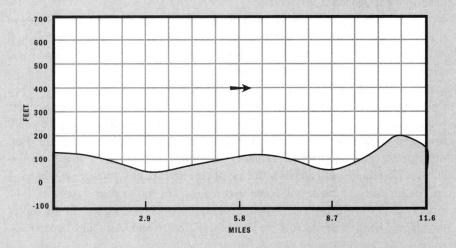

the airport beyond a small pond with cattails and (usually) Canada geese. It's a fairly nice stretch of woods here, and it makes up for the initial suburban feel.

About 1 mile later, cross Aviation Boulevard, and continue to the Benson-Hammond House, home of the Anne Arundel County Historical Society. Built in the 1830s and the only structure left from the farming period of a postcolonial settlement, the house now serves as a farm museum. A short post in front of the museum reads "East Coast Greenway."

At 1.25 miles stands a grove of pines, the dominant trees around the airport. You'll also see cattails, a reminder that this is marshy Chesapeake watershed area. At 1.3 miles, cross a little driveway that parallels Aviation Boulevard and heads into the BWI General Aviation Facility, and continue to the Maryland Aviation Administration at 1.8 miles. The area becomes very boggy, and you'll see more cattails and marshland. You'll come to Dorsey Road at 2.9 miles and Newport Road at just under 3.3 miles. Going straight here takes you to the B&A Trail (see page 12); to stay on the BWI, go right toward the sign reading BWI OVERLOOK. You'll soon enter arguably the nicest stretch of the trail.

Immediately to the left is busy Aviation Boulevard, but you'll quickly turn away from the road and head into the woods, where you'll see red oaks, tulip poplars, and of course the dominant pines. Even though you're deep within the woods, planes roar overhead, maybe only a couple of hundred feet or so above the ground. It's an amazing dichotomy: serene woods shattered by screaming jet engines, retreating to serenity again, and on and on. In all, this wooded stretch lasts 0.7 miles. On the other end of it, at 4.2 miles, a field opens to the right; this makes a great spot to sit and watch the planes—if you're awed by jets, don't pass up this opportunity. They come roaring over the tree line in descent and zoom past, barely a hundred feet in the air. Only air traffic controllers and runway directors get a better view. In addition to this perfect natural place to watch the planes, you may want to stop at the Tom Dixon Jr. Aircraft Observation Area just ahead at 4.3 miles; the trail runs to the left of the parking area, which includes benches and a playground.

At 4.4 miles, you'll reach Dorsey Road, which parallels the trail. When you reach Arundel Avenue at 4.7 miles, cross over Dorsey Road and go left. You'll pass a VFW hall on the left at 5.25 miles. Just beyond is the BWI Plaza if you need a quick pit stop for food or drink.

Continuing on, the trail turns into one of many boardwalks; these wooden walkways denote environmentally sensitive wetland sections. At just over 6 miles, you'll come to another nice wooded area away from the roads where again you'll have a good view of planes taking off, but they're fairly high at this point. Pass through a large pine grove, and then cross a 900-foot boardwalk at 6.7 miles.

At 7.2 miles, you'll come to the metal CAR RENTAL RETURN sign; if you hang out for a moment, a plane will come roaring over the hill to your right—you'll be directly under it and can see its belly from a pretty close distance. At the top of the hill at 7.6 miles, head left at the Rental Car Return and Maryland Department

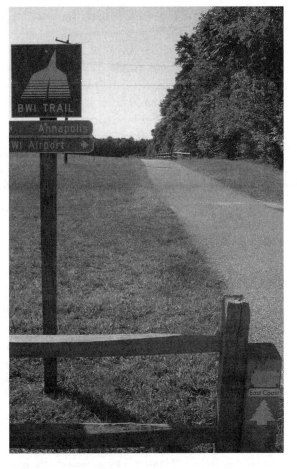

of Transportation (MDOT) headquarters sign. On the bridge, as you go over MD 170, look for the bicycle icon to the right; when you see it, head down the ramp, passing thick woods—again, mostly pine—to the left. You'll see the Northrop Grumman building to the right on the other side of MD 170.

At 8.2 miles, you'll see the Light Rail tracks to the left, in a nice section full of sycamore and tulip poplar with water on both sides of the tracks. You'll soon see a big marsh, often filled with herons, geese, and ducks on the left. At 8.7 miles, you'll come to a sign pointing to Amtrak/ MARC parking in front of the Maryland Aviation Administration Kauffman Building; go right across the street to a long wooden boardwalk. Stop for a moment on the boardwalk—this is one of the nicest spots on the trail. Herons often wade here, the vegetation is abundant and aquatic, and the marsh itself is ringed with pines.

When you climb the big ramp over I-195 at 9 miles, you'll have a decent view of the entire airport to the right; but the view is not all mechanical—a wildflower meadow sits to the right at 9.2 miles. The trail splits at 9.4 miles; head left in the direction of the sign pointing toward Andover Park (heading right will take you on a half-mile spur that includes a pedestrian bridge over MD 170, but it ends at the MDOT headquarters). At Andover Park, you'll find a pasture observation area and an equestrian park, as well as the continuation of the loop that will take you back to the Linthicum Light Rail station.

At 9.7 miles, cross over two small sections of roadway (Elm and Elkridge Landing roads). Once on the other side, you'll see the BWI Light Rail station. There's parking here too, and you can alter the hike length and configuration by parking here instead of at the Linthicum station. Or you can park at one station, walk to the other, and ride the Light Rail back; this will essentially cut the hike distance in half.

Continuing on the trail, at 10 miles you'll come to an open area that runs up a hill and into a field, where you'll see some old farm equipment, a reminder of what the area looked like before the airport was built. From the late 18th century until 1947, when construction began on today's Thurgood Marshall BWI (formerly Friendship International Airport), farmers cultivated the land for tobacco and grains as well as fruits and vegetables. At the Andover Overlook at the top of the hill, you can see the layout of the entire airport—runways, arriving and departing planes, and control towers. Take time to rest on the benches here; sitting in this pastoral setting and looking off into the distance gives a nice feeling of bring removed from the hectic everyday world.

Just beyond you'll come to the Andover equestrian area—not surprisingly, you'll see horses in the field in front of the farmhouse. Just off the trail you'll see another jarring juxtaposition—the "propel" sculpture, which is part of the Maryland Millennium Legacy Trail Art Project. The sculpture, made of stainless steel, weighs over a ton, and its curves reflect the uniqueness of the area. Within the sculpture you can see shapes reminiscent of rolling fields, clouds, waterways, and industry.

Follow the asphalt path until it turns into a sidewalk in front of Lindale Middle School at 10.8 miles; at 11 miles you'll reach Hammonds Ferry Road. Take a left; you've now made a complete loop back to the sidewalk where you entered the trail.

NEARBY ACTIVITIES

The 1830s Benson-Hammond House on the first part of the BWI Trail houses the Anne Arundel County Historical Society and serves as a farm museum. It is open Thursday through Saturday from 10 a.m. to 6 p.m.; (410) 760-9679, **www.aachs.org.**

For a more nature-oriented hike that will take you through habitat varying from marsh to mature forest, head to the Severn Run Environmental Area (see page 26). Follow I-97 south to Benfield Boulevard west (Exit 10), and take the first left onto Najoles Drive and then the first right onto Dicus Mill Road. A well-defined trail heads out from Dicus Mill where it crosses over the Severn Run. You can fish for perch, bass, and trout from this point. The trail is open year-round from dawn to dusk.

DOWNS MEMORIAL PARK

IN BRIEF

Enjoy a heady combination of mature forest, boggy marshland, self-guided nature trails, golden sand beach, and stunning water views.

DESCRIPTION

This land, now owned by the Anne Arundel County Department of Parks and Recreation, comes well stocked not only in natural beauty but also in human history. Downs Memorial stands on Bodkin Neck, a peninsula at the confluence of the Patapsco River and Chesapeake Bay. Deeds to its earliest settlement date to 1670 and include Charles Carroll, a signer of the Declaration of Independence, among its initial landowners.

After entering the park, immediately turn right into the first parking area. You'll find two trailheads, one closest to where you've pulled in and the other on the far end of the parking area; take the one closest to the entrance. It begins in the woods under the overhanging sign that reads Eco Trail—Self Guided Nature Trail.

This stand of hardwoods contains oak, poplar, beech, birch, sycamore, holly, gum, and sassafras. At 180 feet, you'll see a bench and little sign suggesting that hikers stop and listen to the sounds of the forest. You'll find interpretive signs such as this one all along

KEY AT-A-GLANCE INFORMATION

LENGTH: 3.8 miles

CONFIGURATION: Jagged loop

DIFFICULTY: Easy

SCENERY: Chesapeake Bay, beach, pond, mature trees

EXPOSURE: More shade than sun

TRAFFIC: Light on trails, moderate–heavy at overlooks and pavilions

TRAIL SURFACE: Mostly asphalt

HIKING TIME: 2 hours with linger time on the beach

ACCESS: Cost is $5 per vehicle. Park hours are 7 a.m.–dusk year-round. The visitor center is open Monday and Wednesday–Friday, 9 a.m.–4 p.m.; 11 a.m.–3 p.m. on weekends. The park and all of its facilities are closed on Tuesday; holiday hours vary.

MAPS: USGS Gibson Island; trail maps at Gate House, Information Center, and Web site

WHEELCHAIR ACCESS: Yes

FACILITIES: Restrooms, water, playground, gazebos, picnic, ball fields

SPECIAL COMMENTS: No alcohol, no swimming, dogs must be leashed except in designated areas. For more information call (410) 222-6230 or visit www.co.anne-arundel.md.us/ RecParks/parks/downs park.

Directions

Take I-695 to I-97 South. Leave I-97 at Exit 14, and take MD 100 East to Mountain Road East. When Mountain Road veers off to the right, stay straight on Pinehurst Road, and take a right into the park entrance at Chesapeake Bay Road. The gatehouse will be straight ahead.

GPS Trailhead Coordinates

UTM Zone (WGS84) 18S

Easting 375547

Northing 4329815

Latitude N 39° 6.516337'

Longitude W 76° 26.364620'

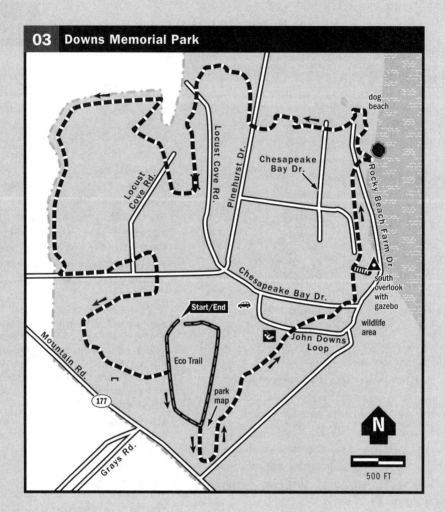

03 **Downs Memorial Park**

dog beach

Locust Cove Rd.

Locust Cove Rd.

Pinehurst Dr.

Chesapeake Bay Dr.

Rocky Beach Farm Dr.

south overlook with gazebo

wildlife area

Chesapeake Bay Dr.

Start/End

John Downs Loop

Eco Trail

park map

Mountain Rd.

177

Grays Rd.

N

500 FT

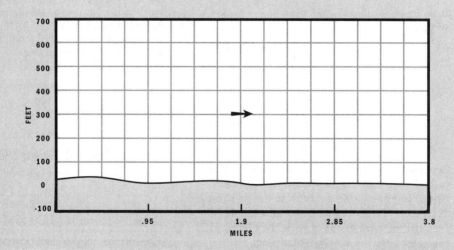

the Eco Trail; they describe the bark, trees, moss, leaves, insects, and animals you'll see as you hike.

At 440 feet, you'll come to a map that, like all others in the park, has a "you are here" marker to help you keep your bearings. The trail splits here; go to the right. You're still on the Eco Trail, and accordingly you'll see more signs; the next one gives a rundown of Maryland's official state tree (white oak), flower (black-eyed Susan), dog (Chesapeake Bay retriever), bird (Baltimore oriole), insect (Baltimore checker spot butterfly), and fish (rockfish).

You'll soon reach an unpaved sand trail; follow it to the asphalt Perimeter Trail, and take a left. You're now off the Eco Trail, but you'll finish the portion you've skipped toward the end of the hike. On the Perimeter Trail, which is close to Pinehurst Road, you'll hear some car traffic; but very soon you'll leave the road behind and follow the trail deeper into the thick woods. Look closely through the dense tree cover to see a chain-link fence that delineates the park boundary. The woods beyond the fence give the trail a remote woodsy feel.

In a half mile, the perimeter trail links with the Senior Trail, which is paved and leads to the left; keep going straight, and you'll soon pass an open play area with a basketball court on the left. The trail opens up as you pass a soccer field. To the left is a wildlife area and to the right an exercise pavilion and bulletin board with illustrations depicting proper stretching techniques.

You'll pass through another stand of trees before the view opens up again and the South Overlook appears. Walk up the wooden boardwalk toward a gazebo that once belonged to H. R. Mayo Thom, a wealthy Baltimorean; his family's estate included this area from 1913 through 1937. The gazebo provides a quintessential Maryland view: the Chesapeake Bay, largest estuary in the United States and boasting the world's largest crop of clams and oysters. If you have some quarters with you, operate the binoculars and view the osprey platform out in the water; you'll also see an oyster nursery below and an aviary and raptor pen inside the buildings behind you. (Next to the raptor pen you'll find "mother's garden," where there's a stone bench constructed in 1915. If you sit on it and make a wish, the wish comes true.)

When you've had your fill of the vista, head down from the overlook and continue toward the beach, where you'll walk among aquatic plants, skimmers, kingfishers, and gulls. You're not allowed to swim, but kick off your shoes and feel the soft golden sand under your feet while you delight in the soothing scene: birds wheeling in the air, water lapping against the rocks, smooth stone and bleached driftwood on the beach.

At the big jumble of rocks, head left toward the paved trail on the other side. Cut in on the dirt path and follow it to a tiny spit of sand and a series of rocks. There, you can walk out into the water a few feet so that there's nothing in front of you but the bay lapping on both sides of the rocks.

At 1.1 miles, you'll see a volleyball net to your left. Head right toward the wood block seats and the North Overlook. If you were standing here in 1822,

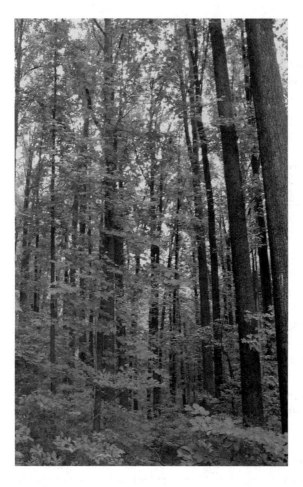

you'd see workmen building Bodkin Island Lighthouse, which stayed in use until 1855. The tower has since crumbled and remains only as a "navigational hazard" on present-day maps.

Just beyond the North Overlook, you'll find a beach where dogs can roam off leash. Heading back to the paved path from the dog beach, you'll see an unpaved trail immediately to the right; it heads through the woods and takes you to a big stagnant pond. Walk under the wooden boardwalk, and then go up for a view of the entire pond. You'll most likely see a few frogs and snakes. Next head back up the wooden ramp to the paved Perimeter Trail, where you'll see picnic benches to the left. Stay to the right, and at 1.25 miles, you'll come to bathroom facilities and a water fountain with pavilions and volleyball nets just beyond.

At 1.4 miles, head uphill to a wide footbridge, where you'll cross over Pinehurst Road; pick up the trail on the other side. Side trails to the left will take you to tennis, basketball, and handball courts, but keep going straight, cutting back into the woods away from all the facilities. On either side of trail, you'll see tall, straight oaks as well as holly trees. You'll come to one more stand of picnic benches and open play areas before you hit a valley of marshy aquatic plants to the right. Here, at 1.8 miles, you'll cross over the southern tip of Locust Cove and head into a Natural Area. Head right toward the trail split; this puts you deep into the Natural Area and parallels Locust Cove on the right. Thick woods, mostly pines and oaks, dominate this area, and spongy, green moss lines both sides of the trail. Moss also fills the occasional cracks where roots have broken through the pavement.

At 2.1 miles, take a little gravel path off the main trail. It takes you close to the water and then loops back to the paved Perimeter Trail. You'll soon come to the park boundary and see a few private houses pop into view through the woods on the right. In this increasingly boggy and marshy area, clumps of moss and trees with lichen-covered trunks attest to how low the elevation is here; you're barely above sea level. Invariably, both sides of the trail will be muddy, and you'll appreciate the fact that the trail is a bit raised in this section.

At 2.7 miles, the trail crosses over Pinehurst Road. Your car is just ahead, but to continue the hike, head right when you see the gatehouse. The Perimeter Trail parallels first Pinehurst Road and then Mountain Road. Cut along an unnamed, unpaved trail at 2.9 miles to stay deeper in the woods and lose the sound of the occasional car going by (though it's not terribly busy). You'll see three separate unpaved trails; take the one in the middle. It can be easy to lose, but as long as you continue in more or less a straight line, you'll link back up with the Perimeter Trail soon enough; even if you do stray off the path, you won't need to bushwhack—the vegetation is relatively sparse.

Head left on the Perimeter Trail, and at 3 miles, you'll see a bench on the left and an unpaved trail behind it immediately to the right; follow it to a V. Take the right side; it will allow you to link up with the Eco Trail where you first began. Even though you've already been on this section, you're now heading in the opposite direction, and you'll soon link up with the section you skipped originally. At 3.2 miles, take a left where the trail splits, and finish hiking the Eco Trail. About midway down this section, you'll be walking on an old farm road once traversed by horses and carriages and later used by farmers and lumberjacks.

You'll see rare chestnut trees as well as the ubiquitous oaks and hickories on this section of the trail. At 3.4 miles, you'll come to Chesapeake Bay Road; take a left to return to the other side of the parking area from where you began the hike.

NEARBY ACTIVITIES

Plenty of opportunities exist for fishing or picnicking with the whole family at one of the many pavilions inside the park. Check out the Victorian-style garden behind the south overlook as well as the nearby raptor pen and aviary. Children may be interested in the Rocky Beach Farm Youth Group Camping Area; pick up a brochure at the visitor center. If you haven't had your fill of bay-view parks, visit nearby Fort Smallwood Park. Long owned by Baltimore City, Fort Smallwood was taken over in 2006 by Anne Arundel County Recreation and Parks and has seen a major upgrade in facilities. Take Mountain Road west to Hog Neck Road north to Fort Smallwood Road east.

04 SEVERN RUN ENVIRONMENTAL AREA

KEY AT-A-GLANCE INFORMATION

LENGTH: 1.6 miles

CONFIGURATION: Out-and-back with loops

DIFFICULTY: Easy

SCENERY: Severn Run, wetlands

EXPOSURE: Mostly shade

TRAFFIC: Light

TRAIL SURFACE: Sand, packed dirt

HIKING TIME: 45 minutes

ACCESS: Dawn–dusk

MAPS: USGS Odenton

WHEELCHAIR ACCESS: No

FACILITIES: None

SPECIAL COMMENTS: There are other hiking options available in the Severn Run NEA, but they are not contiguous. I've chosen this hike because its many intersecting paths allow for more exploration. Additional short hikes can be found off New Cut Road heading northwest toward Quarterfield Road and at the end of Indian Landing Road; from Benfield, go south on Veterans Highway as it turns to Generals Highway. Then go left on Indian Landing. Severn Run NEA sits within a flood area.

GPS Trailhead Coordinates

UTM Zone (WGS84) 18S

Easting 358764

Northing 4327558

Latitude N 39° 5.143068'

Longitude W 76° 37.978942'

IN BRIEF

Make your way around a little-known and underappreciated spot of beauty tucked between major highways.

DESCRIPTION

Even residents of the immediate area might not know of Severn Run Natural Environmental Area's existence, though they have no doubt driven right past it innumerous times. That's because it straddles I-97, Veterans Highway, and other major roads. Its 1,600 acres follow the course of the protected Severn Run in six separate and not always connected tracts. Severn Run has no infrastructure, which might account for its relative lack of use. But this makes it a real unspoiled jewel of a place.

As indicated in Special Comments, this hike is perhaps the easiest to access, and has the most well-defined trails that allow for many configurations. To start, head straight on the Jeep trail. There's a split almost immediately. This is just a small loop, so you can take either direction. At 0.2 miles, cross two footbridges, making note of the low elevation (sea level) and flood potential. However, one thing in favor of soaking up the moisture is the fact that the trail soon becomes almost

Directions

Take I-97 south toward Annapolis to Exit 10, Benfield Boulevard west. Take the first left onto Najoles Drive. As Najoles makes a big rightward curve, the road turns into Dicus Mill Road. Cross the one-lane bridge and look for the little parking areas on either side of the road. After parking, walk back over the bridge and take a left up the Jeep trail.

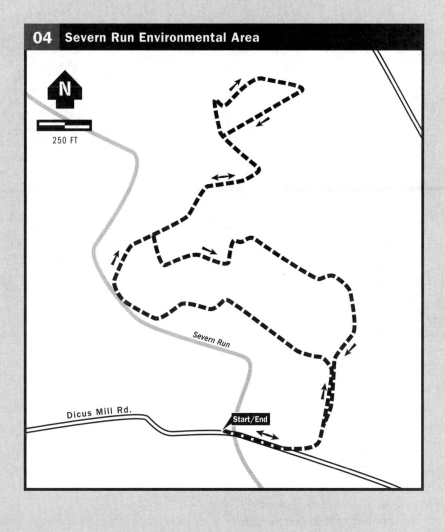

04   **Severn Run Environmental Area**

N

250 FT

Severn Run

Dicus Mill Rd.

Start/End

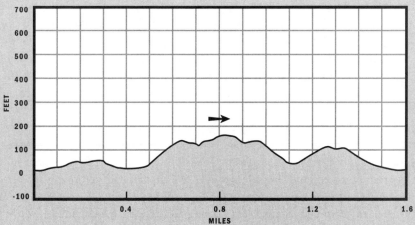

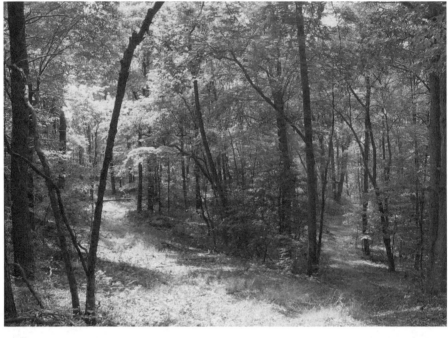

Trail bi-section

entirely sand; it seems incongruous with the initial packed dirt, but it's also part of the charm of the place.

Despite the poor soil, there's a thriving forest of holly, chinquapin oak, poplar, ironwood, sweetbay magnolia, and many other mature hardwoods. Additionally, there's a thick understory; along this short hike, you'll pass several varieties of ferns, adder's tongue, ebony spleenwort, pink lady's slipper, azalea, and trailing arbutus, among other flora.

At the trail split at 0.5 miles, head left to a picturesque spot next to the water. When you've had your fill, head back to the trail and continue left, eventually heading uphill. No doubt you'll notice all the little crisscrossing trails. Come to an overgrown Jeep trail full of tall grasses and young pines. Follow it uphill. Go left when the trail splits again; you'll have nice views of the valley to the left. There's lots of mountain laurel and azalea in this section. Make a U-turn when you reach the top of the hill; ahead of you is actually a parking lot for the I-97 business park.

At 0.9 miles, the trail splits again—go left to where you hiked earlier. You're backtracking now; at 1.1 miles, when you reach the bottom of the hill, rejoin the trail and go left again. This trail split leads you to a different spot from where you were before. Follow the trail around, eventually heading downhill over log steps, until you reach the split at the bottom of the hill at 1.4 miles. Go left and head back to your car. Along the way, you can take the other side of that little loop you came to at the beginning of the hike.

NEARBY ACTIVITIES

Just five exits up I-97 North, you can access the BWI Trail (see page 16). Heading east on Benfield will eventually take you to the B&A Trail (see page 12). Continuing south on I-97 and east on US 50 takes you to Annapolis, arguably the most historical and prettiest state capital in the country. Head over the Severn, and just before the Bay Bridge you'll find Sandy Point Park, which oversees Severn Run NEA and offers great swimming and other amenities. For more information, call (410) 974-2149 or visit **www.dnr.state.md.us/publiclands/southern/sandypoint.html.**

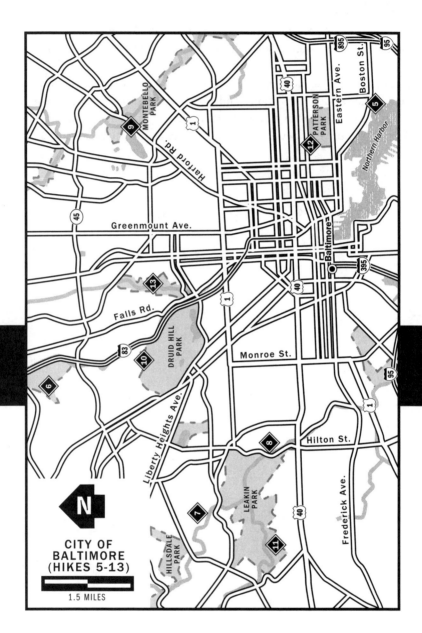

CITY OF
BALTIMORE
(HIKES 5-13)

1.5 MILES

N

CITY OF BALTIMORE

05 BALTIMORE WATERFRONT PROMENADE

KEY AT-A-GLANCE INFORMATION

LENGTH: 4.7 miles

CONFIGURATION: One-way

DIFFICULTY: Easy–moderate

SCENERY: Downtown Baltimore, Inner Harbor, Federal Hill, monuments, historical sites, historical neighborhoods

EXPOSURE: Sunny

TRAFFIC: Heavy

TRAIL SURFACE: Asphalt, brick, concrete, cobblestone, wood

HIKING TIME: 2.5 hours

ACCESS: Always open—use normal caution after dark.

MAPS: USGS Baltimore East

WHEELCHAIR ACCESS: Yes

FACILITIES: Food, water, bathrooms in restaurants and shops along route

SPECIAL COMMENTS: Final plans call for the Waterfront Promenade to extend 7 miles from Canton to Locust Point. As of fall 2008, however, there were still major southern portions unfinished. The section of waterfront from the Ritz-Carlton below the Visionary Art Museum in Federal Hill to the Hull Street Pier in Locust Point is completed only in sections. With a recent economic downturn, expect that this final section may not be complete anytime soon.

GPS Trailhead Coordinates

UTM Zone (WGS84) 18S

Easting 364343

Northing 4348497

Latitude N 39° 16.512909'

Longitude W 76° 34.361908'

IN BRIEF

Join the throngs strolling around Baltimore's tourist meccas, but begin and end where few tourists venture.

DESCRIPTION

From the Korean War Memorial, you'll be more or less paralleling Boston Street to your right. But it's often blocked from view, and in any case, the far more lovely scene is to your left: the Patapsco River as it forms Baltimore's Northwest Harbor. As you make your way toward the Inner Harbor, you'll be reminded of just how lovely and peaceful—yes, peaceful—a major city can be. If it's early morning, your only accompaniment will be walkers, joggers, and loads of ducks.

Canton's development has been nothing short of remarkable, turning an industrial and neglected waterfront into a series of polished marinas and waterfront housing, mixed in sensibly with existing restaurants and shops. With downtown looming to the east, your view to the south is just charming: pleasure craft plying the river, gaggles of ducks paddling around the water, an occasional blue crab crawling its way up the side of a wooden pier or retaining rope, and the iconic

Directions

Take I-83 south until it ends at President Street; go 0.6 miles to Fleet Street at the big curve to the left. Go 0.8 miles to a right onto Boston Street. Go 0.9 miles to a right onto South Ellwood/Korean War Memorial Drive. Park in the lot and head right, toward the water. The promenade begins at the fishing pier at the south end of the Korean War Memorial Park.

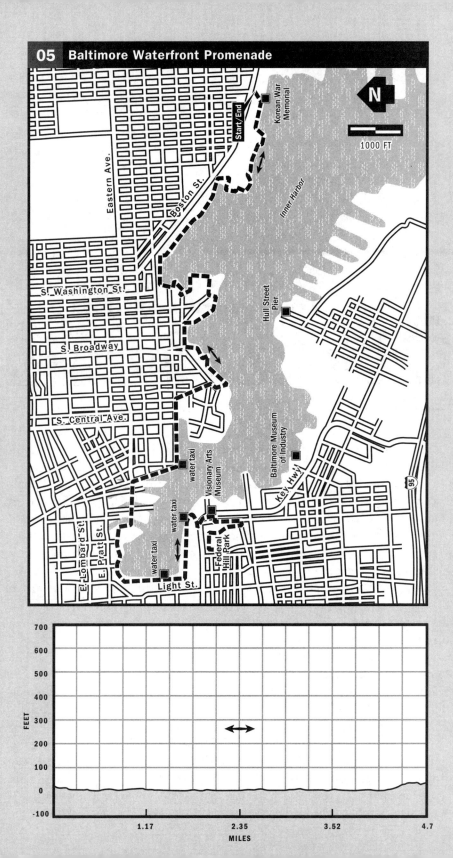

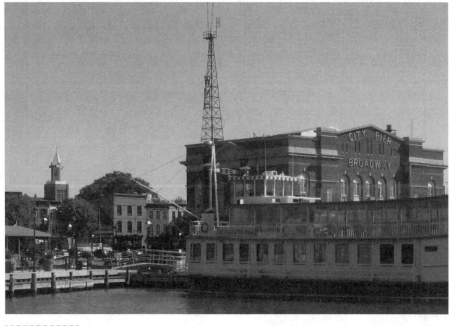

Broadway Pier

Domino's sugar sign; its red glow can be seen at night from almost anywhere in the harbor.

You'll reach Fells Point at 1.7 miles. This historical neighborhood dates back to 1670, but was first incorporated as a town in 1763, becoming part of Baltimore City ten years later. There are still existing houses from that era, and with Broadway Market just a few blocks from the water on South Broadway, you'd be encouraged to poke around this wonderful and beautiful cobblestoned neighborhood. You can see, among other notable historical structures, the house on Aliceanna Street where Frederick Douglass lived while still a slave. It was in this neighborhood where Douglass learned to read and write, starting him on his extraordinary journey to being one of the most influential and important men in the history of the republic.

At 2 miles, in the heart of Fells Point, pass Broadway Pier, home to NBC's long-running acclaimed cop drama, *Homicide: Life on the Street*. When you reach Chester Cove Marina, turn around for a good view of the gold onion domes of St. Michael's Ukrainian Catholic Church, near Patterson Park. You will reach the Frederick Douglass–Isaac Myers Maritime Park and Museum (**doug lassmyers.org** for info) at 2.5 miles, at the intersection of Caroline, Thames, and Philpot Streets. Head north along Lancaster Street, momentarily turning away from the water—no worries; you'll be back soon.

Continuing on, you'll reach the Living Classroom Foundation, where you'll see a sign pointing you to the "pedestrian walkway." The small skiffs in the water to the left here make a pleasing backdrop. Invariably, on nice days people will be sitting on the benches to the right under the shade trees. Despite the heavy boat traffic here, the water is cleaned frequently, and it's a pleasant spot to sit and read, eat, or people-watch. Across the street on Lancaster you'll see new hotels and restaurants.

As you approach President Street, to the right stands the striking memorial to the 1940 massacre in Katyn, Poland; the three-story sculpture is in the shape of a golden flame with bronze figures intertwined. Behind the monument is the Civil War Museum (1850 President Street Station, open Tuesdays through Sundays from 10 a.m. to 5 p.m.); history students will know that it was here, not Fort Sumter, where the Civil War actually began when, on this very spot, a Confederate-sympathizing mob attacked Union soldiers on their way to Washington, D.C.

At just under 2.9 miles, head right to stay on the brick; if you go straight on the wooden boardwalk in front of you, you'll end up on the patio of Victor's Café. Now the downtown financial district and Inner Harbor come into view. The National Aquarium is straight ahead, and to the left, you'll see Federal Hill, your ultimate destination. Pass the water-taxi stand on the left as you parallel President Street. Mature shade trees border the water, and more ducks congregate in this area.

The Baltimore Public Works Museum (open Tuesday to Sunday, 10 a.m. to 4 p.m.) is on the right, housed in a beautiful 1912 brick pumping station. Nearby you'll see a series of Italian flags; you're on the edge of Little Italy. Go left over the bridge at 3.2 miles, and you'll see the sail-themed architecture of the Columbus Center, a national center for marine research, to the right, and the National Aquarium (**www.aqua.org**) straight ahead. As you pass it, the Hard Rock Café and ESPN Zone, the country's first, will come into view.

For a taste of history, visit the USCG *Cutter Taney* sitting in the water to the right. It's the only remaining survivor of the attack on Pearl Harbor; you can go on board and check it out. Walk to the second bridge over the water, and follow that to the left. Cross the pedestrian bridge at the Hard Rock Café at three quarters of a mile. You'll come straight to the World Trade Center, which is the country's tallest pentagonal building; the 27th floor offers an unmatched view of Baltimore's harbor and skyline. If you want to ride out into the harbor, you can rent a paddleboat just below the World Trade Center. (For my money, I'd rather put in with the Canton Kayak Club, **www.cantonkayakclub.com**.)

At just under 4 miles you'll come to the Pratt Street Pavilion, a popular place for shopping and dining—here you can find almost anything you might want to eat or purchase in either the Pratt Street Pavilion or the adjacent Light Street Pavilion. The open space between the two provides an outdoor stage for a variety of performances—music, juggling, dancing, and magic shows. The performers are often quite good, making it worth a stop to check out whatever's going on. But use common sense; obviously a large, stationary crowd offers lots of opportunities for pickpockets.

The USS *Constellation* Museum, in the water at 4 miles, comes next (April 1 to October 31: 10 a.m. to 5:30 p.m.; November 1 to March 31: 10 a.m. to 4:30 p.m.). The crowds begin to thin out a bit after the Light Street Pavilion, and you'll have unobstructed views of the aquarium to the left across the harbor. To the right you'll see the visually striking Baltimore Area Visitor Center (BAVC), which complements the nautical theme built into the architecture of the Columbus Center and the Aquarium. About a half mile straight up Conway Street to the right of the BAVC stands Oriole Park at Camden Yards, still widely regarded as one of, if not, the nicest stadiums in Major League Baseball.

The popular Maryland Science Center (**www.maryland sciencecenter.org**), with its massive *Tyrannosaurus* in the window, looms straight ahead. When you reach the Science Center at 4.2 miles, head left, keeping the water on your left; the crowds thin even more here. Pass a merry-go-round to the right, exactly across the harbor from the World Trade Center. Next is Rash Field, where you might catch an open-air acrobat practice. The promenade essentially ends here as you reach the Rusty Scupper Restaurant. There is more brick waterfront beyond as it wraps around the Ritz-Carlton, but it doesn't feel quite so public here. From this section to Hull Street is more of a patchwork of sidewalk and crumbling waterfront. It's certainly not so terrible to make your way along the water (at the very least, you'll pass the unique Baltimore Museum of Industry in another half mile). But to complete the hike as described here, cross the parking lot at the Rusty Scupper and then cross Key Highway beyond and follow the sidewalk to the left as it passes the American Visionary Art Museum (open 10 a.m. to 6 p.m., Tuesday through Sunday, **www.avam.org**).

After the museum, continue on the sidewalk, heading right and then left until you soon reach the edge of Federal Hill Park. Turn up the hill and follow the stairs to the top. Federal Hill has been a popular spot ever since the founding of Baltimore in 1729. About 4,000 people crammed in here for a feast in 1788 to celebrate the ratification of the U.S. Constitution by the State of Maryland. During the Civil War, Union troops fortified Federal Hill and trained their guns on the city. The site officially became a park in 1880.

There are great views up here. These include the neighborhood of Federal Hill; bear witness to the craze of building rooftop decks on these narrow row homes, many built in the 1700s. M & T Bank Stadium, home of the Ravens, sits about a mile in the distance. Keep circling around on the sidewalk until you catch a glimpse of where you've just walked. Standing next to the antique cannons, the 15-star American flag, and the monuments to Colonel George Armistead and Major General Samuel Smith, gives you an unparalleled view of the harbor.

NEARBY ACTIVITIES

Your best bet is to stop at the Baltimore Area Visitor Center, which is open daily from 9 a.m. to 6 p.m.. Call (410) 837-4636 or (877) BALTIMORE, or visit **www .baltimore.org**.

CYLBURN ARBORETUM

IN BRIEF

Take in a stunning array of flowers and trees on the grounds of a beautiful 19th-century mansion.

DESCRIPTION

Construction on the Italianate Cylburn Mansion began in 1863, but it wasn't completed until 1888, when Jesse Tyson, a wealthy Baltimore businessman, moved in with his much younger bride, Edyth Johns. After Jesse died in 1906, Edyth remarried, and she and her husband lived in Cylburn until 1942, when the house became the property of the Baltimore City Department of Public Welfare. In 1954, the Board of Recreation and Parks created the Cylburn Wildflower Preserve and Garden, which was later renamed Cylburn Arboretum.

The grounds of Cylburn are pretty any time of year but are especially glorious in mid- to late spring. There are no fewer than 13 separate gardens that range from Victorian-designed formal spaces to backyard vegetable gardens and a plot devoted to alpine plants. All of this flora goes a long way toward attracting birds. More than 170 species have been spotted at Cylburn, including bald eagles.

From the parking area, cross the entrance road and head down the gravel path, passing the signs for the bog, Circle Trail, and

KEY AT-A-GLANCE INFORMATION

LENGTH: 2.2 miles

CONFIGURATION: 2 intersecting loops

DIFFICULTY: Easy

SCENERY: Trees and flowers, an Italianate mansion

EXPOSURE: Mostly shaded

TRAFFIC: Moderate on trails, heavy in gardens and mansion, especially in spring and summer

TRAIL SURFACE: Dirt, asphalt

HIKING TIME: 45 minutes, longer for poking around gardens, mansion

ACCESS: The grounds are open every day of the year 6 a.m.–9 p.m., except in winter, when the gates close at dusk. Maryland Transit Administration (MTA) bus runs just outside Cylburn. For a complete schedule, call (866) RIDE-MTA or visit www.mtamaryland.com.

MAPS: USGS Baltimore West

WHEELCHAIR ACCESS: Mansion only

FACILITIES: Restroom and water in the mansion; portable toilets and water outside as well

SPECIAL COMMENTS: To schedule a trail, garden, and/or museum tour, call (410) 367-2217.

Directions ⟶

Take I-83 to Exit 10, Northern Parkway west. Take the first left onto Cylburn Avenue, and continue until it ends at Greenspring Avenue. Take a left onto Greenspring Avenue and then another immediate left into Cylburn Arboretum. Follow the road to the parking area on the left.

GPS Trailhead Coordinates

UTM Zone (WGS84) 18S

Easting 357386

Northing 4357108

Latitude N 39° 21.099494'

Longitude W 76° 39.308910'

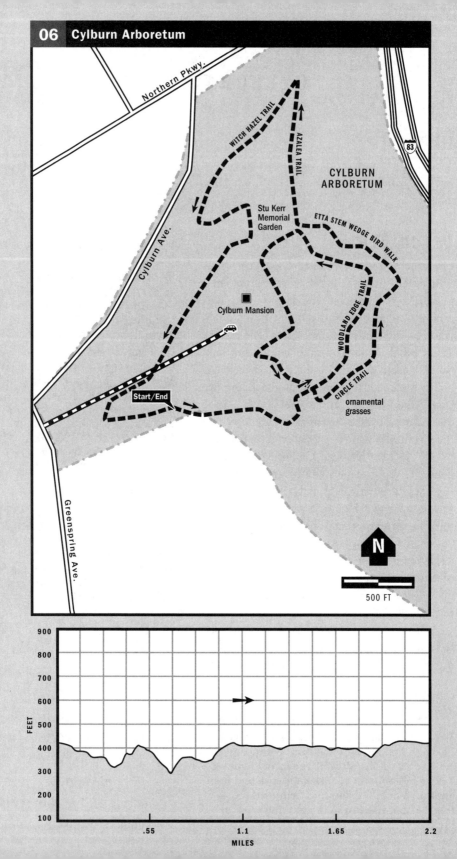

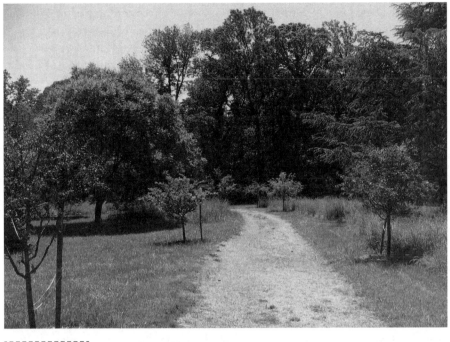

Woodland Edge

Elizabeth E. Clark Azalea Path. When you see the Circle Trail to the left, take it. Lined with a series of stone benches, the Circle Trail runs through the woods, but not very deep. A trail split follows soon; go right. At a quarter mile, take a right downhill to the Etta Stem Wedge Bird Walk, a pleasant little diversionary trail that runs parallel to the Circle Trail but deeper into the woods. When you rejoin the Circle Trail from the Etta Stem Wedge Bird Walk, you'll most likely scatter unsuspecting squirrels and birds at the feeder at the intersection of these two trails (as well as three others). Take a quick detour right onto the Azalea Trai. Railroad ties will ease your way when this path begins its gradual descent down the hill.

At the next trail split, continue on the Azalea Trail. At 0.6 miles, you'll see the Witch Hazel Trail, a nice little detour worth taking. The trail has lichen-covered granite all around it. You'll reach the Woodland Edge Trail at 0.8 miles; take it to the right. Go 0.1 mile, passing the Circle Trail, and head out to a paved area. Here, take a right.

Now on the paved road, walk behind some maintenance buildings and into an open area. Down the hill to the right are some beautiful wildflowers. When the road heads downhill at 1 mile, where you see a little parking spur to the left, head left and follow the tree line through a very wide lane of grass. At 1.2 miles, at an enormous hickory tree, cross the entrance road on the left. Now across the road, turn left and follow the tree line; look out for a trailhead, which you'll find at 1.3 miles (roughly where the entrance road splits and where you took a right to park). Thin tree trunks placed on the ground on both sides of the path make the trailhead easy to spot. Initially, cedar chips cover the trail, but after 250 feet, the trail emerges. Follow the tree line onto the Woodland Edge Trail.

At a trail split, take a left and then another left at 1.4 miles. At the Ryer Garden, take a right and cross over the Circle Trail. Go straight ahead on the Woodland Edge Trail to a thicket of bamboo. The trail here crosses over a little footbridge at a bog. You'll see the mansion to the left. Along the trail you'll see poplars, Japanese maples, oaks, gums, and birches, among other trees.

At 1.8 miles is the point at which you headed to the Azalea Trail earlier. This time, take a left, passing the bamboo and heading toward the mansion. Pass a honeybee apiary on the right and the Stu Kerr Memorial Garden, with its little red schoolhouse, on the left. Nearby you'll see lots of stone and metal sculptures. On Saturday mornings in June and July, children ages 3 to 6 can enjoy a nature story hour here. On the right is the Garden of the Senses, where you'll see shooting stars, celandine poppies, white trilliums, blue phloxes, pawpaws, weeping cherries, and several different types of magnolias.

In fact, several gardens dot the area, and it's worth your while to stop and take them in. Passing the nature museum on the right, on the paved road heading toward the mansion, you'll find the Shady Garden, on the left just before the mansion. In front of the mansion is a circular driveway ringed by marigolds and black-eyed Susans with a centuries-old black walnut tree in the middle.

NEARBY ACTIVITIES

Just down I-83 is Druid Hill Park, where you'll find tennis and basketball courts, a public swimming pool, a disc-golf course, the Baltimore Conservatory (displaying thousands of plants and flowers in a lovely glass pavilion), and the Maryland Zoo. Go south on I-83 to Exit 7 and head west on Druid Hill Park Drive to the park entrance, off Swann Drive.

GWYNNS FALLS PARK 07

IN BRIEF

Adjacent to and connected with Leakin Park, this section of the Gwynns Falls Trail runs through one of the largest unbroken urban forests in the United States. Follow the falls several miles through its most scenic sections to Leon Day Park and back.

DESCRIPTION

Walk away from Clifton Avenue and head straight into the woods. Initially very tall oaks flank the wide trail, but after 300 feet the trail turns to cedar chips; you're now deep in the woods. Ignore the cut to the right and continue down the hill straight ahead until you can see Gwynns Falls; be careful—this downhill section of the trail is very rocky and it's easy to twist an ankle. When you reach the falls, head left and walk downstream.

This is a little-used section of trail, and it's narrow and covered in spiderwebs. But at 0.4 miles, the trail rises above the falls and gets much wider. Enormous beech trees abound, along with lots of sassafras, holly, oak, and walnut. You'll reach Windsor Mill Road at 0.5 miles. Take care crossing the road and head left on the other side. Take a quick right into the Windsor Mill parking area.

The area is named for the old Windsor Mill, just one of many flour and textile mills

KEY AT-A-GLANCE INFORMATION

LENGTH: 5.1 miles

CONFIGURATION: Out-and-back with 2 loops

DIFFICULTY: Easy–moderate

SCENERY: Gwynns Falls, mixed hardwoods

EXPOSURE: Half and half

TRAFFIC: Light–moderate

TRAIL SURFACE: Packed dirt, crushed rock, and asphalt

HIKING TIME: 2 hours

ACCESS: Dawn–dusk; Maryland Transit Administration (MTA) runs buses to Gwynns Falls Park; for a complete schedule, call (866) RIDE-MTA or visit www .mtamaryland.com

MAPS: USGS Baltimore West

WHEELCHAIR ACCESS: No

FACILITIES: None (bathrooms and water at Winans Meadow Trailhead section of Gwynns Falls Trail—see Leakin Park hike, page 61).

SPECIAL COMMENTS: For a hike along the Gwynns Falls Trail from Leon Day Park to the trail's terminus, see page 45. For more information about the trail, visit www .gwynnsfallstrail.org or call (410) 396-7946.

Directions

Take I-83 to Exit 6, North Avenue west. Go 3.5 miles and turn right onto North Hilton Street. Go two blocks and turn left onto Bloomingdale, which soon becomes Clifton Avenue. Continue 1.3 miles where Clifton swings around abruptly to the right at a guardrail; park here. You'll see a sign to the left marking the trailhead, "Windsor Hills Conservation Trail."

GPS Trailhead Coordinates

UTM Zone (WGS84) 18S

Easting 354111

Northing 4353315

Latitude N 39° 19.016905'

Longitude W 76° 41.539092'

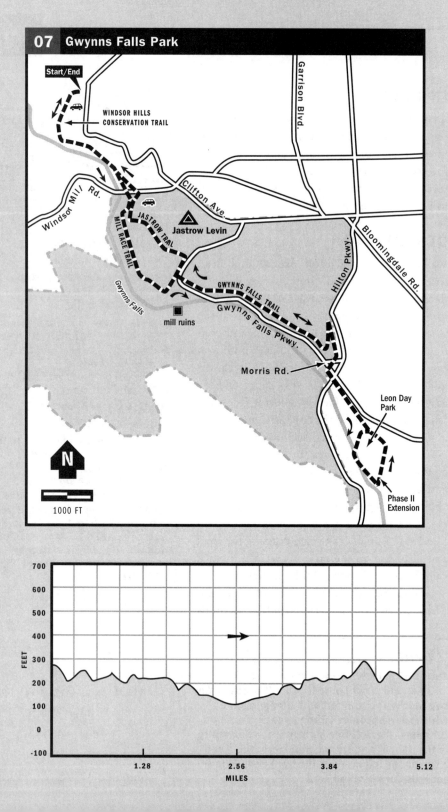

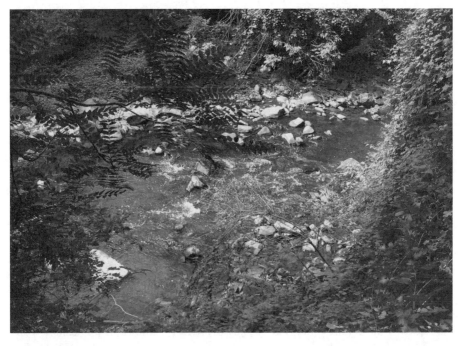

Gwynns Falls

built along the Dead Run and Gwynns Falls in the early 1800s. The trail surface becomes crushed stone on the Mill Race Trail, named for the waterwheels that once conveyed water five mills downstream to Calverton (present-day Rosemount). You'll see the Jastrow Trail immediately to the left, but stay straight—you'll return on the Jastrow Trail. An informational sign points out the three distinct tree levels along the trail: oak, hickory, tulip poplar, beech, and black walnut form the canopy; redbud, dogwood, serviceberry, and spicebush form the midlevel; and laurel, rhododendron, azalea, mulitflora rose, may applejack-in-the-pulpit, and fern fill the understory.

This is a very pleasant section. Even though Windsor Mill Road is not far away, the falls below easily drowns out traffic noise. To the left, the thickly wooded hill rises precipitously; here the beech and walnut are especially enormous and old, somewhat amazing considering the lumber needs of the growing city over the last few centuries.

At 0.8 miles, cross over a little footbridge that is covered alternately with rock, metal, and plastic. Just beyond lie pure thick woods. Occasionally, views open up on the right and all you can see are the tops of trees—no roads and no buildings, despite being in the middle of the city. You'll see mill ruins to the right at 1 mile. You have several options here: Jastrow Trail to the left, Stream Trail to the right, and the Gwynns Falls Trail straight ahead. The out-and-back Stream Trail is little different from the Windsor Hills Conservation Trail you took originally, and since you'll take Jastrow coming back, go straight.

For almost the next mile, the scenery doesn't change much, but it's consistently stunning; every time it opens up, you'll have phenomenal views of the stream valley below, especially in winter. In summer, you'll see nothing but a riot of green, and in autumn, yellow, orange, and red dominate. At 1.8 miles, you'll hit asphalt as the trail parallels Morris Road and Hilton Parkway. Unfortunately, you'll lose the forest here, but it's not an unpleasant walk by any stretch.

At just under 2 miles, you'll reach Franklintown Road. Take a left and go under the Hilton Parkway bridge. Follow the signs to Leon Day Park. You'll see a Gwynns Falls Trail sign to the left just before you go under the bridge. Cross Franklintown Road and pick up the asphalt on the other side; Gwynns Falls sits in a buffer of trees to the right. At 2.2 miles, cross over a wooden footbridge and come to Leon Day Park, named in honor of the West Baltimore resident and Negro League baseball star who was inducted into the Baseball Hall of Fame in 1995. A loop circles the park so you can go in either direction. On the far side of the park, at 2.5 miles, you'll see a railroad bridge and a small truss bridge. The path continues there and marks the beginning point of the Phase II Extension of the Gwynns Falls Trail. Just beyond the bridge is Western Cemetery.

Loop the park; on your return trip, you'll reach the three-way trail intersection at 3.7 miles. This time, take the Jastrow Trail to the right. (The short connector trail between the Gwynns Falls Trail and the Jastrow Trail is indicated as the Girl Scouts Trail on the old Phase I Trail Guide, but there are no signs on the trail to indicate that). When you see Chesholm Road straight ahead, take a left up the hill on the asphalt, which soon crumbles into dirt and grass; this is the Jastrow Trail (250 feet after turning up the Girl Scouts Trail).

The Jastrow Trail rises uphill above the stream valley to the left. At just over 4 miles, you'll pass the Jastrow Levin campsite, a youth group campground and picnic area, on the left. The trail here is much tighter and wilder than the major sections of the Gwynns Falls Trail. You'll see lots of midlevel growth, and you'll have to duck under vines a few times. At 4.3 miles, Windsor Mill Road reappears; railroad ties on the trail will ease the steep descent. As soon as you reach the bottom of the hill, you'll rejoin the Mill Race Trail at the Windsor Mill parking area. Head right, cross over Windsor Mill back to the Windsor Hills Conservation Trail, and back to your car.

NEARBY ACTIVITIES

Within 10 miles, plenty of other hiking and recreation opportunities abound. Head south on Hilton Parkway from Gwynns Falls Park to MD 40 west and continue to Patapsco Valley State Park. Go east on Hilton Parkway to Liberty Heights to Druid Hill Park, home of the Maryland Zoo, among other attractions. Also on Hilton Parkway, just before Liberty Heights, is Hanlon Park and Lake Ashburton; although not a hiking destination, the view of downtown over the lake is fantastic—and something of a local secret.

GWYNNS FALLS TRAIL FROM LEON DAY PARK TO CHERRY HILL PARK 08

IN BRIEF

Follow a greenway trail through West Baltimore. Bracketed by wooded and waterfront parks on both ends, the middle section is entirely urbanized, running through some of Baltimore's lesser known but more interesting neighborhoods.

DESCRIPTION:

Since the publication of the first edition of *60 Hikes within 60 Miles: Baltimore*, the Gwynns Falls Trail has been designated as both part of the East Coast Greenway and the Chesapeake Bay Gateways Network. It has also become a focal point for city activities; check out the Web site for a calendar of happenings—it's wonderfully packed with hikes, art shows, and cultural festivities of all kinds.

John Smith mapped the Gwynns Falls in 1608, though the Susquehannock and Algonquian Indians had been nearby for centuries. Smith said the stream tumbled over "felles," or falls, which explains the sometimes confusing local practice of naming streams and rivers as "falls" (see Jones Falls, Gunpowder Falls). The stream itself was named for Richard Gwinn, who established a trading post here in 1669. In 1904, the Olmstead brothers laid out a series of parks and open spaces to be included in their plan for the Greater

KEY AT-A-GLANCE INFORMATION

LENGTH: 11.1 miles
CONFIGURATION: One-way
DIFFICULTY: Moderate
SCENERY: Gwynns Falls, city neighborhoods, waterfront parks
EXPOSURE: More sun than shade
TRAFFIC: Moderate–heavy
TRAIL SURFACE: Asphalt, cement
HIKING TIME: 4 hours
ACCESS: Many of the parks along the route are open dusk–dawn. The trail is always open but best avoided after dark. There are Light Rail stops as well as bus service at many points along the route. For a schedule, call (410) 539-5000 or (866) RIDE-MTA, or visit www.mta maryland.com.
MAPS: USGS Baltimore West, Baltimore East, Curtis Bay. A printable trail map is available at www .gwynnsfallstrail.org.
WHEELCHAIR ACCESS: Yes
FACILITIES: Many establishments along the route offer food, shelter, phone, and bathrooms.
SPECIAL COMMENTS: This is a hike for the urban adventurer, often running along city sidewalks through neighborhoods, substations, even industrial parks.

Directions

Take I-83 to Exit 6, North Avenue west. Go 3.5 miles and cross North Hilton Street. The very next left is Morris Road (a detour for Franklin town Road). Follow Morris until it ends at Franklintown and take a left. The first right, under the bridge, is the parking lot for Leon Day Park.

GPS Trailhead Coordinates

UTM Zone (WGS84) 18S
Easting 355860
Northing 4351425
Latitude N 39° 18.013093'
Longitude W 76° 40.297959'

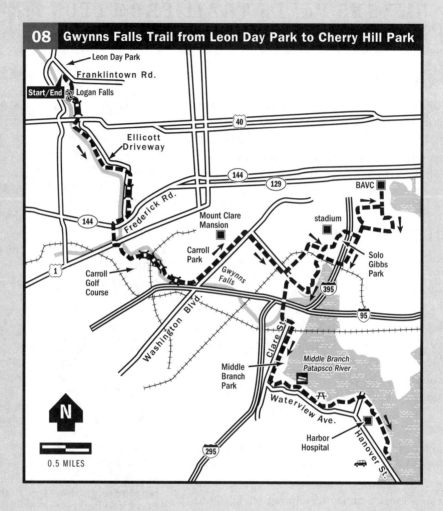

Gwynns Falls Trail from Leon Day Park to Cherry Hill Park

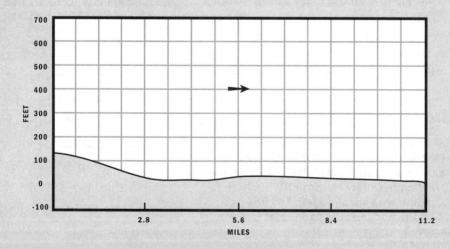

Baltimore Public Grounds. The Gwynns Falls Trail (GFT) resurrects much of that plan.

This portion of the hike begins at Leon Day Park, named in honor of the West Baltimore resident and Negro League baseball star who was inducted into the Baseball Hall of Fame in 1995. The park boasts new facilities, including playgrounds, lighted sports fields, and restrooms. Go 0.3 miles to the other end of Leon Day where you'll cross under a steel bridge and enter CSXT property, which for the next 1.5 miles is very nicely wooded with the Gwynns Falls to the right down the hill and large rock outcroppings up the hill to the left. Though you won't see it, beyond the hill is Western Cemetery, more than 250 years old and incorporated in 1846. Cross under a bridge at 0.6 miles and look for the informational sign and benches at 0.8 miles. The sign will tell you that this section was once known as "Baltimore's Niagara Falls." You'll be tempted to laugh at the hyperbole, but the water pouring over the rocks is nice nonetheless. Though with this pleasing scene, there's no mistaking the strange dichotomy around you: the pretty Gwynns Falls, set in thick woods full of beautiful sweet gum, hickory, and maple sometimes despoiled by a dumped furnace or plastic tubing.

However, there's no question that things are on the upswing; the more trail users, the better things will become. The trail council hosts clean up days, as well. The presence of the informational signage along the GFT is part of the charm. The signs usually contain images of what the place looked like 100 or 150 years ago—it's interesting to look at a spot and see the changes (or better yet, that very little has changed). One such location is at 1.2 miles, at the triple-arched Baltimore Street Bridge, constructed in 1932.

Cross over Baltimore Street, following the Ellicott Driveway, a once mill-race then vehicular road, now closed to traffic and crowded with thick woods. At 1.8 miles, take a right at Frederick Road (there are GFT signs at all sections where it's not abundantly clear which way to go). Cross over the CSX line as well as Gwynns Falls on a bridge and head left at Dukeland. Cross Hurley at 2.2 and take a left, crossing the falls once again. Initially, there's a car grave-yard to the left, but it soon becomes quite wooded again, and coming soon is one of the most interesting and scenic sections of the entire trail: a series of three steel bridges crisscrossing old stone abutments of the former Brunswick Street Bridge.

Long before the bridges, it was this area where native Indians crossed the stream. A fourth bridge comes soon after, and you'll head under the wagon pass of the old Carrolton Aqueduct, the B&O's first bridge, constructed in 1829. The trail soon skirts the outer edge of Carroll Golf Course and becomes very urban soon after, passing the renovated Montgomery Business Park to the left (not like the other green parks you've passed, but a very impressive building), paralleling Washington Boulevard.

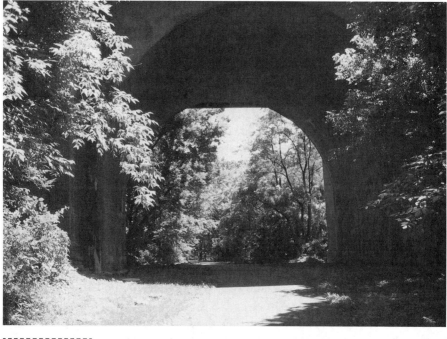

Railroad overpass

    Enter Carroll Park at 3.7 miles; aside from many recreational opportunities, the park is most famous for being the home of Mount Clare Mansion, circa 1760, Maryland's first house museum and one of the oldest colonial Georgian houses in Baltimore. (For info on visiting: **www.mountclare.org** or call [410] 837-3262). When you see three wooden poles in the path, take a right crossing Washington and onto Bush Street. The trail is delineated as a well-marked bike route in the street. Obviously, if you're walking, use the sidewalk parallel. Warning: this will no longer feel like a hike, but rather a city stroll. Further warning: if you follow the length of the GFT, it will remain urbanized for quite a while. Nevertheless, you'll pass through some historic and interesting city neighborhoods.

    First up is the Camden-Carroll Industrial Area. Follow the Bike Route signs to a left onto and then straight up Ridgely Road. Cross railroad tracks and take a right onto West Ostend Street, again following Bike Route and GFT signs. You're on the edge of downtown, passing M&T Bank Stadium, home of the Ravens, on the left. Take a right onto Warner Street across from the stadium. Once you cross the railroad tracks, you'll see signs for the GFT pointing straight as well as left. If you've had enough urbanity and want a return to green, go straight. If you want to do the whole trail, head left. Assuming you've headed left, pass under I-395 and through Solo Gibbs Park, a small community park in Sharp-Leadenhall, a neighborhood that is more than 200 years old and home to the city's first African-American enclave.

Take a right on Henrietta Street, and then a left on Williams Street to Light Street. Follow Light to the Baltimore Area Visitors Center (BAVC) at the Inner Harbor at mile 6.4, where you can find out anything and everything about what to see and do. (If you're really up for a vigorous day, ask about the guided Heritage Walk, which leaves from the BAVC and connects 20 historic sites and museums near the Inner Harbor.)

Coming back to the GFT, take a right on Lee Street and then a left on Sharp Street, going through Otterbein. A mid-19th-century neighborhood of orderly row houses and flower boxes, it's a true success story. Locals might remember Otterbein as the site of the $1 houses, sold to those willing to settle and revitalize. These days, those same houses fetch in the six figures. Follow Sharp Street to a right on Stockholm Street and go once again under I-395 to a left back onto Warner Street. Take a left onto Ridgeman Street and then another quick left into a little wooded area, still following the Bike Route signs.

Immediately go over a steel bridge, crossing short tentacles of the Middle Branch of the Patapsco River. Cross another bridge; you'll see the Greyhound Bus Terminal nearby, but you're waterside, sort of "underneath" the city. If you've done any downtown driving and have entered the city from I-95 on the I-395 ramp, you'll be familiar with the view. It's an odd feeling watching a large great white heron lope off across the Patapsco, bounded by a grove of wildflowers, underneath the swirl of interstate ramps.

When you pass under I-95, you'll be crossing the Gwynns Falls again, near where it empties into the Middle Branch of the Patapsco River. Take a left onto Clare Street, passing through the Westport Electric Substation. Take a right onto Kloman Street when you hit the railroad tracks. Pass the Westport Light Rail stop and take a left when you reach Waterview Avenue. If you've had enough urban adventuring, you'll be relieved as you enter Middle Branch Park. There's a wildlife observation boardwalk to the left that ends at a viewing deck at 9.5 miles. Surrounded by milkweed, cattails, goldenrod, and wildflowers, you'll see many water birds about: herons, gulls, ducks, and geese, as well as less familiar common snipe, ring-necked pheasant, Savannah sparrow, and tree sparrow—a somewhat incongruous but pleasing sight against the backdrop of the city skyline.

Go left onto the asphalt from the wooden boardwalk and pass another observation deck soon, then the Cherry Hill Marina, home of the Baltimore Rowing Club (**www.baltimorerowing.org**, [410] 355-5649). Follow the path as it winds along the water, passing picnic benches and shade trees, and go under the Vietnam Veterans Memorial Bridge. The Broening Boat Ramp is just beyond, yielding to a lovely little section that winds along the edge of the Patapsco. Despite trash here and there, bird life flourishes; the Baltimore Bird Club has sponsored outings in the area.

To the right is Harbor Hospital, buffered by a hill of wildflowers. The trail ends at the fishing piers near Hanover Street. There's a path that leads under the road, and there are plans to link it with the BWI and B&A trails to the south as a continuation of the East Coast Greenway. (Across the Hanover Street Bridge is Reedbird Island Park, a little-known peaceful Baltimore green space.)

There's parking available at Harbor Hospital to make the GFT one-way: take I-95 to Exit 54, Hanover Street. Go over the Hanover Street Bridge and turn left at Cherry Hill Road or Reedbird Avenue. The parking lot is at 3001 South Hanover Street.

NEARBY ACTIVITIES

Too numerous to list here—ask for help at the Baltimore Area Visitors Center on Light Street at the Inner Harbor. You'll find enough nearby activities to keep you occupied for a long, long time.

HERRING RUN PARK–
LAKE MONTEBELLO

 09

IN BRIEF

Stroll around the busy urban retreat of Lake Montebello and then plunge into the thick woods surrounding Herring Run, a forested marvel surrounded by dense population.

DESCRIPTION

A $20 million restoration to Lake Montebello, which removed sludge buildup from the chemically treated water and added landscaping and road improvements, was completed in 2007. New plantings, roadwork, and an iron-barred fence around the lake have really spiffed up the place. Also added was a median (complete with flowers and ornamental grasses) that separates cars from the hiking and biking lanes, each clearly delineated.

Backtrack where you came in by car, head down the hill, and cross Harford Road at the light at the intersection of Montebello Terrace, Harford Road, and Chesterfield Avenue (you'll see St. Francis of Assisi Church across the street). Once you've crossed, head left down the hill on the paved trail. Hooper Field, ringed by mature trees, opens up to your right. This path continues to descend until Harford Road is high above you to the left. At 1 mile, you'll come to a T-intersection, with the

KEY AT-A-GLANCE INFORMATION

LENGTH: 3.7 miles (5.6 miles with extension)

CONFIGURATION: 2 loops connected by an out-and-back

DIFFICULTY: Easy–moderate

SCENERY: Lake Montebello, Herring Run

EXPOSURE: More sun than shade

TRAFFIC: Heavy around lake, light–moderate at Herring Run

TRAIL SURFACE: Asphalt, grass

HIKING TIME: 1.5–2.5 hours

ACCESS: Dawn–dusk

MAPS: USGS Baltimore East

WHEELCHAIR ACCESS: Yes, to Belair Road

FACILITIES: Bathrooms, water

SPECIAL COMMENTS: The water of Herring Run has been deemed unclean by the Baltimore City Department of Health; walking near the water poses no threats, but stay out of the water itself. On a happier and more obscure note, the country's first monument to Christopher Columbus sits in Herring Run Park, on Harford Road between Walther Boulevard and Argonne Drive.

Directions

Take I-83 to Exit 9 to Cold Spring Lane east. Follow Cold Spring Lane to Harford Road (0.5 miles past Morgan State University) and turn right; after you enter Herring Run Park, turn right onto Lake Montebello. Once you've entered the park, you can only head left; there's plenty of parking on the side of the street roughly one-quarter of the way around the lake.

GPS Trailhead Coordinates

UTM Zone (WGS84) 18S

Easting 363869

Northing 4354855

Latitude N 39° 19.944613'

Longitude W 76° 34.768724'

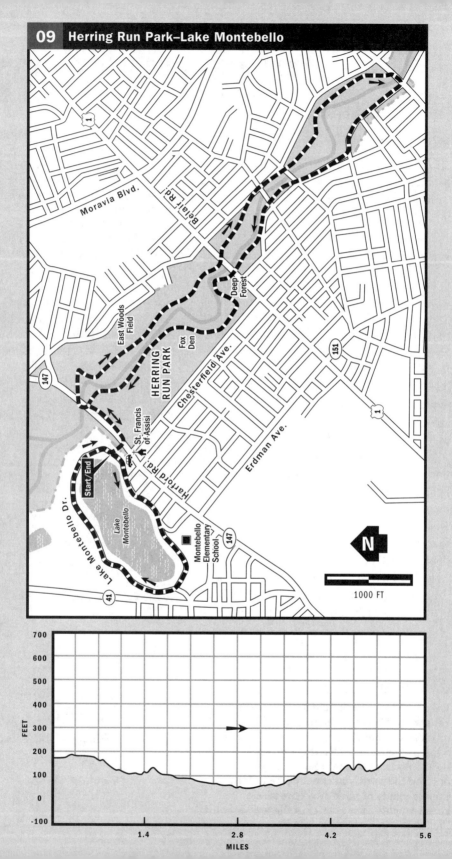

Herring Run

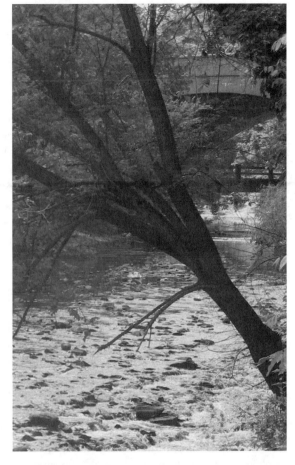

Harford Road Bridge to the left; take a right. Herring Run is on your left inside a stand of woods.

At 1.1 miles, the water comes into better view, but unfortunately trash can spoil the view, especially after a heavy rain, which speaks to the fragile nature of such urban runs as Herring. Even so, the water sounds soothing. Also, the path where you're walking is generally tidy, which seems to suggest that the problem isn't necessarily people throwing their garbage here, but rather rainwater picking up city trash and carrying it into the water.

At 1.3 miles, you'll enter the woods, well away from city traffic. Hearing swiftly moving water to the left and seeing thick woods on either side is heavenly. You'll soon come to a little stone bridge. To the right are some beautiful rock formations, creating natural cavelike shelters. Just beyond to the left you'll see a sign informing you that you are in Fox Den. Old oaks and maples dominate this truly magnificent, isolated, idyllic, stretch of forest. The trail remains wide and paved, with lots of underbrush and trees towering above on either side—a perfect example of how truly beautiful this entire area was, is, and can be.

At 1.5 miles, you'll enter a section appropriately called Deep Forest. At 1.9 miles, the trail begins to head left. You'll see woods in front of you. Row houses come into view behind the woods as you enter Orlinksy Grove. Here the trail follows the natural curve of the run itself and then opens up as a field comes into view on the right. Straight ahead is Belair Road; if you head left, you'll see a little dirt path to the water. This is a good place to stand—the water flows clear and absolutely free of trash. On either side, the water moves quickly over a series of rocks, while straight ahead it runs smoothly past a rock outcrop on the other side.

In the first edition of *60 Hikes within 60 Miles: Baltimore,* I suggested heading left on Belair, picking up the trail on the other side of Herring Run, and making your way back to Lake Montebello. However, I always regretted not continuing the hike along the green space surrounding Herring Run. I must admit that the following portion of the hike isn't nearly as nice as what has come to this point, so turning back now isn't such a terrible idea. However, continuing on, as described here, isn't so terrible either. It's certainly more urban here, and there is no real trail for much of the following walk, but you can hug the tree line, and there's still much green space, including many little cut paths through the vegetation toward the water. If you turn around now, the total hike will be 3.7 miles.

But assuming you've decided to keep going beyond Belair Road, you'll see residential homes to the right and thick woods to the left. Come to and cross Mannasota Avenue, then Brehms Lane. There's a playground to the left. Again, the scenery is more urban, but you can still head down to the water on some cut trails. At 2.6, there are ball fields and portable toilets. When you reach Sinclair Lane at 3 miles, turn around. Cross and head left on the other side, where you'll find more of the same: ball fields, playgrounds, and cut paths.

Once you reach Belair Road again, the hike resumes the beauty of the first part. Back in the woods on the other side of Herring Run from where you were before, at 2.6 miles, you'll cross a raised bridge over a small tributary. To the left you'll see a yellow pump house. There are sporadic arrows painted on trees, but disregard these and stay on the path, which is easy to follow.

At 4.5 miles, you'll pass a sign that reads WILDLIFE HABITAT: THIS BRUSH PILE PROVIDES PROTECTION FROM WEATHER AND PREDATORS FOR MANY SMALL BIRDS AND MAMMALS. This section is called Second Tributary, and the path opens up as the trail swings around to the right, passing ball fields to the left. A series of brick duplexes to the right pops up in the clearing up the hill. At a sign telling you this area is called East Woods Field, take the small dirt path into the woods, paralleling the paved path below. This dirt path rises up the hill and soon links again with the paved path at 4.8 miles; taking this path allows you to stay in the woods, which is nice if it's a hot day. When you come back onto the paved trail, Herring Run will be straight ahead. Head to the right on the paved trail and cross over First Tributary. The path runs much closer to the water on this side than it did on the outbound side. A series of rocks in the water gives off a pleasing sound, almost enough to drown out the sound of traffic, which you'll hear again as soon as you approach Harford Road. When you reach the bridge, walk under it; you'll see restrooms and a water fountain to the right. This is a popular area for dog walkers. Loop around and walk under the next arch of the bridge back to the path you took into the park.

Heading back to your car on the portion of the lake loop you haven't yet done, you'll see the green-roofed, brick Montebello State Hospital looming on the hill. Soon after you'll see tidy Baltimore row houses to the right. Just before reaching your car, a series of evergreens planted in neat rows appears on the right, while cattails dominate the lakefront on the left. Loads of birds and butterflies shuttle between these two oases.

NEARBY ACTIVITIES

A city-owned public golf course is in Clifton Park, just a half mile south of Lake Montebello on Harford Road. A half mile north is Morgan State University. If you have the opportunity, try to catch a performance by the university's world-famous choir, which has earned international acclaim (information: [443] 885-3598; **www.msuchoir.org**). For good eats and a bit of shopping, head to the revitalized Belvedere Square; from Lake Montebello, go south on Harford, take an immediate right on 32nd Street, and another quick right on Hillen Road. When it turns into Perring Parkway, take a left onto East Belvedere Avenue and you'll reach Belvedere Square in 3 miles; on Friday nights in the summer, enjoy live music outside from 6 to 9 p.m. For more information, visit **www.belveresquare.com.**

10 JONES FALLS TRAIL

 KEY AT-A-GLANCE INFORMATION

LENGTH: 6.4 miles

CONFIGURATION: Out-and-back with lake loop

DIFFICULTY: Easy–moderate

SCENERY: Druid Lake, Druid Park (Maryland Zoo, Baltimore Conservatory), Round Falls

EXPOSURE: More sun than shade

TRAFFIC: Moderate–heavy

TRAIL SURFACE: Asphalt

HIKING TIME: 2.5 hours

ACCESS: Dawn–dusk. The Woodberry Light Rail Station is just past the I-83 overpass on Union Avenue (see Directions). Maryland Transit Administration buses run to Druid Hill Park; for a schedule, call (410) 539-5000 or (866)RIDE-MTA, or visit www.mtamaryland.com.

MAPS: USGS Baltimore East, Baltimore West; printable map at www.jonesfalls.org

WHEELCHAIR ACCESS: Yes

FACILITIES: Restrooms, water, playground, gazebos, picnic, pool, tennis and basketball courts

SPECIAL COMMENTS: For more information on the trail, call (410) 396-0730 or visit www.jonesfalls.org.

- -

GPS Trailhead Coordinates

UTM Zone (WGS84) 18S

Easting 357969

Northing 4354655

Latitude N 39° 19.779596'

Longitude W 76° 38.871961'

IN BRIEF

Take in the first phase of the Jones Falls Trail through wooded Druid Hill Park.

DESCRIPTION

When complete, the Jones Falls Trail (JFT), Baltimore's newest greenway—and one of its finest—will stretch 12 miles from the Inner Harbor in the south all the way to Robert E. Lee Park just over the city line in Baltimore County. The trail will more or less follow the course of Baltimore's main north–south waterway, Jones Falls.

It's an ambitious plan, and long overdue. Having kayaked the Jones Falls before, I can attest to the paradoxical nature of this river: it can be exceedingly beautiful in spots and then terribly neglected in others. It is, in essence, a perfect microcosm of Baltimore itself. Because it runs right down the middle of the city and eventually makes its way into the harbor, its condition goes a long way toward determining the health of the city's natural spaces overall. A hiking and biking trail running along its course can only do more to raise the profile of this once and potential future jewel.

- -

Directions ⟶

From downtown or south: Take I-83 North to Exit 8, Falls Road. Follow Falls Road for 2 blocks and make a left onto Union Avenue. Go 0.4 miles and make a right onto Clipper Road. Make an immediate left onto Clipper Park Road, then another left onto Parkdale Avenue. Park on the street. The trailhead is at the end of Parkdale.

From north: Take I-83 South to Exit 9A, Cold Spring Lane. Make a left onto Cold Spring, follow it to Falls Road, and make a right. Go 0.7 miles and make a right at Union Avenue. Follow directions above from Union.

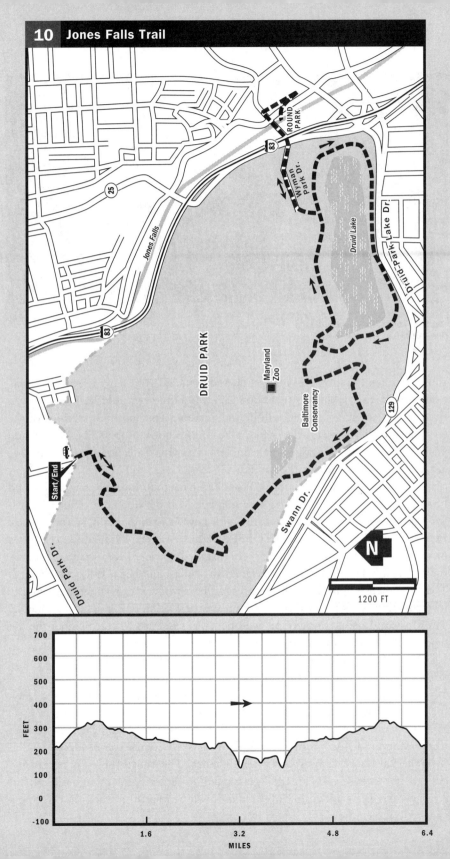

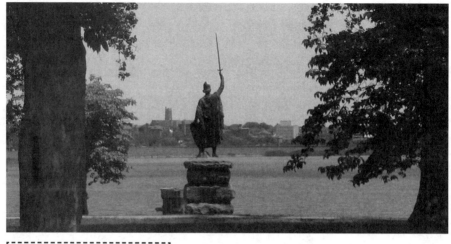

Wallace statue, fronting Druid Lake

As of Spring 2009, only the first phase of the trail was complete. Phase 1 runs from Penn Station to Woodberry and is included in its entirety here. Stay tuned for further additions that promise even more great hiking. In the meantime, major portions of what will be the northern and southern sections of the completed trail are included in other hikes in this book: Robert E. Lee Park and Cylburn Arboretum for the north and the Gwynns Falls Trail and Baltimore Waterfront Promenade for the south.

Begin the hike in Baltimore's Woodberry neighborhood, an attractive and historical mill area housing the new Clipper Mill development, which beautifully mixes historical mill structures with new environmentally sound homes. Entering Druid Hill Park at the end of Parkdale Avenue, you'll come to a series of switchbacks at 0.2 miles; these were installed to meet accessibility standards for people in wheelchairs. It's an impressive display, and beautifully constructed. The trail then winds through picturesque hardwood forest, some particularly lovely sections of which are crowded with mature tulip, oak, poplar, and maple. The area can be something of an eye-opener to residents who remember the old days when this part of Druid Hill was something of a no-go zone.

You'll come to the outer edges of a disc-golf course, one of the more popular courses in the area (watch for errant discs). At just under 1 mile, the trail swings close to a road before making a U-turn back into the deep woods. Look for an old circular stone shelter on the right. Follow the path as it skirts the edge of a bus parking lot for the zoo. The trail then swings around near the entrance to the Maryland Zoo (information: [410] 396-7102; **www.marylandzoo.org**) and then the Baltimore Conservatory at 1.3 miles. The conservatory is one of the city's better-kept secrets; an 1888 glass pavilion serves as the main building, but two new pavilions added in 2004 make this a wonderful attraction, offering a chance to see exotic plants and flowers.

Baltimore has had many nicknames over the years, including Mobtown for the population's penchant for fomenting . . . well, mobs; Charm City, the current nickname; and Monument City, a popular name in the 19th and early-20th centuries for the city's profusion of commemorative sites. Name the person, and there is probably a monument somewhere to him or her in Baltimore.

As you begin to make your way toward Druid Lake, you'll see four of these monuments in quick succession, and their eclectic nature truly is a testament to Baltimore's love of monuments. First, look for a memorial to George Washington. It will be facing away from you, but you will see PRESENTED BY THE FAMILY OF NOAH WALKER etched in the back. When you reach this monument, make a U-turn left and follow the path to the lake loop, at 1.9 miles. Head right, passing the small marble monument to Christopher Columbus. The inscription etched in the marble reads, CRISTOFORO COLUMBO. THE ITALIANS OF BALTIMORE, 1832. As you continue around the lake, next up is a very impressive statue of a man in chain mail, shield by his side, sword raised above his head—this is William Wallace, "Guardian of Scotland." He stands atop five massive granite boulders. The statue was originally presented by William Wallace Spence on November 30, 1893, and was rededicated on August 22, 1993, by Baltimore's Society of St. Andrew. Last is a memorial to artist Eli Siegel, founder of aesthetic realism. His likeness is cast onto a bronze plate that has been set into a large rock.

Druid Lake is a pretty and popular place for city residents to get some exercise on its 1-mile loop. Ringed with aquatic plants, the lake provides a home to a multitude of ducks, geese, and red-winged blackbirds. Founded in 1860 and listed on the National Register of Historic Places, 674-acre Druid Hill Park was created with revenue collected from a penny tax on nickel horsecar fares. In the 19th and early-20th centuries, couples in love would head out onto the lake in rowboats. A lot has changed since those days, but the lake remains just as lovely. Still used for city drinking, the water looks clean and fresh. The fountain that sat dormant for more than ten years was restored to working order in June 2004, and multicolored lights below the surface now accompany its sprays at night.

At 2.4 miles, you'll reach the iconic "Moorish" or "Turkish" Tower, a squat white-marble structure with club-shaped windows. From here you can see Wyman Park, the bell tower of Gilman Hall on the Johns Hopkins University campus, and the old brick Stieff Silver building, among other notable landmarks. Being in this spot in late March and early April yields a special treat: the hill below is completely covered in yellow tulips.

After making almost a complete circuit of the lake, take a right at 2.9 miles onto the trail, where you'll see a red metal bicycle and signs pointing you forward to the Jones Falls Trail (up the hill a bit from the lake). In another 0.2 miles, you'll pass the Druid Park pool on the left; for info, call (410) 396-6477.

Cross I-83 (below you) at 3.2 miles. Once on the other side, you'll see the Stieff Silver building to your left. You'll see signs pointing you toward JHU, Wyman Park, and the JFT to Inner Harbor. Follow the JFT signs as the trail

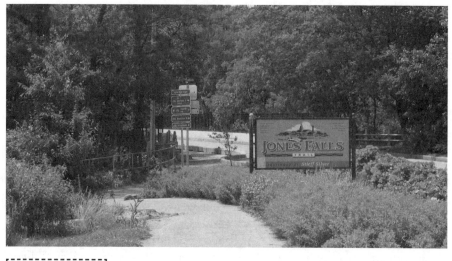

JFT at Boy Scout Park

goes through another series of switchbacks. At the bottom of the hill, cross Fallsway and go to the viewing deck for Round Falls at 3.6 miles, a scenic view indicative of the Jones Falls's potential (and current) splendor.

At this point, I'd recommend turning around. The JFT continues here, but it parallels Fallsway past a not terribly pleasant collection of industrial buildings until it emerges onto Maryland Avenue near Penn Station. That said, the Baltimore Streetcar Museum ([410] 547-0264; **www.baltimorestreetcar.org**) is just a half mile down Fallsway and is certainly worth a visit.

Instead of following your incoming route and heading left at the lake, go right to complete the only section of the lake loop that you haven't yet done. Beautiful old oaks and tulip poplars spread their branches over the asphalt. Beyond them sit benches and picnic tables. This is where one of the fireworks scenes was filmed in Barry Levinson's movie *Avalon*.

NEARBY ACTIVITIES

Apart from the cultural attractions, swimming pool, and disc-golf course listed previously, you'll also find tennis and basketball courts in Druid Hill Park. Also, near the hike's end at Boy Scout Park, you're only a few blocks from Johns Hopkins University and the Baltimore Museum of Art, just down Wyman Park Drive.

LEAKIN PARK

IN BRIEF

Have several "I can't possibly be anywhere near a city" moments along this amazingly wild and isolated trail through one of the largest unbroken urban forests in the United States.

DESCRIPTION

If you haven't been here before, the end of I-70 might come as something of a shock. An interstate that runs more than 2,000 miles all the way to Cove Fort, Utah, has its eastern terminus rather abruptly in a circular Park and Ride lot and a forest beyond. Originally, plans had called for the extension of the highway through both Leakin and Gwynns Falls Parks; opposition groups formed, and after a four-decade battle, plans for the highway extension were shelved and the parks spared. We are the lucky beneficiaries today.

Follow the well-marked Gwynns Falls Trail around the Park and Ride and into the Franklintown neighborhood of West Baltimore. This historic area dates back to the mid-18th century. Do note that the trail does disappear for a bit here and you'll have to use the road shoulder. However, the trail soon picks up on the other side of the road and plunges into mature forest. Along the way, you'll pass two important historical structures: a gristmill in operation from 1761 to 1934, and the Franklintown Inn, dating to the 1800s.

At 1.4 miles, come to a series of switchbacks that take you to Franklintown Road. You'll reach Leakin Park's Winans Meadow

KEY AT-A-GLANCE INFORMATION

LENGTH: 6.5 miles

CONFIGURATION: Out-and-back with loop

DIFFICULTY: Moderate

SCENERY: Mature forest, Dead Run and Gwynns Falls, historical structures

EXPOSURE: Mostly shaded

TRAFFIC: Light on Leakin Park trails, moderate on Gwynns Falls Trail, moderate–heavy near parking area and pavilion in park

TRAIL SURFACE: Packed dirt, exposed roots, rocks, asphalt

HIKING TIME: 2.5 hours

ACCESS: Dawn–dusk. The Maryland Transit Administration (MTA) runs buses along Windsor Mill and to the I-70 Park and Ride. For a complete schedule, call (866) RIDE-MTA or visit www.mtamaryland.com.

MAPS: USGS Baltimore West; Leakin Park trail maps are available at the Winans Meadow parking area.

WHEELCHAIR ACCESS: Gwynns Falls Trail portion

FACILITIES: Restrooms, water at Winans Meadow parking area

SPECIAL COMMENTS: For information on Leakin Park happenings, visit www.leakinpark.com.

GPS Trailhead Coordinates

UTM Zone (WGS84) 18S

Easting 353279

Northing 4351332

Latitude N 39° 17.936826'

Longitude W 76° 42.091963'

Directions ——————————➤

Take I-695 to Exit 16, I-70 East/Park and Ride. Park where the expressway ends and look for the Gwynns Falls trailhead.

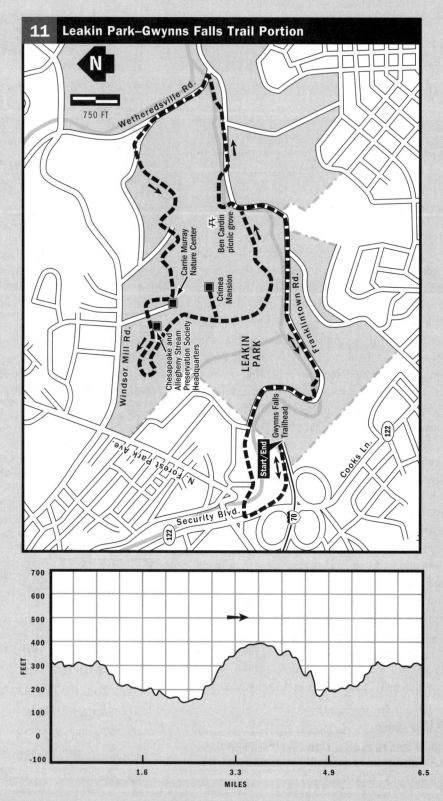

11   Leakin Park–Gwynns Falls Trail Portion

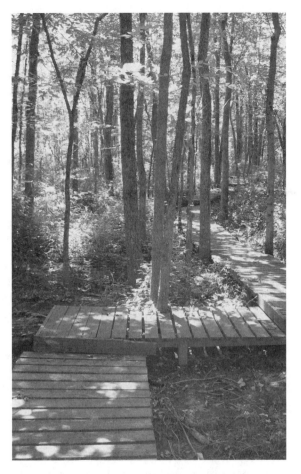

parking area soon after. Here, you'll see where the Gwynns Falls and the Dead Run meet. In colonial times, the Gwynns Falls marked the boundary between the Iroquoian and Algonquian-speaking tribes. At this time, around 1800, Baltimore was the nation's third-largest city, and growth and industrialization came quickly. This swath of natural beauty miraculously managed to survive. Unfortunately, Leakin Park eventually became synonymous with crime, but it has been restored, is vigorously maintained, and is now a true urban retreat.

Despite this, you might initially have a sour taste in your mouth as you head right on the paved path at the parking area—you're likely to see a lot of trash on either side of the trail as well as in Dead Run to your left. You might find this depressing and have some desire to give up. Don't—pleasures await you farther down the trail.

At 1.9, you'll see a footbridge over Dead Run to the left, but head straight. Despite the trash in the river, Dead Run actually sounds nice because it is swift and full of rocks. At 2.3 miles, cross over a pretty steel bridge; immediately merge left onto Wetheredsville Road, which is closed to traffic. Grass and weeds have begun their job of reclaiming the road. Immediately head uphill into the woods and turn right on the dirt "Stream Trail." Over the road below is the broad and lovely Gwynns Falls; your view will be mostly unimpeded in winter.

When you come out of the woods at the intersection of two paved roads, head left toward the sign for the Carrie Murray Nature Center—you're now on Hutton Road, which is also closed to traffic. Straight ahead you'll see a sign for the Gwynns Falls Trail, and immediately to your left, you'll pass a greenway meadow, where, depending on the season, you'll see milkweed, fiddlebug nymph, Queen Anne's lace, goldenrod, and monarch and swallowtail butterflies.

Walking up Hutton Road, you'll be mostly in the shade and see lots of rocks and moss on either side of the cracked asphalt. You'll see signs for the Wetland Trail and Nature Center. Head into the woods and walk along the boardwalk through a stand of smaller, newer trees—mostly oaks and beeches. You'll be thankful you're on a raised boardwalk as you cross over small streams, marshy aquatic plants, mud, and poison ivy.

Soon, the boardwalk ends and the trail becomes dirt and moss. Here comes one of those moments that if you were dropped here from a plane, you would never guess you were in the middle of an industrialized city. All you can see are sky and trees; portions of the hit movie *The Blair Witch Project* were shot here, and the thick forest makes it easy to see why.

The trail then leads uphill and becomes a loose collection of exposed roots and rocks. You begin to zigzag up and down—mostly up—until you come to a clearing and the Carrie Murray Nature Center at 3.1 miles. The nature center was named for the mother of Orioles Hall of Famer Eddie Murray. If it's open, it's worth going inside. Most interesting is the rehabilitation center for injured birds of prey; the center also provides a nice display of reptiles.

Moving away from the nature center, turn right at the paved trail and go up and over the hill. You'll see a small parking area to the right and a dirt footpath across from it on the left; follow the path into the woods. You'll see white blazes on this trail, which is very dense and well shaded, mostly by tall oaks, and again you'll feel as if you can't possibly be anywhere near Baltimore. The blazes soon turn red, and you'll see a sign pointing to the Ridge Trail, but go straight. To the left you'll see pavilions, picnic benches, a parking area, playground, volleyball net, and tennis courts. This part of the trail is called the Norman Van Allen Reeves Memorial Trail. You'll see a boarded-up chapel to the left; colorful wildflowers surround it in spring and summer.

When the trail emerges from the woods onto a paved road and parking lot, turn left and cross over the train tracks through the open field; head left, and follow the tracks to the Chesapeake and Allegheny Steam Preservation Society Headquarters, which was constructed to look like an old train depot. Circle around the tracks, keeping the woods on your right. This area is exposed, but to your right you'll see a wildflower meadow loaded with milkweed.

At 3.9 miles, follow the dirt road into the woods, which will bring you to a clearing. Follow the tree line until you come to a paved road, and take a right; stone buildings appear on your right. Keep walking and soon on your left you'll see the carriage house, chapel (which you passed earlier), caretaker's house, and honeymoon cottage of the Crimea Mansion, now the headquarters of Outward Bound.

Crimea was built in the mid-1800s by Thomas Winans, who made a fortune in Russia overseeing construction of the transcontinental railroad for Czar Nicholas I. He called the estate Crimea after the Russian peninsula of the same name. The owners, who were known Southern sympathizers, tried to discourage Union troops from entering their estate by constructing a faux fort with fake cannons. It didn't work; the troops of General Benjamin Butler cut up the orchard for firewood, arrested Winans's father, Ross, and locked him away in Fort McHenry.

With the mansion in front of you, backtrack and turn left on the gravel road at the little parking area at 4.2 miles. Head downhill in the woods; to the right you'll see some absolutely magnificent huge old white oaks. Be careful— the trail is rocky here, and it's easy to twist a knee. After about a hundred yards, you'll see a foot trail to the right; take it and it will lead you to that magnificent stand of white oaks.

The trail gets a little tighter here, and a few sections are washed away from erosion. Get ready for the next "I can't believe . . ." moment. When you come to a T-intersection, head left. You'll soon arrive in a big clearing with picnic benches and a pavilion, the Ben Cardin picnic grove at 5.1 miles, named after the Baltimore congressman and now Maryland senator. Walk downhill toward the patch of wetlands next to the pavilion. You might see mudflat dragonflies, red-winged blackbirds, and periwinkle. Walk along the paved path and cross over Dead Run on the bridge to the parking area at Winans Meadow. Backtrack on the Gwynns Falls Trail to I-70.

NEARBY ACTIVITIES

On the second Sunday of each month from April to November, the Chesapeake and Allegheny Steam Preservation Society runs trains for passenger pleasure rides from 11 a.m. to 3:30 p.m. For info: (410) 448-0730; **www.alslivesteam.org**. The Gwynns Falls Trail intersects with Leakin Park trails at Hutton Street.

12 PATTERSON PARK

KEY AT-A-GLANCE INFORMATION

LENGTH: 2 miles

CONFIGURATION: Loop

DIFFICULTY: Easy

SCENERY: East Baltimore, historic structures, duck pond

EXPOSURE: Sunny

TRAFFIC: Moderate–heavy

TRAIL SURFACE: Asphalt

HIKING TIME: 45 minutes–1 hour

ACCESS: Open 24 hours a day year-round; take due caution after dark. Maryland Transit Administration (MTA) buses run on streets bordering the park on all four sides; for a complete schedule, call (866) RIDE-MTA or visit www.mtamaryland.com.

MAPS: USGS Baltimore East; online park map at www.pattersonpark .com/Images/lgRunMap.jpg

WHEELCHAIR ACCESS: Yes

FACILITIES: Water fountains, ball fields, tennis and basketball courts, playgrounds, swimming pool, skate center

SPECIAL COMMENTS: The Pagoda is open Sundays from May–October, 12 p.m.–6 p.m., with free music Sunday nights from May–August. For information, call (410) 276-3676 or visit www .pattersonpark.com.

GPS Trailhead Coordinates

UTM Zone (WGS84) 18S

Easting 363348

Northing 4350237

Latitude N 39° 17.443907'

Longitude W 76° 35.074968'

IN BRIEF

Enjoy a renewed urban oasis, 137 acres in Baltimore's oldest public park.

DESCRIPTION

Often referred to as "Baltimore's Backyard," Patterson Park has hosted residents since 1669, and became a public park in 1827. Previously, it served an important defense function. During the War of 1812, as the British were burning the nation's capitol, entering North Point, and bombarding Fort McHenry, they were stopped at Patterson Park's Hampstead Hill, where the sight of 100 cannons and 20,000 troops made them head back toward the harbor and their waiting ships. After the park's formation, it became a fortification yet again, during the Civil War.

The park ran into some hard times again during the 1980s and early 1990s when it became synonymous with drug activity. Neighborhood revitalizations and booms in the housing markets of nearby Highlandtown and Canton, however, renewed interest in the park as a place of recreation and a true urban oasis has been created. The "Friends of Patterson Park" gets the primary credit for the park's renaissance. You'll pass the organization's white brick headquarters as you head left from the trailhead.

Directions

Take I-83 south until it ends at President Street. Continue straight on President Street and then left onto Eastern Avenue and go approximately 25 blocks to Patterson Park Avenue; turn left and park on the side of the road. The trail starts between the two concrete pillars where Lombard Street ends at Patterson Park Avenue.

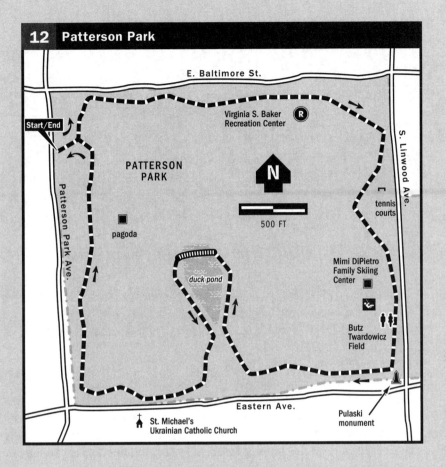

12 Patterson Park

E. Baltimore St.

Start/End

Virginia S. Baker
Recreation Center ®

PATTERSON
PARK

N

500 FT

S. Linwood Ave.

tennis
courts

Patterson Park Ave.

pagoda

duck pond

Mimi DiPietro
Family Skiing
Center

Butz
Twardowicz
Field

Eastern Ave.

✝ St. Michael's
Ukrainian Catholic Church

Pulaski
monument

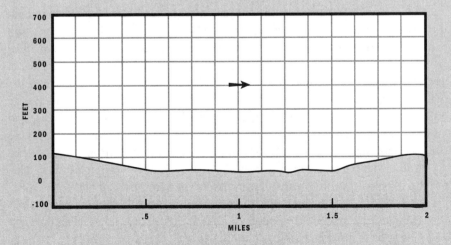

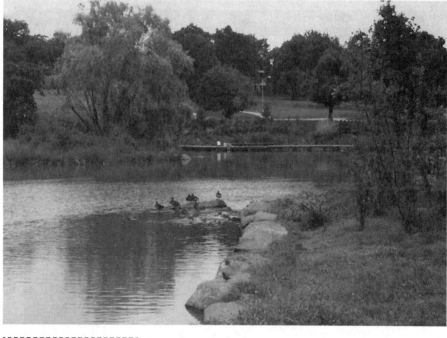

Ducks in Patterson Park pond

You'll see a fountain straight ahead; take a left where the giant shade trees tower over the benches. Baltimore's ubiquitous row houses ring the park, and you will have views of East Baltimore from several points in the park, especially the higher ground near the trailhead. Open, well-maintained, trash-free fields border the first part of the trail. At a quarter mile, take a left when you see the Virginia S. Baker Recreation Center, and then take a quick right onto the narrow paved path, which runs alongside mature maple and white oak. (For activities at the rec center, call [410] 396-9156.)

At just under 0.4 miles, take a left and another quick left 50 feet later, heading down a sycamore-studded hill. You'll see ball fields to the right farther down the hill. Take the next right onto a narrower path, which descends slowly until level with the fields. You'll see a bench here, surrounded by more shade trees, and at 0.5 miles you'll come to tennis courts on the left. Stay on the paved inner path, passing the water fountain to the left. When you see the red Tudor-style building straight ahead, take a left; you'll pass by playgrounds, swing sets, and an Olympic-size pool (it's a bargain to swim here—just $25 to join for the whole summer and day passes only $1.50; call [410] 396-3838 for info).

You'll come to the Dominic "Mimi" DiPietro Family Skating Center (a blue building) next—for info on skating admissions and lessons, call (410) 396-9392. Take a left here. When you reach the grass buffer near the street, across from the tennis courts, take a right; you'll pass the Butz Twardowicz Field to the right and a portable bathroom to the left.

At 0.8 miles, you'll come to a ring of iron bars protecting an impressive concrete monument to the "Father of the American Cavalry," General Casimir Pulaski, fronted by an enormous American flag and flanked by tall evergreens; go right. At 0.9 miles, you'll come to another water fountain. On the next pretty, serene stretch you'll walk uphill past lots of mature trees. At 1 mile, you'll see a laminated map of the park on a bulletin board. Head up three concrete steps to the black asphalt that winds through trees and heads toward the interior of the park.

You'll soon reach a catch-and-release duck pond; it requires a fishing license. Take a right to circle the pond. While many ducks and geese congregate here, more than 50 bird species, and another 100 varieties, have been spotted in Patterson Park, mostly members of the thrush, warbler, and sparrow families but also some birds rarely spotted in the area, such as the gadwall, blue-winged teal, and merlin. Visit the park's Web site and **www.baltimorebirdclub.org** for more information on birding at Patterson Park.

Cross over the pond on the boardwalk, winding through a large concentration of cattails and lily pads. The boardwalk, which is just under a tenth of a mile long, ends at the stone wall that encircles the pond. At 1.3 miles, when you've made a full circuit of the pond, take a right and then head straight toward the white asphalt and row houses. At 1.4 miles, turn right and you'll soon be standing in front of the gold-tipped onion domes of St. Michael's Ukrainian Catholic Church. Follow the path to the right as it heads uphill and take a left when you reach the wider path. You will see playgrounds and a pavilion to the right.

At 1.7 miles, you'll pass a monument to German composer Conrad Kreutzer to the left and see the octagonal, four-story Chinese Pagoda up the hill on the right. Charles Latrobe designed the structure, which was originally known as the Observation Tower, in 1890. This striking hybrid of Oriental and Victorian design, graced by beautiful stained glass, sits on Hampstead Hill and provides scenic views of downtown and the harbor. These views help explain the line of cannons, marked 1814, in front of the pagoda. These cannons delineate the chain of fortifications that once ran from the harbor all the way to Johns Hopkins Hospital and helped repulse the British. After walking around the pagoda, head left and you will see the concrete pillars where you began your hike straight ahead. Note the lovely fountain to the right and the water fountain just off the path.

NEARBY ACTIVITIES

The Inner Harbor, with its multitude of things to see and do, is just half a mile to the west via Eastern Avenue or Lombard Street. Take Eastern Avenue to Albemarle Street to taste the great food that can be found in Little Italy and Greektown, which is just east of Patterson Park and Highlandtown; if you're in the area in June, be sure to go to the annual Greek Festival. Just south is Fells Point, a National Register Historic area, first incorporated in 1773; you'll find plenty of shopping, food, history, and people-watching in this fascinating neighborhood.

13 JHU-WYMAN PARK-STONEY RUN TRAIL

KEY AT-A-GLANCE INFORMATION

LENGTH: 7.2 miles

CONFIGURATION: Out-and-back

DIFFICULTY: Easy–moderate

SCENERY: Mature hardwoods, Stoney Run, Johns Hopkins University

EXPOSURE: A bit more shade than sun

TRAFFIC: Moderate on trail, moderate–heavy at Wyman Dell, playgrounds, and university

TRAIL SURFACE: Dirt, asphalt, cement

HIKING TIME: 2.5 hours

ACCESS: Trails are always open, although signs at Wyman Park and the playground near Cold Spring declare the parks open during sunlight hours only. The Maryland Transit Administration (MTA) bus runs several stops along the southern portion of the route; for a complete schedule, call (866) RIDE-MTA or visit www.mtamaryland.com.

MAPS: USGS Baltimore West, Baltimore East

WHEELCHAIR ACCESS: No

FACILITIES: Playground, ball field, campus, museums

SPECIAL COMMENTS: Hiking at dusk in the middle of June yields an incredible concentration of fireflies.

- -

GPS Trailhead
Coordinates

UTM Zone (WGS84) 18S

Easting 359905

Northing 4354340

Latitude N 39° 19.628305'

Longitude W 76° 37.520821'

IN BRIEF

Begin near and on the campus of America's oldest research institution. Then escape the city without leaving it as you hike through a wooded riparian buffer in historic Roland Park.

DESCRIPTION

The hike begins directly across from the entrance to the Baltimore Museum of Art (BMA), a wonderful museum that's always worth a visit. From across Art Museum Drive, head down the stone steps to the Dell, a treasured green space and a hub of activity. Follow the path as it loops around the Dell, and then exit at the far end up the stairs on the other side of where you entered.

Back on street level, follow the sidewalk across Wyman Park Road (the BMA will be on your right). Follow the signs for the Jones Falls Trail. Soon, Johns Hopkins University appears on the right, specifically Mason Hall. Head up the first stairwell and onto campus. Take a left between Hodson and Clark halls. The beautiful Federalist architecture of the campus opens up—even the newer buildings (some only a few years old) copy the style of the university's oldest buildings, which date to the 19th century. The university was incorporated in 1867 and received a bequest of $7 million from its namesake upon his death in 1873. At the time, it was the largest philanthropic donation in American history. The

- -

Directions

Take I-83 to Exit 9, Cold Spring Road east. Follow to a right on Charles Street (Rt. 139 south). Pass JHU on the right; pass 33rd Street, and take a right on Art Museum Drive. Park on the street.

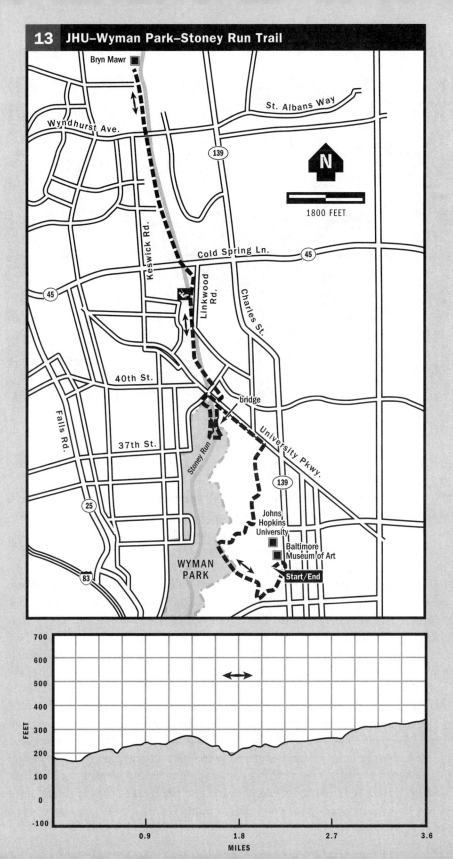

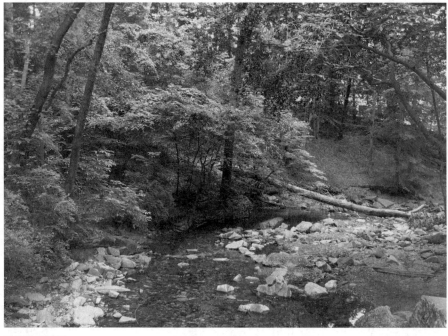

Stoney Run

medical school and hospital, across town, are consistently ranked the country's—even the world's—finest.

You can pick your own route through the picturesque campus, but you'll want to keep heading northwest (in essence, straight and left until you reach University Parkway). For an easy route, pass Ames and Latrobe halls, head left up the stairs, and pass Krieger Hall. The Eisenhower Library appears on the right, with venerable Gilman Hall on the left. Go down the stairs at Mergenthaler and Remsen halls. Take a right after Remsen, then a left onto the main path. At the athletic center, take a right and then a left at University Parkway at roughly 1.1 miles, depending on your exact route. The National Lacrosse Hall of Fame appears on the left (plans have been floated to move the museum, however).

When you get to San Martin Road, cross and take a left. At 1.5 miles, you'll see a little path aside wooden posts. After 0.1 mile, a little path heads down the hill to the right. Follow it to Stoney Run, and then cross over on the bridge. Crows, sparrows, jays, vireos, blackbirds, and an oriole or two flitter overhead. Rabbits, squirrels, and chipmunks scurry over the trail, and abundant ducks, frogs, and snakes live at the water's edge. Be on the lookout for night herons on the water.

Head straight up to a well-worn path and take a right (a trail also heads left for about 0.75 miles before petering out), staying on it as it heads up the hill and back to University Parkway. Cross University at the light to the right, and head down Linkwood Road (just before 39th Street). You may be disappointed when you see that Stoney Run is a small trickle contained within cement in this section of the trail, but don't despair—it gets better soon.

You've now entered Roland Park, one of Baltimore's most distinctive neighborhoods. The setting of Barry Levinson's *Avalon,* it's an eclectic mix of Queen Anne, English Tudor, Georgian, and Shingle architecture. Developed in the 1890s by City Beautiful designer George E. Kessler and Frederick Law Olmsted, the neighborhood continues today as an oft-studied example for urban planners on how to create a community that naturally conforms to its geological contours. Part of Roland Park's charm is its vast amount of greenery, with gardens, centuries-old trees, and of course, Stoney Run, which runs through its heart.

You'll soon see the trail appearing as well-trod packed dirt, with a nice buffer of woods—oak and tulip poplar mostly—shading both sides of the water. Cross Stoney Run on the footbridge, and follow the trail as it winds out of the woods and through a thick stand of bamboo before crossing a concrete bridge. To the left you'll see a series of private houses and community gardens, all immaculately maintained. Cross Overhill Road and pick up the trail on the other side, where it winds along the edge of the tree line, blocking the houses from view. At 2.2 miles, there's a popular playground to the right. Linkwood Road to the east is sufficiently far away, across a green field, and thick trees shield Wickford Road, to the west, entirely from view, making this a pleasant spot for kids to play, and for family picnics.

Passing the playground, you'll soon come to a chain-link fence and Cold Spring Lane beyond it. Cross Cold Spring at 2.5 miles and head left; take a right at 200 Cold Spring, and pick up the trail in the woods at the far end of the little parking area. The trail begins as a bed of cedar chips before reverting to packed dirt. Several varieties of oak and maple, as well as hickory, poplar, sassafras, ash, and the occasional walnut, shade the trail here. You'll also see a thriving understory filled with berry bushes, morning glories and trumpet vines, honeysuckle, and staghorn sumac, among other vegetation. Stoney Run flows to the right over loads of small rocks. Birds, rabbits, and squirrels shuttle between the woods and the water's edge.

The trail emerges into an open field as the surface returns to cedar chips. Just beyond, at a large cut to the left up to Wilmslow Road, you'll see a community bulletin board announcing area happenings and opportunities to help the Stoney Run Association with cleanups and other activities.

At 3.3 miles, cross Wyndhurst Avenue and pick up the trail on the other side as it plunges back into the woods. The trail rises above Stoney Run, and across the water you'll soon see tennis and basketball courts as you pass property owned by the Friends School (the oldest continuously operating school in Baltimore, founded in 1784) and then Gilman School. After another 0.2 miles, the trail ends at the back of a building that is part of the Bryn Mawr School campus; you have to turn around here.

On your return, when you get to Wilmslow Road, cross to the other side of Stoney Run and follow the trail there until you cross back just before Cold Spring. When you get back to San Martin, you can either retrace your steps or find a different route through campus. I'd recommend going left at University and then right at Charles, passing the campus ellipse, and then taking a right on Art Museum Drive. This route gives you access to the wonderful BMA sculpture garden at the corner of Charles and Art Museum Drive.

NEARBY ACTIVITIES

On the campus of Johns Hopkins University, you'll find the Homewood House Museum ([410] 516-5589; **www.museums.jhu.edu/Homewood**), the Baltimore Museum of Art ([443] 573-1700; **www.artbma.org**), and the National Lacrosse Hall of Fame ([410] 235-6882, ext. 122; **www.uslacrosse.org/museum**). The Roland Park Historic District, which is located between Belvedere Avenue, Falls Road, 39th Street, and Stoney Run, includes the country's first shopping center, a Tudor collection of storefronts that is the prettiest strip mall you'll ever see.

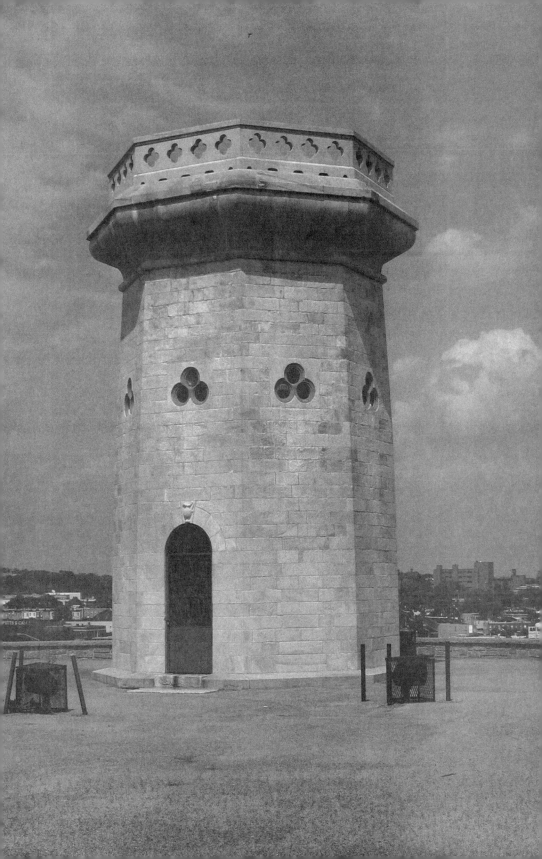

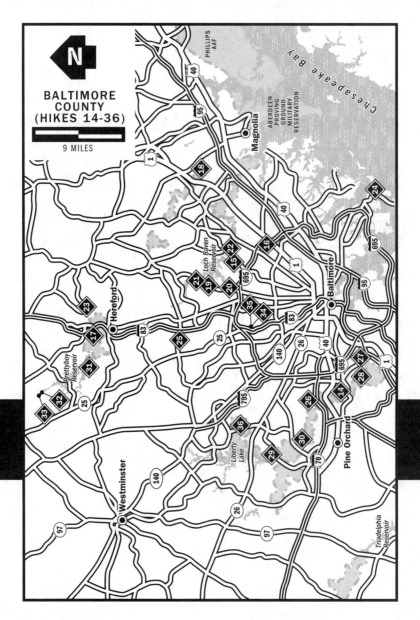

BALTIMORE COUNTY

14 BANNEKER HISTORICAL PARK– NO. 9 TROLLEY LINE TRAIL

KEY AT-A-GLANCE INFORMATION

LENGTH: 3.9 miles

CONFIGURATION: Two-way out-and-back

DIFFICULTY: Easy

SCENERY: Historic sites, Cooper Branch, abundant birdlife

EXPOSURE: Slightly more sun than shade

TRAFFIC: Moderate

TRAIL SURFACE: Asphalt on Trolley Line Trail, packed dirt at Banneker

HIKING TIME: 1.5 hours

ACCESS: Dawn–dusk, year-round

MAPS: USGS Ellicott City, trail maps for Banneker property inside the museum (open Tuesday–Saturday, 10 a.m.–4 p.m.)

WHEELCHAIR ACCESS: Yes, on Trolley Line Trail

FACILITIES: Restrooms, phone, and water at museum

SPECIAL COMMENTS: The trails around the Banneker property can easily be explored on their own, and the No. 9 Trolley Line Trail can be taken alone too, but combining them allows for a number of possible configurations.

GPS Trailhead
Coordinates
UTM Zone (WGS84) 18S
Easting 346834
Northing 4348187
Latitude N 39° 16.170316'
Longitude W 76° 46.531641'

IN BRIEF

Take in historic sites with a big dose of nature. Along the way, enjoy a good meal and shopping in Ellicott City.

DESCRIPTION

The No. 9 Trolley Line Trail follows the route of the old trolley line built by the Columbia and Maryland Railway in the 1890s to establish rail service between Baltimore and Ellicott City. The No. 9 Trolley ran until 1955. Several artifacts from the old line can still be spotted along the trail.

Beginning at the terminus of Edmondson Avenue, the trail runs first through the town of Oella; named for the first woman to spin cotton in America, it was home to cotton-mill workers for generations. The first residents built their homes of stone a few years before the War of 1812, while those who settled here in the years leading up to the Civil War used brick. Oella bustled until 1972, when Hurricane Agnes swept through the Patapsco Valley and destroyed much of the town; sadly, it never fully recovered. A nice wooded buffer flanks the trail, with the Cooper Branch of the Patapsco River running on the left.

Directions ⟶

Take I-695 to Exit 14, Edmondson Avenue west. Take Edmondson until it ends at Chalfonte Road. The trail begins at the end of Edmondson. To drive directly to the Banneker Museum: Take I-695 to Exit 13, Frederick Road, toward Catonsville. Go 3 miles and turn right onto Oella Avenue; continue half a mile to the Banneker Historical Park and Museum gates, on the left. Park in front of the museum; the trailhead begins behind the museum, past the botanical conservation area.

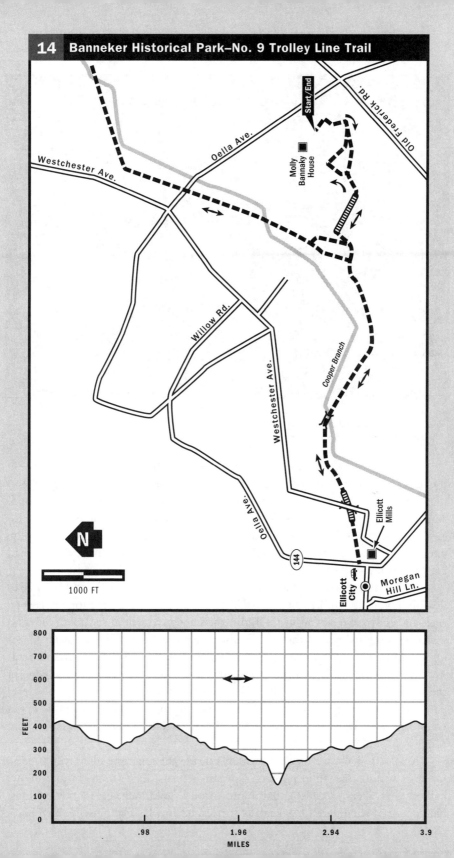

Start/End

Old Frederick Rd.

Oella Ave.

Westchester Ave.

Molly Bannaky House

Willow Rd.

Westchester Ave.

Cooper Branch

Oella Ave.

Ellicott Mills

144

Ellicott City

Moregan Hill Ln.

N

1000 FT

800
700
600
500
FEET
400
300
200
100
0

.98   1.96   2.94   3.9
MILES

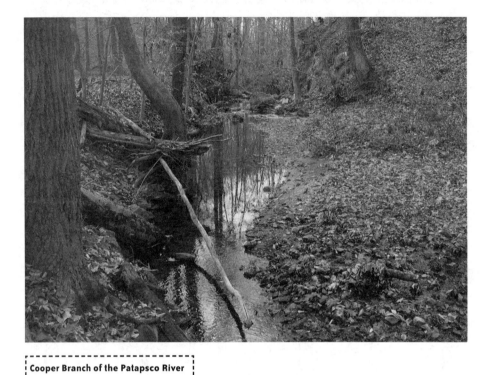

Cooper Branch of the Patapsco River

Quickly cross Oella Avenue. At 0.7 miles, you'll pass a big white house on the left; head up the hill to make your way to the Benjamin Banneker park and museum. You'll see a little creek to the left and a bunch of bamboo just beyond. The trail naturally continues downhill, but look for a sharp right up the hill. You'll reach the hilly rise, and you'll see a stream valley below. If you see the paved trolley-line path again, you've missed the trail—turn around and head back up. White-tailed deer abound in this area, so be on the lookout.

At 0.8 miles, cross a stream on a small wooden boardwalk, and then head downhill. Parallel the stream and you'll soon come to a small section of crushed rock and railroad ties. Cut to the right, then keep straight ahead to a field, and then cut right again into the botanical-conservation area. There are no blazes on the short, nubbly trees and tall walnuts, but you should have no trouble finding the trail, especially as it turns to cedar chips and then leads to the edge of the woods and the Banneker Museum about 500 feet beyond. There are several paths here, so you may find yourself on one other than those described here, but you'll find your way to the museum with little trouble in any case, reaching it at roughly 1.1 miles.

A wildlife-habitat checklist, available inside the museum, alerts you to look for spicebush plants, tulip poplars, Christmas ferns, Eastern bluebirds, yellow-bellied sapsuckers, warblers, Baltimore orioles, goldfinches, cedar waxwings, blue jays, red-shouldered hawks, box turtles, and owls. The museum also has a

"Birds of the Banneker Historical Park Birding Checklist" for more experienced bird-watchers. This brochure lists 60 birds, including four different finches, five sparrows, three owls, and four woodpeckers.

Benjamin Banneker, the foremost African American man of science in the early years of the United States, lived his entire life on the land where the museum now sits. Open since 1998, the museum and park continue to grow and develop. The Molly Bannaky House, a circa-1850 stone farmhouse, has been fully restored and now houses a library and meeting room. Other structures of interest on the property include an archeological dig area, a nursery, the Banneker Ice Pond, and the Lee Family Farm Ruin. Banneker was born a free black in 1731 and lived until 1806. His life's accomplishments included constructing a wooden striking clock and a projection of a solar eclipse; helping survey the land for Washington, D.C.; publishing six almanacs; and exchanging antislavery correspondence with Thomas Jefferson. The museum does an excellent job illuminating the life and contributions of this underappreciated figure in American history, and it is definitely worth a long visit.

When you've finished your museum visit, turn around and head back from where you came. Retrace your steps until you come to the cut where you earlier headed right; this time, follow the railroad ties down the hill, past the chain-link fence to the right marking the Banneker property boundary. The paved path beyond the fence is the Trolley Line Trail again; head left on it.

Back on the trolley line, you'll see Cooper Branch again to the right as you walk downstream. To the left sits a marshy area, surrounded and protected by a fence. The sound of water spilling over the big rocks in Cooper Branch provides a pleasing accompaniment. To the left rises a big hill studded with beeches and Christmas ferns. It's easy to see the natural contours of the valley and the ease with which the trolley ran through here. On first glance it appears that no blasting was necessary in the construction of the line, and judging by the size of the nearby oaks, little of the surrounding area was disturbed.

You'll cross Cooper Branch on an old stone bridge, a relic from the trolley line; your path doesn't change because the water runs underneath the trail. The legacy of rock blasting soon becomes clearer; you'll see jagged rocks, covered in fern and moss, jutting toward the trail from the left. Walk under a power-line cut, and be sure to look up for the hawks and turkey vultures that frequently glide above. I saw no fewer than two dozen of them circling around in the sky.

More jagged, moss-covered rocks, decorated here and there with sumac, crowd the trail until it turns into a long wooden boardwalk at 2.2 miles. In this area, look for the dangling cables tethered to the rocks; these used to support the trolley's electrical service. The boardwalk runs under the Westchester Avenue bridge. Although the bridge is a few hundred feet above your head and Westchester Avenue is only a narrow, two-lane road, you might feel a bit unnerved walking under this noisy steel bridge when cars go over. You can spot a stone column for the original bridge, ending below the current bridge.

You'll reach Ellicott City at just under 2.4 miles, and you'll see a sign that reads HISTORIC ELLICOTT CITY NO. 9 TROLLEY LINE TRAIL with a parking area just beyond. From this vantage point, it's easy to spot the remnants of the old train bridge over the Patapsco to the left. The trail soon ends; swing around and go down the wooden stairs lined with a row of Eastern red cedar. You'll see the brick trolley shop to the left, open and serving the public since the mid-1800s. Once down the stairs, you'll come to Ellicott Mills, established in 1772. The original rail line that ran from Baltimore, completed in May 1830, ended at this point. Railroading is prominent here, as Ellicott City boasts America's first railroad station; the same building now houses the B&O Railroad Museum, which is open Monday through Saturday, 10 a.m. to 4 p.m., and Sunday, 11 p.m. to 4 p.m.; information: (410) 461-1944; **www.borail.org.**

Because downtown and Main Street are right in front of you, why not take advantage and eat, shop, or browse? When you're ready to go back to your car, head back up the stairs to the trail and retrace your steps. This time, when you reach the Banneker property at 3.1 miles, pass by it and continue straight to Edmondson Avenue.

NEARBY ACTIVITIES

Assuming you've already spent significant time in the Banneker Museum and checked out Ellicott City's many attractions, you might want to experience the great hiking at nearby Patapsco Valley State Park. The Hollofield Area of the park (see page 284), with its ball fields, camping, playgrounds, equestrian trails, picnic areas, and, of course, hiking trails, can be reached by taking a right on Rogers Avenue from Frederick Road/Main Street in Ellicott City; turn right on MD 40, Baltimore National Pike. You'll come to the park entrance a couple of miles on the left before you reach the river.

CROMWELL VALLEY PARK WITH LOCH RAVEN ADD-ON

IN BRIEF

An opportunity for pleasant hiking within 371-acre Cromwell Valley Park, as well as adding a more strenuous Loch Raven extension. Keep your eyes open for abundant wildlife.

DESCRIPTION

Cromwell Valley Park (CVP) has a long history, first settled some 300 years ago. Nowadays, thanks to conservation efforts by the county and state as well as the generosity of families that owned the farms that now make up CVP, it exists mostly as an educational park, focusing primarily on farming, history, and nature. Programs demonstrating animal husbandry and organic farming provide educational opportunities year-round. This means that the park is often busy, but the trails remain largely uncrowded.

From the parking area, walk toward Cromwell Bridge Road and take the crossing over Minebank Run, which eventually flows into Loch Raven Reservoir not far to the east. Take a right on the blue-blazed Minebank Trail, which parallels the Minebank Run. Near the water, look for belted kingfishers and great blue herons.

You'll pass many mature trees including maple, walnut, tulip poplar, locust, oak, and sassafras. Staghorn sumac, Queen Anne's lace, and goldenrod flank an old property-line fence to the left. These native species

---

Directions ————————————➤

Take I-695 to Exit 29A, Cromwell Bridge Road. Go left (west) at the light, and enter the park to the left at 0.9 miles (2002 Cromwell Bridge Road). Follow the road all the way until it ends at a gravel parking area.

ⓘ KEY AT-A-GLANCE INFORMATION

LENGTH: 6.8 miles

CONFIGURATION: Combination

DIFFICULTY: Moderate–strenuous

SCENERY: Mature woods, Minebank Run, plentiful wildlife

EXPOSURE: More shade than sun

TRAFFIC: Light

TRAIL SURFACE: Packed dirt, short stretches of asphalt and gravel

HIKING TIME: 2.5–3 hours

ACCESS: Sunrise–sunset

MAPS: USGS Towson; trail maps are available at the information kiosk near the parking area. Online: www.cromwellvalleypark.org/map.

WHEELCHAIR ACCESS: No

FACILITIES: Restrooms and water in park office

SPECIAL COMMENTS: This hike leaves Cromwell Valley Park and includes several miles in adjoining Loch Raven Watershed property; if you prefer an easier or shorter hike, stay entirely within the park. As of summer 2008, the gates at Willow Grove and Sherwood farms close each evening at sunset and open at sunrise. Vehicles in the park after sunset may be locked in overnight.

GPS Trailhead Coordinates

UTM Zone (WGS84) 18S

Easting 366753

Northing 4364315

Latitude N 39° 25.084212'

Longitude W 76° 32.874556'

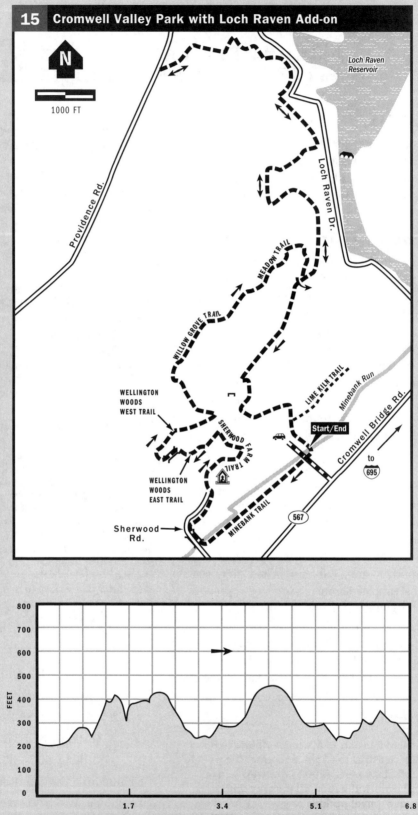

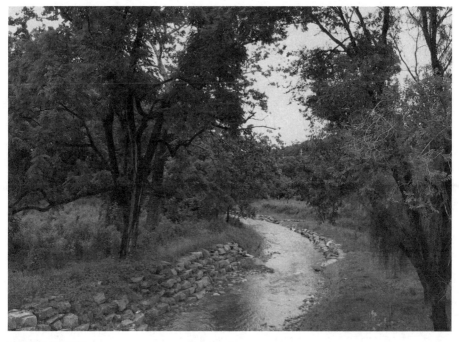

Minebank run

compete with invasive kudzu, porcelain berry, devil's tear thumb, barberry, and multiflora rose. Park volunteers, in league with the Ecosystem Recovery Institute, continue efforts to rid the park of these damaging plants. As the park is actually composed of three separate farms, you'll see divisions such as the fence as well as a grove of beautiful willow trees. All of the foliage here makes the area a haven for birds. In all, CVP hosts hundreds of bird species; for a complete list, visit **www.cromwellvalleypark.org/wildlifeAndBirding/fullBirdList**.

At 0.5 miles, you'll cross a feeder stream before coming to Sherwood Road. Take the bridge across Minebank Run and then follow the road. Do not take the left turn, but stay on the road continuing in the direction indicated by the Sherwood Farm sign. You'll pass the Cromwell Valley Community Supported Agriculture (CSA) site, an organic farm that sells shares to its produce (for more information visit **www.cvcsa.org**). At 0.8 miles, head left, going the wrong way past a "Do Not Enter" sign and through an alley of stately shade trees. This leads to the park office (the beautiful 1935 Sherwood House). When the horseshoe road of the park office begins to slope rightward, cut left toward the woods; you'll see a sign for the orange-blazed Sherwood Farm Trail. Take it into the woods.

This area is a riot of mature hardwood with a thriving understory. The trail splits immediately; leave the wide cedar chip trail and go left onto the narrower packed dirt Wellington Woods East interpretive trail, marked by green signposts. You'll come to a rightward cut at 1.1 miles; continue straight. You'll quickly come to a very discernible trail to the right followed immediately by a Y; take a left and

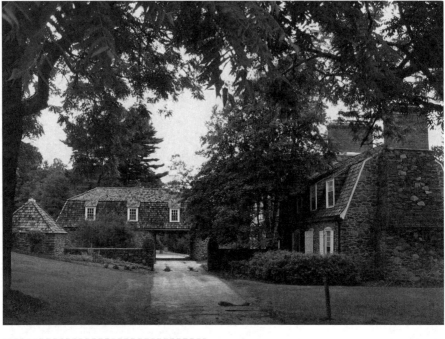

Sherwood House (ca. 1935), the park's office

you'll see a red #1 signpost—this is the Wellington Woods West Trail. Cross a footbridge and follow the trail along the top of a fairly narrow, very rocky ridge. It soon swings to the right on a bed of moss and reaches the edge of the park property. The trail splits again at a red #11 post; take a left and you'll see a green #1 at the split by an enormous oak. These numbered posts correspond to a nature guide that the park office hopes to reissue after some updating.

The path runs over little rippling hills dotted with ferns, a very nice spot. At the next trail split, at the #5 post, go left. You will parallel a little stream to the right and walk uphill along a ridge. You'll hear lots of birds singing as you hike, and you may also see some of the multitude of animals the park hosts. Abundant white-tailed deer live in the park, along with beautiful and elusive red foxes. Other animal residents include beaver, opossum, raccoons, woodchucks, muskrats, several varieties of squirrels and shrews, voles, chipmunks, and mice—ready meals for red-tailed hawks and kestrels. CVP also hosts many reptiles and amphibians including frogs, toads, turtles, skinks, and salamanders, as well as more than a dozen different snakes. A word of warning: the northern copperhead, one of Maryland's two venomous snakes, lives in the park; in the unlikely event that you do see one (look for the telltale diamond-shaped head), give it wide berth.

As you continue on the trail, you'll notice large chunks of Cockeysville marble, remnants of the marble that was heated to produce lime in large kilns in the early 1700s. A couple of the kilns still exist and can be seen near the parking area.

At 1.7 miles, you will see a series of steel cables heading up to a very tall antenna; head right, cross the stream, and go straight up the hill. Cross the intersecting path and continue straight on the wide trail; at the top of the hill, you'll see more offshoot paths—just continue straight on the red-marked Willow Grove Trail. Be on the lookout—this area is especially good for spotting red foxes. Pass through a grove of mountain laurel, and at 2.2 miles, you will connect with the yellow-marked Meadow Trail.

At 2.3 miles, take a right; you'll see the edge of Loch Raven Reservoir through the woods. At 2.7 miles, you'll come to a T-intersection on a path that's very wide even though you're still deep in the woods. To stay entirely in Cromwell Valley Park, or if you're short on time, take a right; otherwise, take the left to continue hiking within the Loch Raven watershed on a 3.3-mile out-and-back. If you take the out-and-back, you'll soon pass a section of woods filled with pristine beech trees. The trail swings around to the right and then crosses a stream; climb the hill to get a very nice view of the stream valley to the right. When you reach the T-intersection near the edge of the reservoir, at 3.1 miles, take a left. Go past a leftward cut and continue straight; at the T-intersection at 3.5 miles, take another left and you'll come to Providence Road at 4.3 miles. If you turn around and backtrack, you'll reach the cut where you took a left at 2.7 miles inside the park; you've now completed 6 miles of the total hike.

After another 0.1 mile, take the little cut to the right; you'll come to a trail split in about 1,000 feet. Go right up the hill onto a narrow footpath, which winds through a pretty area filled with close vegetation and hanging vines. At the next T-intersection, take a left. After you pass a couple of benches on the left, take a right into an open field, a great songbird locale. At the trail split at the edge of the field, go left; when you reach the gravel park road, at 6.7 miles, take a right and your car will be just up ahead, on the other side of the white house. (You'll pass by the white Lime Kiln Trail, an 0.2-mile trail, that runs past the lime kilns, if you want to see them.)

NEARBY ACTIVITIES

Take I-695 to Exit 27B to visit Hampton National Historic Site, a stately home that was once the largest mansion in the United States. Built with a fortune amassed during the Revolutionary War and once the northernmost slave-holding plantation in the country, it still boasts extensive gardens. (Information: [410] 823-1309, **www.nps.gov/hamp.**)

16 DOUBLE ROCK PARK

KEY AT-A-GLANCE INFORMATION

LENGTH: 2.25 miles

CONFIGURATION: Loop

DIFFICULTY: Easy

SCENERY: Stemmers Run, mature mixed hardwoods

EXPOSURE: Mostly shaded

TRAFFIC: Light

TRAIL SURFACE: Packed dirt, gravel

HIKING TIME: 1 hour

ACCESS: Dawn–dusk

MAPS: USGS Baltimore East

WHEELCHAIR ACCESS: No

FACILITIES: Restrooms at the edge of the woods, 0.1 mile from trailhead. Pavilions, ball fields, restrooms, and water at the official park entrance off Glen Road (take Harford Road south, cross Putty Hill Avenue, take a left onto Texas Avenue, go about a mile until Texas Avenue ends at Glen Road, and continue into the park entrance).

SPECIAL COMMENTS: The official park entrance, described above in Facilities, doesn't provide the best access to the trails; instead, follow the directions below to the park entrance sign, where there is no official parking area, but street parking is allowed.

GPS Trailhead

Coordinates

UTM Zone (WGS84) 18S

Easting 368898

Northing 4359237

Latitude N 39° 22.359524'

Longitude W 76° 31.320298'

IN BRIEF

Enjoy a very isolated spot where Stemmers Run meanders over a slew of rocks in the heart of heavily populated Parkville/Overlea.

DESCRIPTION

The Parkville Recreation Council manages the Double Rock recreational area, which provides a green haven within the urban sprawl of the surrounding neighborhoods and nearby Beltway. You can easily miss it—and you'll be wowed by the very wild feel of its trails.

Look to your left at the trailhead, and you'll see a large garden that is open to the public. People who want to plant in the garden must obtain a permit; for information call (410) 887-5300.

At 0.1 mile, turn right off the gravel at the wooden bathroom building and head into the woods; two tall white oaks and a wooden marker with yellow blazes mark the footpath here. Take a right, and you'll immediately notice how mature the forest is, with oak, poplar, and maple soaring overhead. These fantastic foliage trees make autumn a wonderful time to hike this trail. Ferns also abound all around the trail. You'll see a little gulley to the right with a hill beyond. As you descend and the woods rise on either side, you will find it very easy to forget that you are anywhere near civilization.

Directions ⟶

Take I-695 to Exit 31, Harford Road south; go 1.8 miles and turn left onto Putty Hill Avenue. Go 0.2 miles and turn right onto Fowler Avenue; park where Fowler Avenue ends at Hiss Avenue. The trail starts just behind the brown Double Rock Park sign.

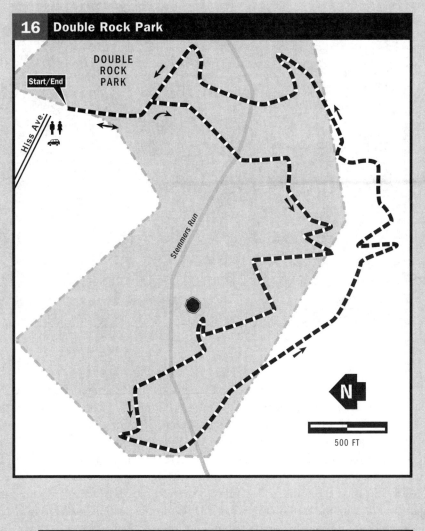

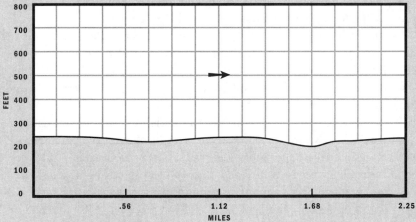

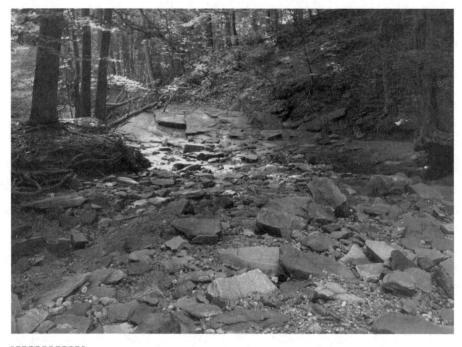

Stemmers Run

At 0.3 miles, turn right at the blue blazes and cross Stemmers Run using the rocks as convenient stepping-stones. (All the water crossings on this hike can be easily negotiated using the many rocks that lie in Stemmers Run.) Bear slightly to the left and follow Stemmers Run as it winds around to the left. You'll see big fish darting around in the water below where it pools and a beautiful area of striated rock above, where the water trickles through. You'll see more blue blazes straight ahead on the trail. At 0.4 miles, head left, crossing Stemmers Run once again and pick up the trail on the other side. Continue heading right, pass by the red-blazed cut into the woods to the left, and follow the blue blazes as they wind up the hill and rise above Stemmers Run and the valley.

At 0.7 miles, you'll see a huge rock outcropping to the right. This perch makes a wonderful place to sit and absorb the beautiful scene below: Stemmers Run spilling over huge chunks of rock. It's a little slice of Appalachia in the crowded Baltimore suburbs—quite literally, since the park's western boundary delineates the city line.

Head back up the hill and continue to the right on the blue-blazed trail. At 0.8 miles, the blazes turn to yellow at the dam (to the right) on Stemmers Run. You'll see an immediate split to the red trail, but stay on the yellow. On this section of the trail, Stemmers Run is now fronted by posts strung with a steel cable. As the trail gradually heads uphill, it begins to parallel a chain-link fence, which marks the park border. The trail winds its way between tall oaks, and at 1.2

miles heads downhill and up rather quickly; be especially careful on a muddy or snowy day since this section can be quite slippery.

At 1.4 miles, the trail heads downhill and ends at the water. Head left as the water snakes around and then splits; take a right over the water at 1.5 miles. Once you're on the other side, go left and then quickly right; you'll see yellow blazes again. Many fallen trees block the trail here, and you'll have to negotiate a few obstacles; be on the lookout for the snakes and turtles that find shelter in the crooks of the prone branches (you don't have to worry too much about poisonous snakes).

As the trail becomes increasingly tight and overgrown, keep a sharp eye out for a faded white blaze on an oak tree to the left. If you miss it, you'll come to a clump of vegetation, at 1.6 miles, where the trail ends abruptly; just turn around and look for the white blaze to the right. It's a mere 200 feet from the trail end. This white-blazed section was clearly once a maintained trail, but it doesn't see heavy use anymore; the blazes are faded and the trail is generally grown over. Most of the white blazes are on beech trees, so look for those. It's easy to lose, but if you keep heading uphill, you'll see occasional white blazes and white arrows to keep you on track. The underbrush is minimal, so you won't have to do much bushwhacking. At the top of the hill, you'll see an arrow pointing to the left; it isn't much of a trail, but if you just head in that direction anyway, you'll very quickly merge onto the well-maintained blue trail again. Take a right onto the blue trail.

At 1.7 miles, you'll see a pavilion to the right and you will come to a Y-intersection just beyond; head right. After a few hundred feet, you'll see an orange post on the left. Go to the left; you're now on a gravel and sand road that leads to an open field and the back of the garden plot you saw at the trailhead. Go left and follow the gravel trail back to your car.

NEARBY ACTIVITIES

If you've built up an appetite, you won't have any problem finding something to eat. Go either direction on Harford Road for a multitude of dining options. For more hiking, head south on Harford Road to Lake Montebello–Herring Run Park (see page 51) or continue past Herring Run for a round of golf on the public course in Clifton Park, between Harford Road, Belair Road, and Erdman Avenue—for info: (410) 243-3500; **www.bmgcgolf.com.**

17 GUNPOWDER FALLS STATE PARK (HEREFORD AREA): GUNPOWDER NORTH-SOUTH CIRCUIT

KEY AT-A-GLANCE INFORMATION

LENGTH: 13.2 miles

CONFIGURATION: Loop

DIFFICULTY: Moderate–strenuous depending on length

SCENERY: Gunpowder River, Prettyboy Dam, varied flora, rock formations

EXPOSURE: Shade

TRAFFIC: Moderate

TRAIL SURFACE: Packed dirt, rock

HIKING TIME: 6–7 hours

ACCESS: Sunrise–sunset

MAPS: USGS Hereford

FACILITIES: Restrooms at the south side of Bunker Hill Road

WHEELCHAIR ACCESS: No

SPECIAL COMMENTS: Several bridges and parking areas make it possible to vary the length of this hike. Be aware, however, that the bridge at Bunker Hill Road has been washed away; you can park here, but cannot cross the river. The hike described below begins at the Masemore Road parking area, west of Bunker Hill. Mountain bikes are prohibited on all trails.

GPS Trailhead
Coordinates
UTM Zone (WGS84) 18S
Easting 355493
Northing 4385991
Latitude N 39° 36.689107'
Longitude W 76° 41.002250'

IN BRIEF

Circle Gunpowder Falls at some of its prettiest and most scenic sections.

DESCRIPTION

The wrought iron Masemore Road Bridge was built in 1898. A wooden pole sits just to the left of the bridge, pointing out the white-blazed Gunpowder South Trail. Follow the trail upstream over mossy rocks and fallen tree trunks for 500 feet to the blue-blazed Highland Trail to the left. Head uphill through mountain laurel and along a ridged groove; you'll see a valley dropping off to the right and Bush Cabin Run heading into the Gunpowder River. Although mountain laurel is by far the dominant flora along this hike, if you complete the entire circuit, you'll pass a riot of trees, plants, and shrubs: river birch, cherry, oak, hemlock, dogwood, and hickory among the canopy. Below are Maryland's usual suspects, but you'll also find species that are very rare to the area, including climbing fumitory, hairy ringed sedge, lobed spleen wart, pink lady's slipper, pygmy shrew, and purple fringeless orchid.

At 0.3 miles, it looks like the trail runs straight ahead, but you'll see lots of fallen trees in the way. The trail actually heads to the right and narrows as it leads deeper into

Directions

Take I-83 to Exit 27, Mount Carmel Road west. Go 0.6 miles and take the first right onto Masemore Road. Follow Masemore Road as it winds past Fosters Masemore Mill (built in 1797); look for the parking area on the right at the bottom of the hill. Walk toward the bridge and pick up the trail there.

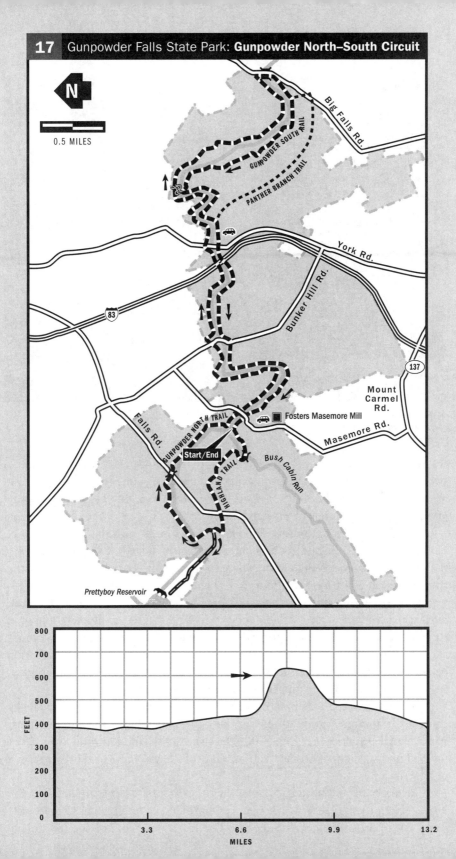

N

0.5 MILES

Big Falls Rd.

GUNPOWDER SOUTH TRAIL

PANTHER BRANCH TRAIL

York Rd.

Bunker Hill Rd.

83

137

Mount Carmel Rd.

Masemore Rd.

GUNPOWDER NORTH TRAIL

Falls Rd.

Start/End

HIGHLAND TRAIL

Bush Cabin Run

Fosters Masemore Mill

Prettyboy Reservoir

800
700
600
500
400
300
200
100
0

FEET

3.3   6.6   9.9   13.2
MILES

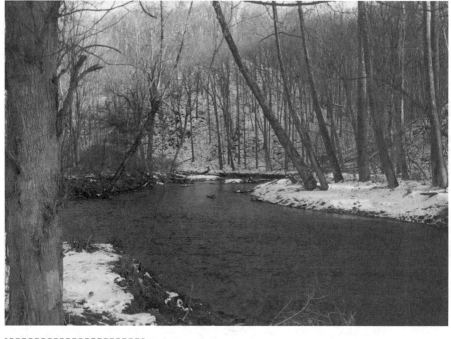

Gunpowder in early fall snow

the woods. When you reach Bush Cabin Run, cross over it to the right. You'll come to a power line cut at 0.5 miles; as you cross it, you may see cows grazing at the farm to the right. Once back in the woods, the trail widens significantly and leads through stands of pine and cedar.

You'll reach the diminutive Falls Road and a small parking area at 1 mile. Cross the parking area and get back on the trail, which leads downhill; you'll see the horseshoe curve of the Gunpowder River straight ahead. At 1.2 miles, the trail splits; head left to reach Prettyboy Dam. The path to the dam is a treat—narrow and winding through and over exposed roots, moss, mountain laurel, mica schist columns, trees with bulbous knots, and hemlocks. If you're hiking in the spring, you can be treated to a variety of wildflowers as well, such as blood-root, Canada Mayflower, columbine, Dutchman's breeches, hepatica, spring beauty, slender toothwort, rue anemone, pink lady's slippers, trailing arbutus, trout lily, violet, and wild ginger, providing an incredible show.

You will reach the dam at 1.7 miles; if it's a summer day and you're lucky enough to catch the dam with one of the valves open, enjoy the cooling spray, which you'll begin to feel some 500 feet away. The dam was built from 1924 to 1933 and was apparently named for a local farmer's horse that drowned in a nearby stream.

Turn around and head back; you'll come to the trail split again at 2.2 miles. Head left and you'll soon reach river level. You'll see lots of little ripples; the rocky river has a series of little bends. The trunks of many of the trees along the riverbank bear telltale beaver gnaw scars. By 2.5 miles, the trail turns into a jumble of rocks, which requires a bit of scrambling. You may think that some major tectonic activity had ceased just before you arrived, and this image of raw nature at work only increases as tree roots spill over the rocks, and spongy moss covers the ground beneath the canopy of mountain laurel.

You'll reach Falls Road again at 2.9 miles; cross the steel bridge and pick up the Gunpowder North Trail. Both the river and trail level out a bit here, making a relatively easy stroll along the riverbanks in the grass. Summer blooms in this area include woodland sunflowers, aster, and goldenrod. You'll come to a little bog at 3.3 miles, and you'll pass through a stand of pines before reaching Masemore Road again at 3.5 miles. Your car is just on the other side of the road, but if you want to continue hiking, stay along the river; the trail will take you through more stands of oak and tulip poplar. Soon, the river becomes quite shallow and you can see a multitude of pretty, light-colored stones in the water. A little farther, the trail runs beneath a limestone rock base some 30 feet in height.

You'll reach Bunker Hill Road at 4.7 miles; you can't cross here because the old bridge washed out, leaving only two stone abutments. Continue along the river, where the trees crowd the riverbanks a bit more, providing some wonderful canopy. Not surprisingly, opportunities for some supreme birding abound: thrushes, vireos, warblers, and woodpeckers populate the forests, while blue herons and kingfishers can be found along the river. Red-tail and red-shouldered hawks circle above in the clearings while Carolina chickadees, indigo buntings, peewees, and phoebes inhabit the trees and shrubs.

Unfortunately, the only unpleasant stretch of this entire hike comes soon. You'll hear it first and then pass under I-83. But you'll quickly leave this area behind. Reach York Road at 5.9 miles; you'll see a parking area across the bridge on the right. Cross York Road and pick up the trail at the break in the guardrail; you'll see a series of white rocks leading toward the river, and blue blazes will quickly follow.

It's initially uphill and down, but it quickly settles down to water level. At 6.4 miles, the trail swings around at a big hemlock, which leans out over the water. Very soon after, you will cross a little stream. The trail begins to feel more isolated here, and the river finally completely overtakes the faint echoes of the traffic on I-83.

At 6.8 miles, you'll pass Raven Rock Falls on the left. It's not a high vertical waterfall, but rather a riffle of rock that ends at the trail. Cross a little stream immediately beyond the falls; the trail soon heads up a little higher on the hill among big rocks, moss, ferns, and more mountain laurel. Some of the schist columns in this area rise about 25 feet. The trail goes a bit deeper into the woods and reaches a trail split at 7.3 miles, right after another stream. Go straight uphill, crossing several deer paths and following the blue blazes; it's a fairly steep climb.

Coming back down the hill, the trail levels out at 7.7 miles and reaches a big river curve at 8 miles. This is a great spot to take in the topography of the area, marked by midsize hills rolling gently to the water; it's typical piedmont Maryland. You'll soon come to a gravel park road; head right, passing a marshy bog. The gravel road ends at Big Falls Road Bridge at 8.3 miles. Cross the bridge and pick up the white-blazed Gunpowder South Trail on the other side. This section is one of the many trout catch-and-return areas.

Now walking upstream, the trail on the south side of the river really hugs the edge of the water and is much more narrow than the other side. At 9.2 miles, the trail splits; the Panther Branch Trail, named for a panther that once lived in a cave visible from the trail, goes to the left and loops into the woods, eventually rejoining the Gunpowder South Trail. If you take Panther Branch Trail, be on the lookout for the remains of two old mills, built in the mid-1700s and destroyed by accidental explosions in 1874. The entire length of the Panther Branch Trail covers 2.2 miles, and taking it will give you a half-mile less of total hike than if you remained on the Gunpowder South Trail.

Taking either option will bring you to the pink-blazed Sandy Lane Trail (0.3 miles in length), which connects Panther Branch Trail and Gunpowder South Trail. Back on the Gunpowder South Trail, go past a stand of holly and a little stream; you'll soon see Raven Rock Falls across the river. At 9.6 miles, you will come to a nice big rock that the trail goes right over. From this vantage point, you're afforded great views of the river in both directions.

The last trail split comes at 9.8 miles. Follow the right turn toward the river; going the other way takes you into the woods over the hill. The trail along the river gets very narrow, becoming at some points just an eroded knife-edge hanging over the water. You should not have trouble keeping your footing if it isn't snowy or icy, but be very careful nonetheless. If you have any fears of slipping and falling into the river, take the wooded option.

Beyond this narrow section, the trail widens and joins the other end of the Panther Branch Trail. Cross the Panther Branch (the waterway); you'll come to York Road just ahead. This section of the trail back to Bunker Hill changes only when it runs away from the river and through forest, where wildflowers and ubiquitous rocks reappear. For the next 3 miles you will follow the same route as before toward the turnaround, just on the other side of the river. The south side between York Road and Masemore Road hosts many more pines than the north side; despite that, the two sides of the river in this stretch generally differ little, and both are beautiful. You will reach Masemore Road and your car at 13.2 miles.

NEARBY ACTIVITIES

To reach Woodhall Winery (**www.woodhallwinecellars.com**), one of Maryland's best, head east on Mount Carmel Road and turn right (north) onto York Road. Follow York Road across Gunpowder River and look for signs to the winery.

GUNPOWDER FALLS STATE PARK:
JERUSALEM VILLAGE TRAIL WITH JERICHO COVERED BRIDGE TRAIL

18

IN BRIEF

Leave from historic Jerusalem Village and follow the floodplain of Little Gunpowder Falls before returning for a trip to the Jericho Covered Bridge.

DESCRIPTION

You can spend hours in historic Jerusalem Village alone, and the fact that some fantastic hiking opportunities abound offers a wonderful bonus. The grist mill, now Gunpowder Falls State Park headquarters, was built in 1772 and continued operations until the last miller died in 1961. Employees of the Gun/Cooper Shop, behind the mill, produced walnut gunstocks for the Maryland militia during the Revolutionary War. Spread out from the mill, all within easy walking distance, stand the Tenant House, Lee Mansion, McCourtney's Store, Spring House, "Dwelling," and the Blacksmith Shop, also built in 1772, where the hike begins. Each historic building tells a fascinating story.

Pick up the trailhead at the edge of the woods behind the blacksmith shop. Initially, this white-blazed trail has cedar chips and packed dirt as it winds through a stand of oak. At the T-intersection at 150 feet, take a left toward Little Gunpowder Falls, which you'll eventually follow upstream. You'll see ruins of the millrace at 0.1 mile. The path is very well maintained, but it feels nicely isolated because it's ridged on both sides.

KEY AT-A-GLANCE INFORMATION

LENGTH: 4.8 miles

CONFIGURATION: Out-and-back with loop, plus added loop

DIFFICULTY: Moderate

SCENERY: Little Gunpowder Falls, wetlands, mixed hardwoods, historic sites

EXPOSURE: Shade

TRAFFIC: Moderate

TRAIL SURFACE: Packed dirt

HIKING TIME: 2 hours

ACCESS: 7 a.m.–dusk

MAPS: USGS White Marsh; trail maps at bulletin board at parking area

WHEELCHAIR ACCESS: No

FACILITIES: Restrooms in park headquarters, open Monday–Friday, 8 a.m.–4:30 p.m.; museum open Saturday and Sunday, 1–4 p.m.; portable bathroom at parking area

SPECIAL COMMENTS: For more information about historic Jerusalem Village, call (410) 877-3560 or visit www.jerusalemmill.org.

Directions ⟶

Take I-695 to I-95 north. Take Exit 74 (MD 152) north toward Fallston. Go 2 miles and turn left onto Jerusalem Road; continue 1 mile to the parking area on the right. The trail starts at the edge of the woods behind the blacksmith shop, to the left of the parking area.

GPS Trailhead Coordinates

UTM Zone (WGS84) 18S

Easting 380391

Northing 4369102

Latitude N 39° 27.791498'

Longitude W 76° 23.422930'

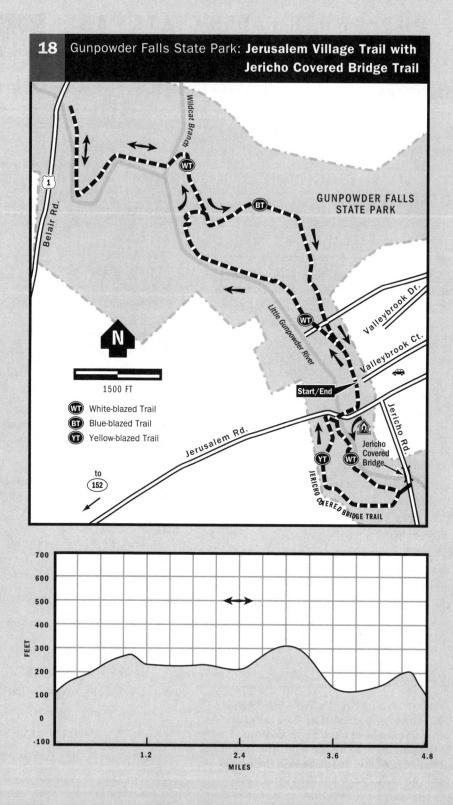

18 Gunpowder Falls State Park: **Jerusalem Village Trail with Jericho Covered Bridge Trail**

N

1500 FT

WT White-blazed Trail
BT Blue-blazed Trail
YT Yellow-blazed Trail

GUNPOWDER FALLS STATE PARK

Wildcat Branch

Little Gunpowder River

Belair Rd.

Valleybrook Dr.

Valleybrook Ct.

Start/End

Jericho Rd.

Jericho Covered Bridge

Jerusalem Rd.

to 152

JERICHO COVERED BRIDGE TRAIL

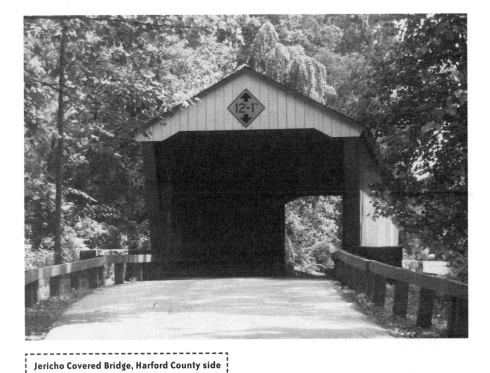

Jericho Covered Bridge, Harford County side

When the trail splits at just under 0.2 miles, with white blazes to the left and blue to the right, stay on the white-blazed trail but take note of the blue, as it will be your return route. The river soon comes into view; it's shallow, very rocky, and roughly 150 feet across. You'll see big chunks of granite, interspersed with ferns, sycamore, and sumac on the hill on the right. Even though the river is not far away on the left, the trail often winds away from it, but the many path offshoots make a quick trip to the river possible.

At just under 0.4 miles, ford a little creek. Beech, hickory, tulip poplar, and red and white oak abound here. As the trail winds uphill, you'll have good views of the river, especially in winter. At 0.5 miles, you will pass a bog on the right filled with cattails, ferns, and wildflowers; towering walnuts and large beeches crowd the bog on every side. The trail is very well maintained; huge trees fall on the trail, but they are quickly cut and pulled to the side. You will see some of them on the edge of the trail, covered in lichen and mosses and sprouting white, flaming red, and orange fungal growth.

At 0.75 miles, pass by the cutoff path leading left toward the water and continue on the white trail as it heads uphill. Once you reach the top, you can either head right on the blue trail to return to your car or stay on the white to continue the hike. At just over 1 mile, come down the hill to Wildcat Branch. Cross it by stepping on the big rocks; the water runs clear and swift toward the Little Gunpowder on the left. On the other side of Wildcat Branch, the trail splits; turn left (the trail to the right ends abruptly). When the trail meets Little Gunpowder River, head right to continue paralleling the river. The trail then heads uphill and winds away from the river; you will pass more millrace ruins on the left. You'll come to a beautiful stretch of river at 1.4 miles; it's rock free and glass smooth for about 100 feet. Unfortunately, you'll begin to hear auto traffic in this area, though you won't be able to see any cars through the thick woods. The trail comes to a disappointing end at Belair Road at just under 1.7 miles at the Harford County line.

Heading back you'll reach the trail split at just under 2.5 miles; this time take the blue-blazed trail instead of the white. You'll be paralleling the edge of the woods at a power line cut. The trail heads to a wide open area and picks up on the other side in the woods, where it heads uphill and becomes very rocky. Cross a little stream and at 3 miles, when the trail splits, head right to rejoin the white-blazed trail. The river comes into view on the right as you go down the hill. The next quarter-mile affords fantastic views of the water. When you rejoin the white-blazed trail, head left toward the parking area. This time, however, instead of returning to your car, go straight toward the mill. Head to the right, cross the bridge on Jerusalem Road, and then cross at the trailhead to reach the Jericho Covered Bridge Trail, denoted by wooden steps, white blazes, and a marker pointing to the covered bridge.

The trail initially follows the river downstream, with thick woods on the hill on the right. At the bend in the river, the trail climbs the hill, giving you a great view. At 0.3 miles from Jerusalem Road, you'll come to the covered bridge; built in 1865, it's the last remaining covered bridge in either Baltimore or Harford County.

On the way back, take the yellow-blazed trail instead of the white. It heads to the left up the hill when the trails split, 250 feet from the road. You'll pass through a stand of tall, thin oaks, and at the top of the hill, red cedar takes over the landscape. You'll see a farm field to the left through the woods. The trail follows the inside edge of the tree line about 10 feet from the field. White-tailed deer love this border area, and you're likely to see loads of them. You'll also see lots of pine, fir, red cedar, and sumac.

At just under 0.8 miles from the beginning of this portion of the hike, you'll come to Jerusalem Road. To avoid walking on the road, which does not have shoulders, head right to pick up the white-blazed trail at the river; then head left. You will rejoin Jerusalem Road at 0.9 miles. Turn right to return to your car.

NEARBY ACTIVITIES

To visit the nationally award-winning Ladew Topiary Gardens, go north from Jerusalem Village to Mountain Road (MD 152) and head left. Follow Route 152 northwest to the dead end at MD Route 146 (Jarrettsville Pike) and go left. Ladew Gardens is approximately 1 mile ahead on your left. For information, visit **www.ladewgardens.com** or call (410) 557-9466.

LOCH RAVEN RESERVOIR: DEADMAN'S COVE 19

IN BRIEF

Find solitude at Deadman's Cove, inside the heavily visited Loch Raven Watershed.

DESCRIPTION

The trail initially runs along an old fire road. It's very wide, and though in the thick woods, it's also well exposed. At first you'll hear lots of traffic noise, but that will quickly disappear. By 200 feet, as the trail heads down a little hill, the sounds of the woods take over. Tall oaks dominate, rising above thick underbrush.

At 0.2 miles, you'll parallel a dry creek bed to the left. Though the trail is still very wide, it's now shaded due to the height of the trees. The grass is tall, so expect a few shin scrapes during summer. By a quarter-mile, you'll see lots of pine along with plentiful white oak, hickory, and sycamore. These woods, like much of the Loch Raven watershed, provide a haven for white-tailed deer, and you're likely to scatter more than a few. Woodpeckers make their homes here too, and the sound of their tree pounding echoes all along the trail. To the left, an interesting wall of trees fronts the creek bed; their uniformity suggests that they were planted here long ago. At just over 0.3 miles, head left and follow

KEY AT-A-GLANCE INFORMATION

LENGTH: 1.7 miles
CONFIGURATION: Out-and-back with short loop
DIFFICULTY: Easy
SCENERY: Loch Raven Reservoir, pine forest, hardwoods
EXPOSURE: Shade
TRAFFIC: Light
TRAIL SURFACE: Packed dirt
HIKING TIME: 45 minutes
ACCESS: Dawn–dusk
MAPS: USGS Towson
WHEELCHAIR ACCESS: No
FACILITIES: None
SPECIAL COMMENTS: Take great care crossing Dulaney Valley Road. There's a bit of a blind curve from the south, and drivers tend to take it too quickly.

Directions ⟶

Take I-695 to Exit 27, Dulaney Valley Road north. Cross Timonium Road and look for the signs for the entrance to Stella Maris Hospice. Roughly a quarter-mile past Stella Maris is the parking area on the left (if you come to the light at Old Bosley Road, you've passed it). The trail starts opposite the parking area across Dulaney Valley Road; it is marked by an orange cable and a sign reading WOODS ROAD CLOSED TO BIKES.

GPS Trailhead Coordinates

UTM Zone (WGS84) 18S
Easting 363036
Northing 4368523
Latitude N 39° 27.323399'
Longitude W 76° 35.516181'

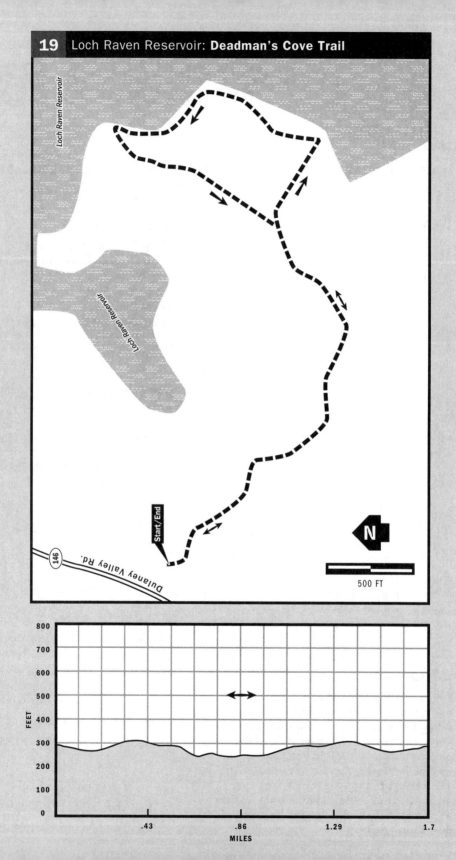

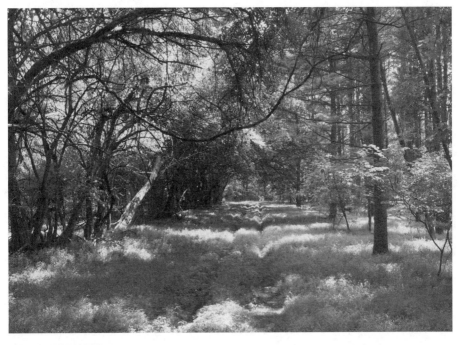

Old carriage road

the tire tracks through towering pines and abundant honeysuckle. Soon after, you'll have your first glimpse of the water through the trees on the right.

As you approach 0.5 miles, a vein of large rocks cuts across the path. When you see a particularly large rock at a trail split, head to the right. The trail gets lost a bit in the tall grass, but the water comes into better and better view, so it's easy to tell where you're going. You'll reach the water at 0.6 miles. Here, you'll have clear, good views across the reservoir—you may see a few people in boats, rowing or fishing. More than likely, you'll have the view all to yourself. The water here is clear, and you'll probably see many fish swimming around at your feet.

Take a left at the water's edge. The trail follows the contours of the waterline. It sometimes gets lost in the undergrowth, especially in summer, and crosses fallen trees branches. But as long as you follow along the water, you'll be fine. At just under 0.8 miles (after you can see the Dulaney Valley bridge over the reservoir in the distance), look for the cut to the left; it runs up the hill from the outermost jut of the land. A rock-studded ravine on the left slopes gently downhill toward the reservoir. The trail rises above the reservoir, which is off to both the right and left (but can only be seen in winter). At a little under 1 mile, you'll reach the trail where you were originally. Follow the trail all the way back to your car.

NEARBY ACTIVITIES

The Fire Museum of Maryland (**www.firemuseummd.org**), the largest such museum on the East Coast, houses 40 pieces of firefighting apparatus dating from 1822. The museum, which also has the largest working telegraph system in the United States, is open weekends May to December; and Wednesday through Sunday, June to August (10 a.m. to 4 p.m. Sunday, 1 p.m. to 4 p.m.); 1301 York Road; (410) 321-7500. Head south on Dulaney Valley Road and turn right onto Seminary Avenue; turn left onto York Road. The Fire Museum is three-quarters of a mile on the left.

Hampton National Historic Site ([410] 823-1309 **www.nps.gov/hamp**), a stately home completed in 1790 and once the largest mansion in the United States, is also within easy driving distance. Built with a fortune amassed during the Revolutionary War, the site boasts extensive gardens on what was once the northernmost slave-holding plantation in the country. Head south on Dulaney Valley Road from Seminary Avenue; go three blocks and turn left onto Hampton Estate Lane. You will see the mansion and grounds entrance on the right.

LOCH RAVEN RESERVOIR: GLEN ELLEN-SEMINARY ROAD

 20

IN BRIEF

Follow the natural contours of the south-eastern edge of Loch Raven Reservoir before ascending the hills above to come back through upland forest.

DESCRIPTION

At the trailhead, you'll see a bulletin board explaining which trails are open to mountain bikes and which aren't. Be aware: these are largely ignored. According to the sign, bikes are allowed only on the wide fire road that begins to the right of where you stand. Even though you are heading left at 200 feet on the narrower dirt path, expect bicyclists.

You'll immediately enter thick woods, full of oak and tulip poplar. The first view of the reservoir comes at 0.3 miles as you begin to parallel a feeder stream to the left. It gets very marshy as the water expands into the main body of the reservoir. The trail is flat and level as it winds through the woods, and the water before you gets wider and wider. Before you momentarily wind away from the reservoir at 0.5 miles, expect to scatter frogs, turtles, and an occasional water snake from the thick underbrush that crowds the edges of the trail.

KEY AT-A-GLANCE INFORMATION

LENGTH: 9 miles

CONFIGURATION: 2 loops with an extended spur

DIFFICULTY: Moderate

SCENERY: Loch Raven Reservoir, upland forest

EXPOSURE: Shade

TRAFFIC: Light–moderate (mostly bicycle)

TRAIL SURFACE: Packed dirt

HIKING TIME: 3–3.5 hours

ACCESS: Dawn–dusk; the Maryland Transit Administration (MTA) runs buses along Dulaney Valley Road and crosses Seminary Avenue; for a schedule, call (410) 539-5000 or (866) RIDE-MTA, or visit www.mtamaryland.com.

MAPS: USGS Towson, stationary trail map at trailhead

WHEELCHAIR ACCESS: No

FACILITIES: None

SPECIAL COMMENTS: Though the majority of the trail traffic is bicycle, cyclists tend to be considerate and usually alert you to their approach.

Directions _____→

Take I-695 to Exit 27, Dulaney Valley Road north. Go five blocks and turn left onto Seminary Avenue (after Meadowcroft Lane); park immediately on the right shoulder in front of the Church of Latter-Day Saints. Carefully cross Dulaney Valley Road and pick up the dirt path paralleling Seminary Avenue; follow the path until it comes out to Seminary Avenue and then quickly ducks back into the woods on the left. Two orange posts strung with a steel cable mark the trailhead.

GPS Trailhead
Coordinates
UTM Zone (WGS84) 18S
Easting 362700
Northing 4365199
Latitude N 39° 25.523801'
Longitude W 76° 35.709422'

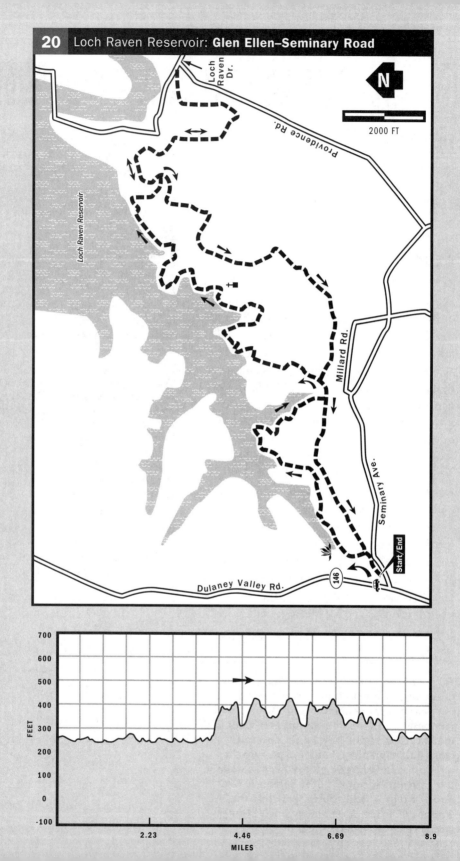

Reservoir Trail

Hundreds of offshoots lead in both directions from the trail; these single-track bike cuts lead to some nice scenery, but they cause severe erosion. Besides, staying on the path yields some fantastic views.

Cross over a small stream at 0.7 miles and then head slightly to the right into a grove of pine trees. This is part of the fire road, and it is accordingly wide— only a thin strip made by tire tracks cuts a path in the middle. After another tenth of a mile, you'll come to a T-intersection. Head right, keeping the water on your left. Keep to the right as the trail heads slightly uphill.

At 0.9 miles, the trail runs to the water's edge.

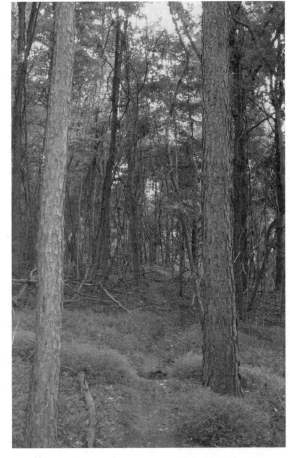

Shaded by mature pines, this nice spot stays cool even on a hot day. For the next half mile, the trail runs along the edge of the reservoir, following its natural contours. At 1.4 miles, the trail moves away from the reservoir and rejoins the fire road; this is the edge of the watershed property, and you'll see a few private homes to the right as you head left.

Immediately cross over a swiftly moving stream filled with big concrete slabs; head uphill. At the split at 1.5 miles, head left; at 1.7 miles, take the narrow foot trail to the left. You'll parallel a very small creek to your left. The reservoir soon comes back into view through the woods. This trail ends at the water's edge and affords some magnificent views of the reservoir. Head back and take a left at the first opportunity (200 feet from the water's edge). For the next 2 miles, the trail literally is the reservoir edge.

Along this section, you'll pass through nice pine groves, over small creeks (where fish and frogs abound), and riparian buffers where lily pads and other aquatic plants grow. At a Y-intersection, head left. Expect to see many white-tailed deer leaping about; indeed, because of the population explosion of deer, controlled hunting has begun as of late 2008. At 2.8 miles and then again at 3 miles, you'll see the remains of two dog burial sites. Another small rock pile with a cross on top sits just beyond. One couldn't wish for a nicer final resting place.

At 3.6 miles, the trail heads abruptly uphill over a clear stream. Rocks and ferns dominate the banks, and trees dangle their roots over the water. As you head up the hill, the ecosystem changes drastically. Alongside the mica-flecked trail, the pines fall away and are replaced by oak, sycamore, maple, and beech. When you reach the top of the hill at 3.8 miles, you'll have a few options. You can continue the hike by heading left and reaching the turnaround point (Providence Road) at just over 5 miles. Or, you can turn right at the fire road to go back to Seminary Avenue and your car, yielding a solid hike of roughly 7 miles.

Admittedly, the scenery doesn't vary much along the fire road between the trail intersection, Providence Road, and the trailhead, but it does provide for a pleasant walk through upland forest. By going to Providence Road before heading back to Seminary Avenue, you'll cross over no fewer than seven rock-strewn, clear streams, and they're often very lovely, cutting banks along the side of the hills.

You have one other option—as you head toward Providence Road, you'll see a red-blazed trail to the left at 4 miles. Surrounded by beech trees, it heads downhill to the water's edge before heading back up to the fire road.

Going back to Seminary Avenue and your car, the trail is very wide and rocky, full of exposed roots, with lots of fallen, decaying tree trunks and ferns on both the right and left. At 7 miles, a few private homes begin to appear on the left. You'll see cleared areas that delineate the edge of the watershed property and the beginning of private property, an occasional stand of bamboo, and some cuts in the woods on the right. More and more backyards appear as you descend the final section of the fire road and return to the trailhead at just under 9 miles.

NEARBY ACTIVITIES

The Fire Museum of Maryland (**www.firemuseummd.org**), houses 40 pieces of firefighting apparatus dating from 1822. The museum, which also has the largest working telegraph system in the United States, is open weekends May to December; Wednesday through Sunday, June to August, (10 a.m. to 4 p.m.; Sunday, 1 p.m. to 4 p.m.); 1301 York Road; (410) 321-7500. Head south on Dulaney Valley Road and turn right onto Seminary Avenue; turn left onto York Road. The Fire Museum is three-quarters of a mile on the left.

Hampton National Historic Site ([410] 823-1309 **www.nps.gov/hamp**), a stately home completed in 1790 is also within easy driving distance. Built with a fortune amassed during the Revolutionary War, the site boasts extensive gardens. Head south on Dulaney Valley Road from Seminary Avenue; go three blocks and turn left onto Hampton Estate Lane. The entrance is on the right.

LOCH RAVEN RESERVOIR: MERRYMAN POINT

IN BRIEF

Follow this popular trail to Merryman Point, where the reservoir spreads out in several directions.

DESCRIPTION

From the parking area, you have several options to begin the hike: the trailhead farthest to the right leads to a narrow path that runs alongside the reservoir, the farthest to the left runs to a fire road, and the second to the left (the one I take) runs along a wide path, but not before going along a narrower path, which will eventually afford nice views of the reservoir and give you the option of linking with the fire road. This, I find, is the most diverse and pleasant route.

Swing around a hill and cross a little creek bed at 0.3 miles. Oak, beech, sycamore, and tulip poplar populate the hillside, and spicebush abounds as well. You'll have an immediate view of the reservoir, which is fed by the many creeks running alongside the hills. Cross one of these creeks at 0.4 miles.

Next, you'll come to a narrow ridge that acts as the trail. It gets so narrow that it even becomes a bit harrowing in places; it wouldn't take much to slip and fall down the hill to the right. If you did, you'd be sliding among the oak and tulip poplar trunks all the way to the edge of the reservoir, some hundred or so

KEY AT-A-GLANCE INFORMATION

LENGTH: 9.8 miles
CONFIGURATION: Out-and-back
DIFFICULTY: Moderate–strenuous
SCENERY: Loch Raven Reservoir, upland forest
EXPOSURE: Shade
TRAFFIC: Moderate
TRAIL SURFACE: Packed dirt, crushed rock
HIKING TIME: 3.5 hours
ACCESS: Dawn–dusk
MAPS: USGS Towson
FACILITIES: None
WHEELCHAIR ACCESS: No
SPECIAL COMMENTS: Parking at the Dulaney Valley parking area is very limited; to park at Warren Road and do the hike in reverse, take I-83 to Exit 18, Warren Road east, and once you've passed Bosley Road, look for the gravel parking area just before the steel bridge over Loch Raven Reservoir.

Directions ⟶

Take I-695 to Exit 27, Dulaney Valley Road north and go 3.5 miles. The parking area is on the left just after Bosley Road and just before the bridge over Loch Raven Reservoir. The trail begins just beyond the parking area at the edge of the woods.

GPS Trailhead Coordinates

UTM Zone (WGS84) 18S
Easting 363549
Northing 4369361
Latitude N 39° 27.781169'
Longitude W 76° 35.168831'

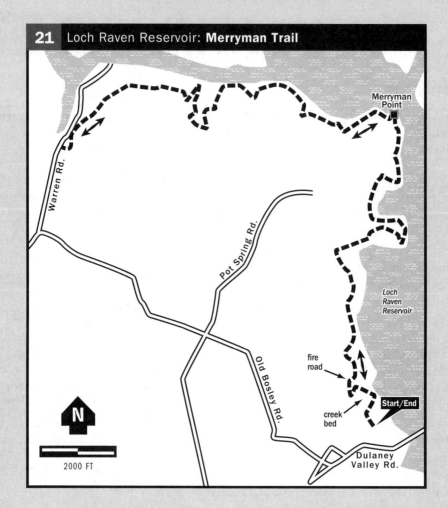

21 Loch Raven Reservoir: **Merryman Trail**

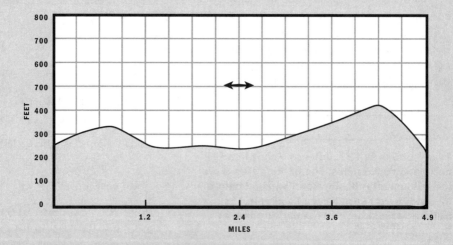

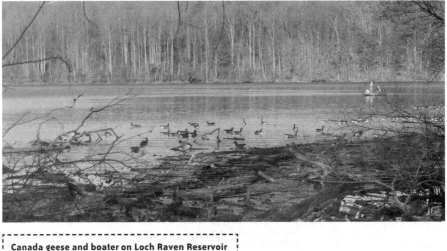

Canada geese and boater on Loch Raven Reservoir

feet down. Be careful to pay attention to where you're walking and don't let the reservoir views and the many birds flitting overhead distract you too much. As you continue along the ridge, your sightline will run along the tops of many of the trees rising up from water level.

You'll rejoin the fire road at 0.6 miles. This wide, more level, crushed rock trail heads downhill and crosses a beautiful little stream. On the other side of the stream, you'll come to a T-intersection; head right as the path runs through a large patch of greenbrier. After roughly 0.75 miles, you'll see the Dulaney Valley Bridge over the reservoir; winter will give you the clearest view of the bridge, which is about a mile away, close to where you parked.

As soon as you spot the bridge, start watching for a little cut path at 0.8 miles. The main fire road trail branches to the left and seems the obvious choice to follow, but if you look closely straight ahead, you'll see the cut path running through a thicket of midlevel growth of thin tulip poplar, grapevine, briers, and spicebush. Taking this path allows you to head to the edge of the reservoir; at one point, the path runs right alongside the water and heads out to a series of large rocks. Since the breeze invariably comes from the east over the reservoir, the water constantly laps against the rocks at your feet. Aside from hearing the pleasing sound, you'll also have a great view over the reservoir.

Moving on, you'll continue to skirt through the woods along the edge of the reservoir, and in many places, a mere foot or two separates you from the water. Come to a thick stand of evergreens and just beyond, at 1.5 miles, a power line cut. A carpet of pine needles lies about, and you can see wide expanses of the reservoir to both the east and west. This is Merryman Point, which gives the trail its name.

At 1.9 miles, cut up the hill and rejoin the fire road, which is essentially a very rocky trail bed, with lots of ferns and oak down the hillside. You'll come to a lovely stretch between 2 and 2.5 miles as you go up and down the hills. The

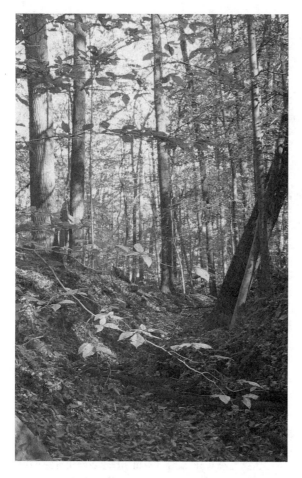

Gulley trail

very rocky, very thickly wooded trail offers constant sweeping views of the reservoir. Cross a creek and then walk around a big cut gulley. At the top of the hill, at 2.7 miles, cross the gulley and pick up the trail on the other side on the right. Back on the fire road, the scenery doesn't change much for the hike's duration, but you'll come to one rather dramatic curve at 3.5 miles, where you'll have to make a steep climb up the hill.

A private home now stands where the path once ran, and you'll have to cut around it. This requires a strenuous climb of about 150 feet before heading back down and rejoining the fire road at 4.2 miles. You'll actually remain at this altitude (just shy of 500 feet) for almost the rest of the hike before gradually descending at the trail's end at Warren Road.

Before you reach the fire road, at 4.7 miles, look through the woods on your right to see the steel bridge on Warren Road that runs over a relatively narrow section of the reservoir. You'll reach Warren Road at 4.9 miles and a parking area across it diagonally to the left; you can park here if the more popular parking area at Dulaney Valley is full. (See Special Comments.)

You could also set up a shuttle to make the hike one way. If you did set up a shuttle, here's how to return to the Dulaney Valley parking area from Warren Road: Go left (west) on Warren Road, turn left onto Bosley Road, and continue until it ends at Pot Spring Road. Take a right and then a left onto Old Bosley Road and continue until it ends at Dulaney Valley. You'll see the parking area on the left.

NEARBY ACTIVITIES

The Fire Museum of Maryland (**www.firemuseummd.org**), the largest such museum on the East Coast, houses 40 pieces of firefighting apparatus dating from 1822. The museum, which also has the largest working telegraph system in the United States, is open weekends May to December; and Wednesday through Sunday, June to August (10 a.m. to 4 p.m.;Sunday, 1 p.m. to 4 p.m.); 1301 York Road; (410) 321-7500. Head south on Dulaney Valley Road and turn right onto Seminary Avenue; turn left onto York Road. The Fire Museum is three quarters of a mile on the left.

Hampton National Historic Site ([410] 823-1309 **www.nps.gov/hamp**), a stately home completed in 1790 and once the largest mansion in the United States, is also within easy driving distance. Built with a fortune amassed during the Revolutionary War, the site boasts extensive gardens on what was once the northernmost slave-holding plantation in the country. Head south on Dulaney Valley Road from Seminary Avenue; go three blocks and turn left onto Hampton Estate Lane. You will see the mansion and grounds entrance on the right.

22 LOCH RAVEN RESERVOIR: NORTHWEST AREA TRAILS

KEY AT-A-GLANCE INFORMATION

LENGTH: 3.7 miles (plus the opportunity for extension—see Nearby Activities)

CONFIGURATION: Out-and-back with short loop

DIFFICULTY: Moderate

SCENERY: Upland forest, rock outcroppings, Loch Raven Reservoir

EXPOSURE: Shade

TRAFFIC: Light

TRAIL SURFACE: Packed dirt

HIKING TIME: 1.5 hours

ACCESS: Dawn–dusk, year-round

MAPS: USGS Towson, Cockeysville

FACILITIES: None

WHEELCHAIR ACCESS: No

SPECIAL COMMENTS: Some fantastic trails offer up spectacular beauty in the extreme western sections of Loch Raven Reservoir. They are tantalizingly close to the hike described here, but unfortunately are blocked off from this hike by the wide arm of Western Run as it flows into Loch Raven Reservoir. See Nearby Activities on page 117 for instructions on reaching them.

- -

GPS Trailhead
Coordinates

UTM Zone (WGS84) 18S

Easting 367754

Northing 4364684

Latitude N 39° 25.292888'

Longitude W 76° 32.181458'

IN BRIEF

A relatively unvisited—and beautiful—section of Loch Raven Reservoir, doing its best impression of Gunpowder Falls State Park's Wildlands.

DECRIPTION

You'll find a number of trail choices all along this hike. Wide and prominent trails parallel each other along the hills. Generally, there are three options: high, middle, and water level. This hike stays fairly level and takes the middle road (a fire road), keeping the reservoir a few hundred feet to the right below. Your first trail level choice comes almost immediately beyond the trailhead, after you've crossed the feeder stream and headed to the right. You can either go up the hill or go straight ahead—go straight, keeping closer to the water. Within 0.1 mile, the edge of the reservoir comes into view.

The scenery is beautiful immediately: sloping hills to the left, studded with mature beech trees, and an abundance of wading birds as the reservoir widens on the right. With lots of rock, moss, and ferns, the area looks a bit more like the wild sections of Gunpowder Falls State Park than typical Loch Raven scenery. You might, however, be a bit startled by a low growling noise in the distance; this is the sound of cars going over the steel bridge on Warren Road. Despite the noise, the bridge's graceful span over the reservoir is a lovely sight.

- -

Directions ⟶

Take I-83 to Exit 18, Warren Road east. Go 1.7 miles to the gravel turnoff area on the right. On foot, cross the road and the trailhead is just on the other side, past the orange cable.

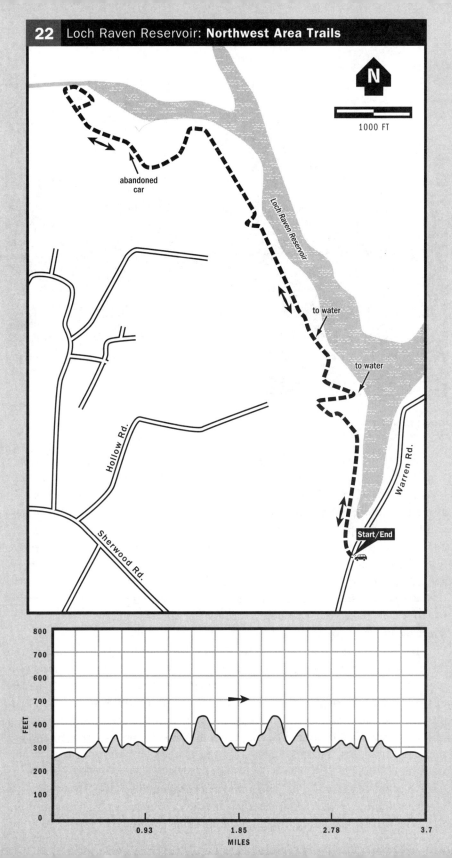

N

1000 FT

abandoned
car

Loch Raven Reservoir

to water

to water

Warren Rd.

Hollow Rd.

Sherwood Rd.

Start/End

800				
700				
600				
700				
400				
300				
200				
100				
0				

FEET

0.93   1.85   2.78   3.7
MILES

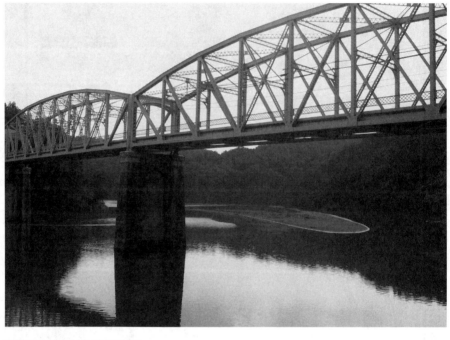

Steel bridge on Warren Road

Follow the contours of the reservoir as well as its feeder streams, making a wide leftward curve around the first one at 0.4 miles. Cross over the little valley stream flowing through a massive metal tube. Once you've crossed, swing around to the right (the leftward path heads to private land). Now, at 0.6 miles, you have three options: left uphill, straight ahead, or right, down to the water. Take the middle path (the left one eventually comes out in the same place you're headed once you round the ridge). But if you want to head to the water, this is a good opportunity to do so. In that case, hug the feeder stream all the way to the reservoir. Just beware: the trail eventually ends, and you'll either have to backtrack or make your way uphill through the forest, neither of which is such a terrible prospect, of course.

Back on the fire road, you'll have yet another opportunity to head down to the water at the next trail split. The same deal applies as before—the trail eventually peters out at the water's edge. Heading along the smaller path to the left of the water trail, you'll come to yet another trail split, 200 feet after the previous one. Continue going straight, rejoining the main fire-road trail, then take a right. The trail heads up and down gradually among moss- and lichen-covered rocks and boulders. There are also towering poplars and pretty little rock outcroppings along the way. These outcroppings rarely give you a clear view of the reservoir, but they tend to be wild and beautiful nonetheless.

Continuing on, the landscape becomes even rockier, and ferns and pines flank the trail. Head straight uphill, among some real pristine forest. You'll be accompanied by mountain laurel, azalea, and lots of birdsong. Follow the trail around another feeder stream, and then, at 1.6 miles, come to the carcass of an abandoned car. The trail continues past it but soon heads out of the reservoir property, so take a right down the hill, in a section full of young, spindly trees. Because you're now off the fire road, the trail gets closer in, as it's not as well used. At 1.8 miles, you'll come to a feeder stream covered by some old railroad ties. Beyond them, the trail dies. Here is the area where Western Run—to the right—cuts you off from the beautiful trails just to the north. Instead of attempting a difficult crossing of Western Run and a serious bushwhack if it's summertime, simply backtrack to your car and make the short drive to those other trails—see Nearby Activities below.

To get back to your car, don't make the crossing on the railroad ties. Instead, turn around and go left almost immediately. Parallel the stream on the left, and then head precipitously uphill, making a little loop here. More pristine beeches abound. You'll reach the portion where you just were in 0.1 mile; take a left here to backtrack.

NEARBY ACTIVITIES

To reach the western trails described previously by car, take Warren Road west back to York Road and take a right. Take a right onto Ashland Road. When Ashland swings to the left and becomes Paper Mill Road, take a right (at Ashland Presbyterian Church) to stay on Ashland. Keep on Ashland until it ends at the Ashland North Central Railroad (NCRR) Trail parking area. Follow the NCRR for a quarter-mile to a rightward cut through an easy and prominent path. This section offers roughly 3 miles of relatively easy but rewarding trails covering the beautiful section of Loch Raven Reservoir south of Paper Mill Road.

23   NCRR TORREY BROWN TRAIL

KEY AT-A-GLANCE INFORMATION

LENGTH: 19.2 miles

CONFIGURATION: One-way

DIFFICULTY: Easy–strenuous

SCENERY: Gunpowder River, Little Falls and Bee Tree Run, forest, riparian buffers, historic structures

EXPOSURE: More shade than sun in summer, reverse in winter

TRAFFIC: Moderate–heavy near parking areas

TRAIL SURFACE: Crushed rock

HIKING TIME: 7.5 hours for entire trail

ACCESS: Dawn–dusk

MAPS: USGS Hereford, Phoenix, New Freedom; virtual map of the Maryland section of the trail can be found at www.johncarterphoto .com/ncrr/virtualmap.html and maps with less detail but with more parking, directions, and facilities information at www.dnr.state .md.us/greenways/ncrt trail.html.

WHEELCHAIR ACCESS: Yes (crushed rock, no asphalt—may be difficult)

FACILITIES: Most parking areas have restrooms; some also include public telephones.

SPECIAL COMMENTS: Plentiful parking areas along the route make choosing shorter or longer lengths easy.

GPS Trailhead
Coordinates
UTM Zone (WGS84) 18S
Easting 360160
Northing 4387046
Latitude N 39° 37.305729'
Longitude W 76° 37.754910'

IN BRIEF

Choose what length hike you want to take and go—logical, well-spaced turnaround points and parking areas make this the perfect trail for anything from a quick walk to an all-day trek.

DESCRIPTION

This popular rail-trail is truly a treasure. Area residents know it as the NCRR (Northern Central Railroad) Trail, but in May 2007 the trail was officially renamed in honor of Dr. Torrey Brown, Maryland's third Department of Natural Resources secretary and the driving force behind development of the abandoned railway, which was initially dedicated in 1984. It is now a national model and hosts more than 850,000 visitors a year. European settlers came here as early as the 1600s and by the mid-1800s established a rail line bisecting the stream valley and linking Baltimore with the northern industrial states. Union troops were stationed here during the Civil War.

The trail actually begins 0.4 miles to the south, at the Ashland parking area; however, the Paper Mill parking area is much larger, and the first 0.4 miles, from Ashland to Paper Mill, really only serve as a preview of what's to come. That said, if you do begin at Ashland, you'll pass some paths that lead to the edge of Loch Raven Reservoir on the right, affording some spectacular views. If

------

Directions ───────────➤

See Maps for directions to individual parking areas. For the Paper Mill parking area (where this hike begins), take I-83 to Exit 20, Shawan Road east. Turn right at York Road. Go 0.3 miles to a left onto Ashland/Paper Mill. The parking area is 1 mile on the left.

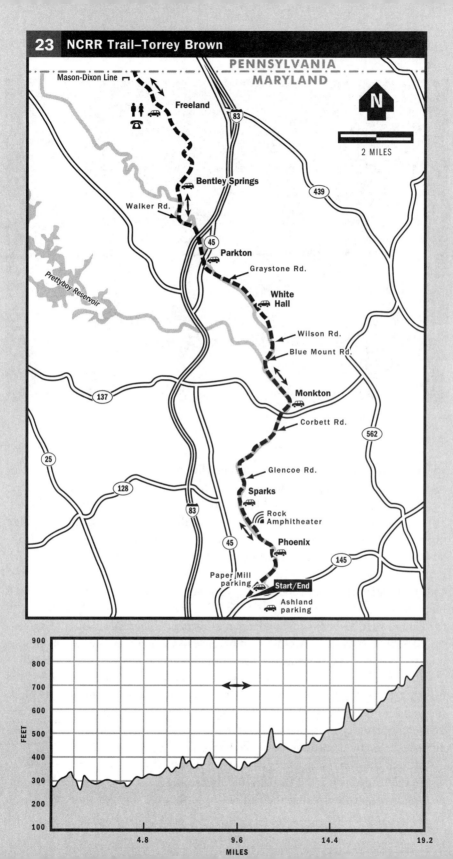

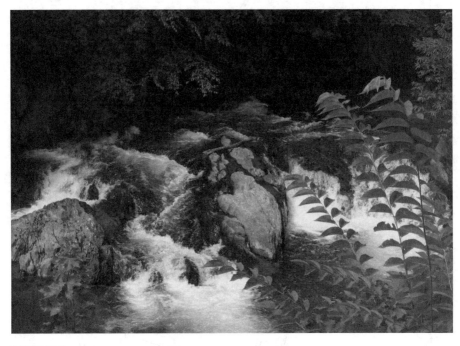

Little Falls

you want to begin from Ashland, follow the directions above, but instead of staying on Ashland Road until it turns into Paper Mill Road, take the first right after turning onto Ashland from York Road. This keeps you on Ashland. Take it until it ends at the small parking area. But from Paper Mill, as you hike northward, you'll notice the 0.4-mile distance disparity between the mileage described here and that posted along the trail. Again, Paper Mill is your much better bet to find parking.

Heading north from Paper Mill, you'll pass the remains of a lime kiln at 0.5 miles. Benches here offer a quick rest. There's a beautiful overlook soon after, with the Gunpowder River flowing underneath (portable toilets also flank the bridge).

The trail is wide but well shaded because of the mature-tree canopy. It may take you a while to get used to the occasional whiz of a passing bicyclist. While you'll certainly see walkers and hikers and even people pushing strollers, the majority of the trail traffic consists of bicyclists. This doesn't necessarily make for unpleasant walking, though, because the trail is wide and flat, providing ample opportunity for wide berths—besides, people who enjoy the trail generally have a happy demeanor, so walkers rarely feel squeezed out.

Reach the Phoenix parking area at 1.5 miles. After another mile, you'll see where the trail was blasted through the limestone; it's easy to imagine the engineering involved in creating the rail bed. Fortunately, enough time has passed that these rock walls are no longer naked and exposed: straggly roots of clinging trees that perch atop the rocks have taken hold, and wildflowers pepper the area, lending splashes of white, yellow, and purple in the summer. At 2.6 miles, be on the lookout for a natural-rock amphitheater to the right, a bit off the trail; it's a stunning spot. You'll reach the Sparks parking area at 3.2 miles. The nature center, located in the old bank building visible from the trail, is open on summer weekends from 10 a.m. to 4 p.m.

Continuing on, the river soon runs out of view for a bit. The scenery doesn't change much over the next couple of miles, but it is consistently pleasant.

The Gunpowder River is never far off; limestone rocks often flank the trail, ferns and wildflowers are abundant, and mature trees abound; each season offers its own charm.

At 5.2 miles is a nice rural scene: there's a bridge over the river, with a barn to the left. This section is particularly beautiful, and because it's between parking areas, it tends to be not very trafficked, either.

Cross Corbett Road (not a parking area) at 5.7 miles. Soon, there's another pretty overlook, at just under 6 miles. The Monkton parking area arrives at 6.5 miles. It's a popular spot, often serving as a meet-up place for tubing and hiking trips. Here you'll find telephones, restrooms, rest areas, a cafe, art gallery, and other shops. Monkton, originally known as Charlottetown, dates to the 1730s. The restored Monkton Train Station serves as a museum, gift shop, and Ranger Station; it's open Wednesday through Sunday, Memorial Day to Labor Day.

Beyond the parking area, at 6.7 miles, there's an amazing sight: the hill to the right appears to be one giant cracked slab of stone, roughly 100 feet in height, at about a 100-degree angle. It looks almost like poured but fractured concrete. At 7 miles, you'll pass a beautiful old collapsed stone building, part of the mid-19th-century settlement of Pleasant Valley. This is a popular put-in spot for tubing. There's a railroad abutment over the river at 8.3 miles. Cross the lily-studded Little Falls twice; this is yet another beautiful stretch of the trail. Abundant blackberries, red raspberries, and black raspberries provide for a feast in summer. Pass some electrical-light signals from the 1930s and arrive at the White Hall parking area at 10.6 miles, roughly halfway up the trail.

As you head north from the White Hall parking area, small trees and the narrow Little Falls to the left dominate the scenery. Cross Graystone Road at 11 miles. Soon after, cross a wooden bridge over Little Falls; you'll see the remnants of railroad tracks on the left. At 11.4 miles, you'll cross the water again and have great views of Little Falls pouring over the rocks below. As you parallel the falls on the left, heading upstream, thick woods and ferns along the hillsides surround you. Come to a put-and-take trout-fishing area and bench at 11.8 miles. Soon after, at 12 miles, you'll find a little overlook area that provides a great view of the clean water spilling over the rocks. A sign here warns about poisonous snakes. Only two such snakes live in Maryland: the timber rattlesnake

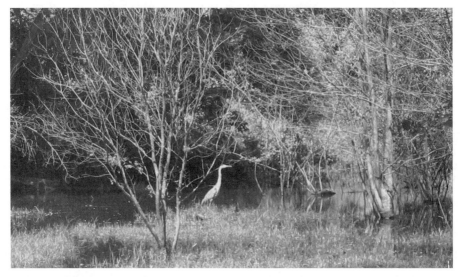

Trailside heron

(extremely rare in this area) and the northern copperhead. Your chances of being bitten by either snake are very slim, but if you do spot a snake, leave it alone.

After crossing a bridge at 12.7 miles, you'll come to the Parkton parking area, which has a small general store on the left and an old train depot on the right. A few private houses appear to the right as you continue on the trail and cross Dairy Road. An exercise course appears on the left, and you'll soon see I-83 ahead; it gets a bit loud for a moment, but you will soon leave the highway behind and regain serenity after you walk under the I-83 ramp.

Cross Walker Road at 14.2 miles; the next parking area is Bentley Springs, a little more than a mile away. Enjoy the shaded stretch of trail beyond Walker Road; first you'll cross water and then the trail opens up, letting you see a farmhouse up the hill on the right. Cross water again at 14.6 miles and come to a shaded bench just beyond. Mountain laurel abounds here, making this a truly lovely spot when the flowers are in bloom.

You'll reach Bentley Road at 15.1 miles; cross Bee Tree Run, and you'll see the Bentley Springs parking area just ahead, with restrooms and a public telephone. At 15.4 miles, the trail gets very boggy, and you'll pass a nice marsh on the left where you're likely to see great blue herons, kingfishers, and mallards. Other prominent fauna along the trail include beavers, monarch butterflies, white-tailed deer, flying squirrels, red foxes, raccoons, black snakes, and Eastern box turtles.

At 16.3 miles, cross Bee Tree Road. Soon after, you'll cross what's left of an old railroad bridge. Watch out for occasional piles of horse manure—this section of the trail is used by equestrians from the nearby camp in Bee Tree

Reserve. You can momentarily get offf the NCRR by taking the path cut into the woods on the right just beyond an informational bulletin board, at 16.4 miles; it leads through the 263-acre reserve.

The trail soon opens up in an area dominated by wildflowers and the trunks of dead trees that now host birds. The trail then plunges back into the woods; in fact, for the next mile, you'll see no sign of humanity aside from the trail and the folks you pass along it. Bee Tree Run, when it comes into view, is narrow and pretty tame in this section; a smattering of ferns winds up the hill on the left.

You'll reach the Freeland parking area at 17.9 miles; the parking area has a restroom as well as a public phone. The Pennsylvania state line is less than 2 miles away. As you walk away from Freeland, you'll see an open marshy area on the right. Soon you'll cross into Oakland, where you'll see a beautiful old barn to the left. As the trail opens up again, you'll get a good sense of the rural nature of the immediate area. At 19.1 miles, the trail begins to resemble the section at White Hall, with blasted rock and clinging tree roots.

At 19.2 miles, you've reached the Mason-Dixon Line, created between 1763 and 1767 to settle a dispute between the Maryland and Pennsylvania colonies. Stones marking the line carry William Penn's seal on the north and Lord Baltimore's on the south. Here you'll find benches and a rest area—a perfect place to relax, eat your lunch, and enjoy that particular thrill one gets from walking from one state into another.

If you're feeling incredibly ambitious, you can keep going. The York County (Pennsylvania) park system picks up where the Torrey Brown leaves off, following the rail bed another 20 miles north into York.

NEARBY ACTIVITIES

For activities near the southern portion of the trail, see the hike profiles for Loch Raven Reservoir: Northwest Area Trails (page 114) and Oregon Ridge State Park (page 128). For the northern reaches of the trail, beyond Whitehall: the 375-acre Morris Meadows Recreation Farm with its Historic Preservation Museum, off Freeland Road between Middletown Road and York Road, features early-American antiques and artifacts. To get there, take I-83 and exit at either Middletown Road (Exit 31) or Freeland Road (Exit 37); for more information, call (800) 643-7056 or visit **www.morrismeadows.us.** If you're into buying antiques instead of just looking at them, head to Monkton, off Exit 27 from I-83, Monkton Road east. To see the national-award-winning Ladew Topiary Gardens, take I-83 to MD 439 (Exit 36), and go east about 6 miles to a dead-end at MD 23; turn right and go about 3 miles to the junction of MD 23 and MD 146 (Jarrettsville Pike). Turn right onto Jarrettsville Pike and continue to Ladew Gardens, about 3 miles ahead on your left. For more information, call (410) 557-9466 or visit **www.ladewgardens.com.**

24 NORTH POINT STATE PARK

KEY AT-A-GLANCE INFORMATION

LENGTH: 3.6 miles

CONFIGURATION: Loop with short spurs

DIFFICULTY: Easy–moderate

SCENERY: Chesapeake Bay, Black Marsh Wildlands, historic structures

EXPOSURE: Slightly more shade than sun

TRAFFIC: Light–moderate

TRAIL SURFACE: Dirt, asphalt

HIKING TIME: 1.5 hours

ACCESS: Trails open November 1–March 31, 10 a.m.–6 p.m. and April 1–October 31, 8 a.m.–4 p.m.

MAPS: USGS Sparrows Point; trail maps at gatehouse

FACILITIES: Portable bathroom at parking area; restrooms, water, and concessions at visitor center (open Memorial Day–Labor Day, Wednesday to Sunday, 11 a.m.–4 p.m.); swimming area and pavilions

SPECIAL COMMENTS: $3 per day-use fee; for excellent information about the history of the park and the area, visit the Maryland Department of Natural Resources Web site, www .dnr.state.md.us/naturalresource/ spring2003/parkprofile.html.

GPS Trailhead
Coordinates
UTM Zone (WGS84) 18S
Easting 376543
Northing 4342250
Latitude N 39° 13.245921'
Longitude W 76° 25.809667'

IN BRIEF

See how things have (and haven't) changed in an area of undeveloped bayfront property where evidence of human habitation dates back 9,000 years.

DESCRIPTION

The white-blazed gravel and grass trail at the end of the parking area spits you back onto the road at the gatehouse after just 75 feet. From there, take an immediate right onto the trail, which is initially shaded by tall, thick trees but opens up at 0.2 miles onto the 232-acre Black Marsh. At 0.3 miles, to the left, you'll come to the Observation Trail, which has light blue blazes and leads you to an overlook where you can view the Black Marsh Wildlands (it's a 0.6-mile round trip to the observation deck and back).

The marsh and forested buffer, protected as a Maryland Wildland and Natural Heritage Area, provides a haven for birds. According to the Maryland Department of Natural Resources, the birds found in and around the marsh include "bald eagles, rare American bitterns, Northern harriers, great horned owls, red-tailed hawks, and elusive black rails. The marsh also serves as home to wading birds such as herons and egrets as well as waterfowl such as canvasbacks, goldeneyes, ruddy

Directions ⟶

Take I-695 to Exit 40, MD 151 south (North Point Boulevard). Go south 3.8 miles and take a left onto North Point Road just after the I-695 overpass. Go 1.8 miles to the park entrance on the left at Bay Shore Road; pass the gatehouse to the parking area on the left. The trail starts at the edge of the parking area.

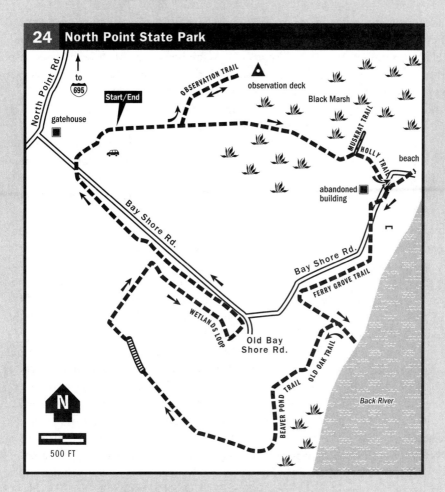

24 North Point State Park

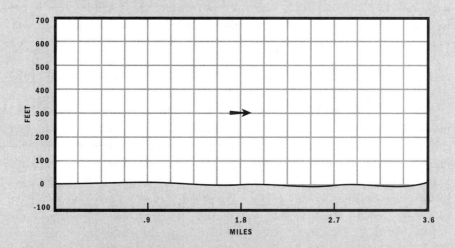

ducks, mergansers, and scaup." For an exhaustive list of the hundreds of birds found in North Point State Park, visit **northpointstatepark.homestead.com/birds .html**. In summer, the white blooms of rose mallows, one of the eight species of rare or endangered plants in the area, cover the entire marsh. You might also see common cranberry, cattail, and swamp milkweed. Many frogs, snakes, skinks and salamanders, and turtles (including the state reptile, the Diamondback Terrapin) make homes in and around the water.

Back on the main trail, cut left at the yellow-blazed Muskrat Trail, at 1.1 mile. This trail brings you to the edge of the marsh, where the remains of a small boat, almost completely overtaken by vegetation, sits by the water's edge. In addition to muskrats, you'll also have a decent chance of spotting beavers, foxes, and otters.

Coming back from the end of the Muskrat Trail, you'll see the purple-blazed Holly Trail about 200 feet to the left. Take the Holly Trail and soon you'll see more sky as things begin to open up. You'll also hear a faint rumble. You'll see red blazes on this section of the trail, but it looks very underused. It's also muddy, tight, and overgrown. Go left at the T-intersection. You'll soon learn what the rumble is and why the sky has come into view: a beautiful little rocky beach, complete with small, lapping waves. Ahead of you sit a lonely lighthouse and the wide, beautiful Chesapeake Bay.

When you're ready to head back, return on the red trail but now continue straight at the T-intersection where you went left earlier. Pass an old cavernous abandoned building posted with NO TRESPASSING. PRIVATE PROPERTY signs; please heed the signs. Once you've passed the building, take a left onto the red-blazed Powerhouse Trail as it widens considerably. A bench at 1.5 miles overlooks the Chesapeake Bay and commands a really nice view. Continue around the edge of the hill overlooking the water; be on the lookout for bald eagles in this area.

After reentering the woods, you will see white blazes again. At 1.6 miles, go left at the blue-blazed Ferry Grove Trail; you'll come to the sky blue-blazed Old Oak Trail at 1.8 miles on the right, but for now, pass it and head toward the water. You'll see a sunken jetty as well as some nice views of the bay. Heading back, take the Old Oak Trail, which is now on your left. You'll be back in the woods, surrounded by oaks and thick underbrush. This trail, which is also very underused, has sections that require minor bushwhacking in the summer. While there are moments in which you'll probably wonder if this is a trail at all, the continued presence of the blue blazes will assure you that you are going in the right direction. This section eventually leads to a better maintained trail.

When you see a blue blaze on a beech tree after 2 miles, head right and pick up Beaver Pond Trail to the left. This wide, exposed trail follows cut grass through an area that provides good habitat for raccoons, gray squirrels, cardinals, great horned owls, red foxes, red-tailed hawks, spotted salamanders, American kestrels, killdeers, plovers, and robins. If you want to make a loop with the hiker-biker trail, take a left when you reach the paved road; it leads to the ultra-busy swimming beach area, trolley house, and visitor center. Here, you'll lose any semblance of solitude, but why not take advantage and go for a swim? If you want to keep your solitude, however, head right when you reach the paved road. You can always drive to the public area after you complete your hike.

If you chose to head right here, you'll pass a grove of black cherry, with white flowers in spring and black fruit in summer. At 2.4 miles, the trail opens up and becomes marshy again. Cross a wooden boardwalk at 2.5 miles and pass a big cornfield on the left as you head to the right. When you see a paved road ahead, take a right into the stubby woods; this is the Wetlands Loop. You'll see an open area on the right with lots of bird feeders. Head left at the V. If you wish to make a complete loop of the wetlands, keep going to the right when you reach the paved road at 2.8 miles; otherwise, turn left onto the road and head back to the parking area. Straight ahead on the road, you will see a bulletin board and the trailhead for the white-blazed Wildlands Loop, a big portion of which you covered at the beginning of the hike.

Heading back to the parking area along the road isn't nearly as unpleasant as it sounds. You'll parallel a cornfield on the left, and a big buffer separates the cornfield from the road. In summer, the sounds of the grasshoppers and crickets will drown out the noise of the cars going by at low speed. You can follow the paved road around to the parking area where you began.

One of the nice things about North Point State Park is that the vast majority of visitors come here for the beach, which means that the trails are fairly free of traffic. When you're finishing hiking, though, you can head down to the beach area for a pleasant diversion. The new visitor center mimics the original Bayshore Park Restaurant, built by United Railways Electric Company in 1906. The nearby large ornamental fountain, originally built in the early 1900s as part of the Bayshore Amusement Park, was in operation between 1906 and 1947. The park included a dance hall, bowling alley, restaurant, gardens, and a pier jutting into Chesapeake Bay. You can still crab and catch catfish, white perch, and striped bass here today. The swimming beach (unguarded) is also nearby, and in between sits Trolley Station Pavilion, a holdover from the days when passengers paid 30 cents to ride the #26 trolley car that ran between Baltimore and the amusement park.

NEARBY ACTIVITIES

The route for British troops to Baltimore during the War of 1812 passed through North Point. Linking nearby Fort Howard (**www.geocities.com/baltforts/Fort_Howard/ index.htm**) and Todd's Inheritance (**www.myedgemere.com/todd's_history.htm**) with this hike provides additional hiking as well as excellent history lessons. Fort Howard is another 2.2 miles south down North Point Road. You'll find Todd's Inheritance a half-mile north of Fort Howard on North Point Road. Thomas Todd settled on this spot in 1664. Retreating British soldiers, defeated at the Battle of Fort McHenry, burned the original Todd home; the house standing here now was built on the original homesite in 1816 and was remodeled in 1867.

25 OREGON RIDGE PARK

KEY AT-A-GLANCE INFORMATION

LENGTH: 4.2 miles

CONFIGURATION: Loop

DIFFICULTY: Moderate

SCENERY: Upland forest, Baisman Run, historic structures

EXPOSURE: Shade

TRAFFIC: Moderate

TRAIL SURFACE: Packed dirt with many sections of exposed roots

HIKING TIME: 2 hours

ACCESS: Dawn–dusk

MAPS: USGS Cockeysville; trail maps at nature center and online at www.baltimorecountymd.gov/Agencies/recreation/countyparks/oregonridgelodge.

WHEELCHAIR ACCESS: No

FACILITIES: Restrooms in the nature center and lodge at main park entrance; take a right at the split in the road to go to the nature center; the park includes a swimming beach, playgrounds, restaurant, and theater.

SPECIAL COMMENTS: The nature center is open every day, except Monday, from 9 a.m. to 5 p.m. No bikes are allowed on the trails; dogs must be leashed.

GPS Trailhead Coordinates

UTM Zone (WGS84) 18S

Easting 354694

Northing 4372885

Latitude N 39° 29.598591'

Longitude W 76° 41.388459'

IN BRIEF

Hike up and down hills in one of the Baltimore area's most popular parks.

DESCRIPTION

Oregon Ridge has become well known around Baltimore for many things: its annual Fourth of July celebration with a performance by the excellent Baltimore Symphony Orchestra, its cross-country skiing trails, a swimming beach, restaurant, and theater. Hiking doesn't usually make the top of the list, and that's a shame because the trails in the park offer a great trek. Unfortunately, a major infestation of gypsy moths wiped out a 20-acre area of 100-plus-year-old chestnut oaks. Clearings took place in summer 2008 and forced trail closures. All trails are now open, but you'll see the devastation at the hike's beginning.

Since you're starting from the nature center, it makes sense to stop in for a moment or two. Inside, you'll find live animals—turtles, red spotted newts, bullfrogs, a bee colony, hissing cockroaches, American toads, crayfish, bullhead catfish, snakes (including the copperhead, the only poisonous snake inhabiting Baltimore County) as well as stuffed owls, fox, elk, European starling, and woodpeckers. You can also walk through a hothouse and see sliders and diamondback terrapins.

Directions

Take I-83 to Exit 20, Shawan Road west. Follow to Beaver Dam Road and follow the signs to the park entrance. Once inside the park, head right at the split in the road to go to the nature center; park in the nature center parking area beyond the bathhouse. The trail starts at the end of the long wooden bridge to the left of the nature center.

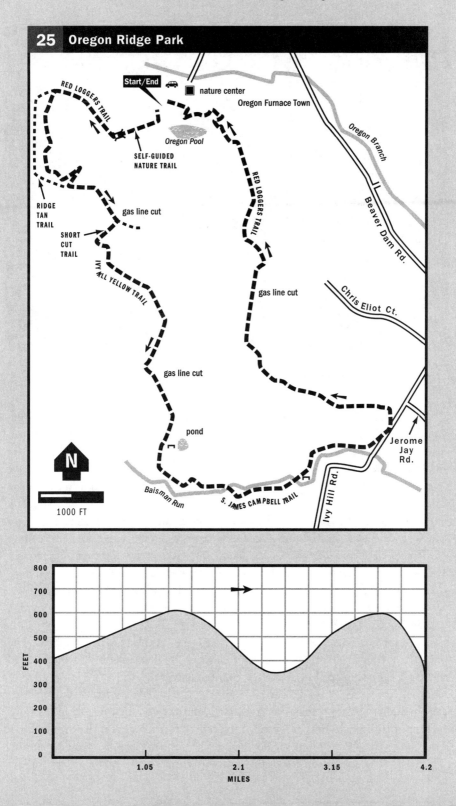

25 Oregon Ridge Park

Start/End

nature center

Oregon Furnace Town

RED LOGGERS TRAIL

Oregon Branch

Beaver Dam Rd.

Oregon Pool

SELF-GUIDED
NATURE TRAIL

RED LOGGERS TRAIL

RIDGE
TAN
TRAIL

gas line cut

SHORT
CUT
TRAIL

IVY HILL YELLOW TRAIL

gas line cut

Chris Eliot Ct.

gas line cut

pond

Jerome
Jay
Rd.

N

1000 FT

Baisman Run

S. JAMES CAMPBELL TRAIL

Ivy Hill Rd.

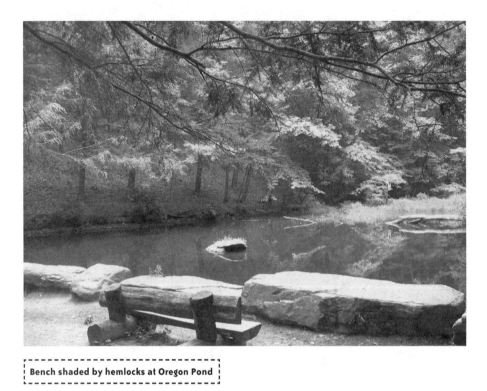

Bench shaded by hemlocks at Oregon Pond

If you're facing the entrance of the nature center, head toward the long wooden bridge to the left to start your hike; stop to pick up a brochure and follow the self-guided nature trail before you cross the bridge. While you're still on the bridge, look out over the valley below to see what's left of the iron ore pit from the mid-1800s; it's heartening to see what 150 years of nature's reclamation has done to restore this area's natural beauty. This mined pit yielded primarily goethite, one of the main ingredients in the manufacture of pig iron. Now you can see American chestnut trees growing here; a plague wiped out more than 95 percent of these trees east of the Mississippi River, making them rare today. You will also see sassafras, black tupelo, two types of wild blueberries, red oak, white oak, ash, red maple, dogwood, tulip, beech, and sarvis trees in the valley. On ground level, you may catch a reflected glimmer of loch raven schist, which contains mica, garnet, feldspar, and quartz crystals.

Head right after the wooden bridge onto the red-blazed Loggers Trail. The name "Loggers Trail" takes on a sad irony, as you'll soon come to the cleared section on the slope of hill above the nature center.

But first, after 900 feet, the trail splits at the tan-blazed Ridge Trail, which takes a higher elevation than the Loggers Trail; the two link after 0.3 miles. This section of trail (including portions of the blue Laurel Trail and the orange Lake Trail) were the areas closed for dead tree removal. At 0.3 miles, you'll begin to parallel a little stream on the right that cuts through the center of the valley;

hills rise on either side of you. At 0.6 miles, the trail begins heading uphill and soon becomes rather precipitous. It's very rocky and very rooty, which makes it tough to hike in ice and snow. You'll come to a T-intersection at 0.8 miles; take a right and head toward the red blazes (to the left is where you would have come from if you took the tan Ridge Trail earlier). Over the last half mile, you've gained more than 250 feet of elevation. Another negative effect of the gypsy moth clearance is that this climb used to at least be shaded, but now, in the full blaze of a summer sun, it is potentially unpleasant.

Come to a gas line cut line at 0.9 miles. You'll actually pass through gas line cuts four times along this hike, and they pleasantly mix things up a bit since they provide sections of high grass that shelter a host of insects, which in turn attract birds. When you enter the woods on the other side, at 1 mile, take a right on the Short Cut Trail, as the Loggers Trail begins to loop back to the nature center.

The Short Cut Trail takes a gradual descent through a grove of ferns before it links with the yellow Ivy Hill Trail at 1.2 miles. Take a right and for the first time, you'll be on level ground. Come to another gas line cut at 1.4 miles, and after 100 feet, you'll be back in the woods.

At 1.6 miles, the scenery begins to change a bit as low-lying bushes and pines make an appearance. Many hawks inhabit this area. The trail descends, heads left, and becomes very rocky again. Many of the rocks at your feet shine with quartz and feldspar. Heavy rains may wash out this section of the trail a bit.

Suddenly you will hear the sound of running water as Baisman Run appears on the right. You'll see a rickety wooden bridge going over the run, but stay on the trail—you'll cross it at places that offer much more secure footing.

Cross Baisman Run at 1.75 miles and come to a T-intersection on the other side; head to the left up the railroad ties to the pond. With a nice wooden bench to sit on and beautiful hemlocks lining the other side of the pond, this is a lovely spot to rest a while. Continuing on, you'll soon see a sign for the S. James Campbell Trail, which also has yellow blazes. Despite the two names, this and the Ivy Hill Trail are actually the same, so if you stay on yellow-blazed paths, you'll be fine. At 1.9 miles, cross the quick-moving but shallow Baisman Run on a series of rocks; take caution if the rocks are submerged—they can be very slippery. You'll most probably get the soles of your boots wet, and even if you step on the stream bottom, the only harm will be that you'll scatter tadpoles, minnows, and skimmers.

When you see a Jeep trail straight ahead up the hill, take a left (the Jeep trail goes out to Ivy Hill Road); a sign points you again to the S. James Campbell Trail. Cross Baisman Run again; there are no rocks here, so you'll get a bit wet. The trail gets tighter and woodsier, but it soon opens up again with thin small trees, some of which have fallen and are lying across the trail; you'll have to hurdle them as you walk beside Baisman Run heading downstream. The sound of the stream belies its size; the many rocks and swiftness of the water make it sound much larger than it is. Cross the stream again at 2.1 miles; this time, there are several large rocks, so you won't have any problem even if the water is high.

Cross yet again about 70 feet later; you might want to stop here and sit on the bench while you listen to the wonderful sounds of nature.

At 2.3 miles, the trail heads uphill to the left as Baisman Run turns to the right; you'll suddenly be thrust into civilization again when Ivy Hill Road appears through the woods to the right. You're skirting the park boundary here, but you won't see or hear much traffic, and you'll soon be heading away from the road again as you go uphill. Like earlier in the hike, it's very steep here, and you'll gain more than 200 feet of elevation very quickly. Go through another gas line cut, and, at 3 miles, you'll come to an intersection and Loggers Trail once again. Head right and go down the hill into a section that is thickly wooded, much more so than the top of the hill on Ivy Hill Trail.

Cross another gas line cut and head toward the lake. You'll see a sign for the nature center and lake access. Go down the hill over railroad ties; if it's swimming season (April to October), you'll hear people playing in the water. At the sign that points to the frog pond, go straight; you'll see a playground on the left, along with volleyball courts. This isn't so much a trail anymore, even though some of the trees here and there bear red blazes; essentially you're walking through the area between the lake and bathhouse. If it's in season, you'll have to exit through the gate and head back to the car, just a few hundred feet ahead to the left; if it's not season, the red blazes run right beside the lake and lead out a door in the wooden fence around the lake area. You'll find concessions, water, and bathrooms here, and the parking area and nature center are just on the other side of the bathhouse.

Before you leave, check out the re-created Oregon Furnace Town, just down the hill to the right of the nature center entrance. This area includes the Tenant House Museum, with historical exhibits on woodsman's tools and the clothing worn by the men who mined the pits here in the 1800s. The 1850 census data shows that approximately 225 people lived here, mostly Irish and German immigrants and emancipated black slaves.

NEARBY ACTIVITIES

The Oregon Grille, at 1201 Shawan Road, offers an expensive but wonderful dining experience; housed in a restored 19th-century stone house, it boasts a five-star rating. You can reach the Maryland State Fairgrounds by taking Shawan Road right and turning right onto York Road. Generally speaking, there's something going on at the fairgrounds all year long, but if you are there in late August or early September, you can enjoy the state fair, which draws people from all over Maryland and adjoining states.

PATAPSCO VALLEY STATE PARK: ALBERTON AND DANIELS AREAS

26

IN BRIEF

Stroll along the Patapsco River, visiting numerous historic sites along the way.

DESCRIPTION

A hike in this portion of Patapsco Valley State Park serves as the best reminder of the thriving nature of the area long before it was a park. Historical structures dot the entire walk.

From the parking area, walk straight beyond the metal gate on the asphalt. Alberton Road used to be a traffic through-road, heading toward the community of Daniels. As a general rule, I'm not a huge fan of hiking on asphalt, but this trail is very peaceful, and very pleasant. It traverses a wide valley, loaded with birds. Thick forest flanks the abandoned road to the right, and the Patapsco River is just on the left; it's full of rocks and runs swiftly. Near the river, sycamores and box elders dominate, but the whole area—up the hills—is studded with beech, dogwood, oak, and tulip poplar. Understory growth includes mountain laurel, redbud, serviceberry, spice-bush, and witch hazel.

At 0.1 mile is a stationary trail map. Skirt left around a private home and quickly return to the trail, which is blazed in white. You'll be walking upstream, and you'll be able to see the CSX rail lines on the other side of the

KEY AT-A-GLANCE INFORMATION

LENGTH: 3.5 Miles

CONFIGURATION: Out-and-back

DIFFICULTY: Easy

SCENERY: Historical ruins, Patapsco River, piedmont stream valley

EXPOSURE: Shaded

TRAFFIC: Light—moderate

TRAIL SURFACE: Cracked asphalt, crushed rock, packed dirt

HIKING TIME: 1.5 hours

ACCESS: Dawn–dusk, year-round

MAPS: USGS Ellicott City

WHEELCHAIR ACCESS: Yes, but may be difficult

FACILITIES: None

SPECIAL COMMENTS: If you possess the complete PVSP trail map, you may notice paths indicated on the map showing a loop route beyond the ruins of Saint Stanislas Catholic Church that empties into the wide space created by the power line cut. However, while paths do criss-cross the area, the loop shown on the map is completely overgrown by thick and prickly vegetation. If you attempt the loop, you're in for an unpleasant trip, especially if it's summer.

Directions ───────────────→

Take I-695 to Exit 17, Security Boulevard west. Take Security past the Security Mall and follow signs to Johnnycake Road. Follow Johnny-cake until it ends, and take a right onto Hollofield Road. Take a left onto Dogwood Road and then an immediate left to the parking area off Alberton Road.

GPS Trailhead Coordinates

UTM Zone (WGS84) 18S

Easting 345387

Northing 4353294

Latitude N 39° 18.914666'

Longitude W 76° 47.608016'

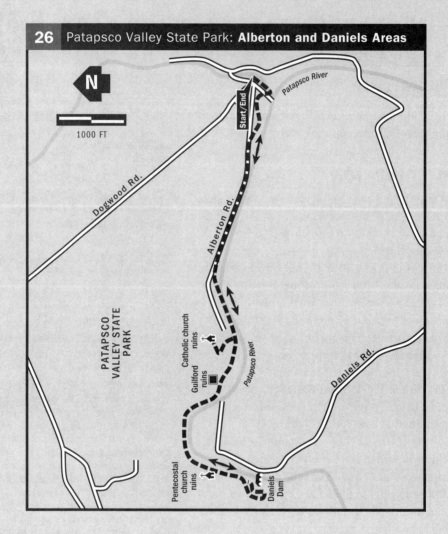

26 Patapsco Valley State Park: **Alberton and Daniels Areas**

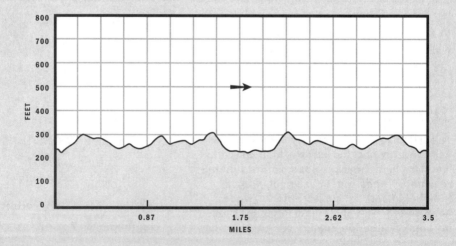

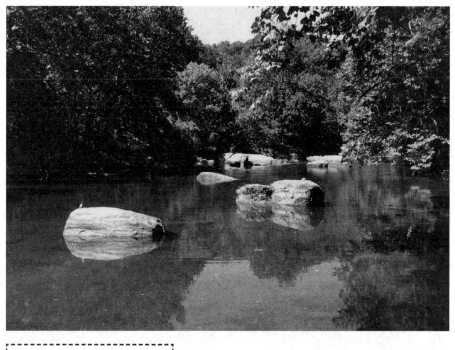

Patapsco River east of Daniels Dam

river. Be on the lookout for belted kingfishers, great blue and little green herons, killdeer, and a variety of ducks. Even bald eagles have been known to make an appearance. Big rocks decorate the river, sometimes changing the water's course. Even more enormous rocks litter the hillsides; they are invariably composed of erosion-resistant mica schist. The best example of these rocks comes at 0.5 miles, where a fantastic column towers over the road.

Be on the lookout for a white-gravel trail at 0.8 miles. Follow it gradually uphill until you see a large wire basket of rocks on your right. Take the path by this basket to the ruins of Saint Stanislas Kostka Roman Catholic Church. Founded in 1879 (the stone structure you'll see was erected shortly thereafter), the church was in use until the town of Daniels was razed in the late 1960s. There's a graveyard behind the church; the large number of children buried there tells of the harsh realities of late-19th-and early-20th-century life.

You'll see paths running away from the church; undoubtedly, you'll also notice that the gravel road you took to get to the church continues up the hill. As mentioned in Special Comments on page 133, you can take any of these other paths, but eventually they all end in thick undergrowth (or residential areas), and you'll have to return the way you came. Instead of slogging it, return to the Alberton Road trail when you've had your fill of poking around the church ruins.

Back on the trail at 1.1 miles, head right and follow it along the river. You'll soon see the remnants of the abandoned town of Daniels, founded in the 1830s as a cotton-milling community. This town was essentially owned by the C. R.

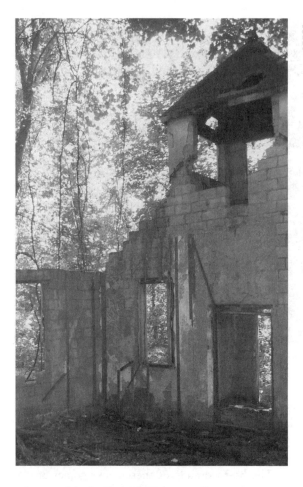

Pentecostal church ruins

Daniels Company, and its residents were mill workers. (This portion of the town, on the Baltimore County side, was actually known as Guilford, but it was in fact considered part of Daniels.)

Continuing along the river, you'll soon come to your best view of the abandoned Daniels Mill across the river. Also here are the still-active CSX bridge as well as the ruins of the old pedestrian bridge.

Just beyond the bridges, to the right at 1.7 miles, you'll see the ruins of the community's Pentecostal church. Dating only to 1940, this church seems to pale in comparison to the older church at the hike's beginning. Just afterward is the Daniels Dam, used to generate power for the mill. Cut left a few hundred feet after the church; the path goes along the river, which brings you closer to the dam. Head up so you're above the dam and looking over it. Pocking the banks near the dam are numerous beaver lodges. The path circles around to the right and then rejoins the main wide trail. Head right to return to your car, reaching it at 3.5 miles. If you head left, in 1.6 miles, you'll reach the portion of PVSP described in this book under Patapsco Valley State Park: Unmaintained Area: Granite–Woodstock (see page 293).

NEARBY ACTIVITIES

Western Run Park is the home of the Diamond Ridge Golf Course. To reach it, head back toward Hollofield Road. Take a left on Ridge Road. The golf course will be on the right. General information: (410) 887-1349; to book a tee time, call (410) 887-GOLF (4653) or (888) 246-5384. If you want to do some shopping, head back out on Security Boulevard and stop at the Security Mall.

PATAPSCO VALLEY STATE PARK: GLEN ARTNEY AREA

IN BRIEF

Take in the best of the Glen Artney Area: two branches of the Patapsco River, mature forest, and Lost Lake.

DESCRIPTION

The trailhead leads onto Soapstone Branch Trail. A long, flat ridge drops off both sides of the trail, with Soapstone Branch to the right and very big beech trees all around. Just before 0.2 miles, the trail heads into a very deep gulley; follow it down to level ground.

At 0.25 miles, you'll see the trail's first purple blaze. Midlevel growth includes mountain laurel and sumac, with oak and beech towering above. This is a good place to consider the drastic contrast between the nearby city and this natural area: Here you are, less than half a mile from a major highway, a Park and Ride lot, residential neighborhoods, schools, and churches, but you can see nothing but thick woods, much of it old-growth.

Near a trail sign, you'll see how the water has cut under a big oak and the root system hangs over. As you move on, huge rocks dominate the trail. You'll make several very easy crossings over Soapstone Branch in this section. At 0.7 miles, up the hill to the right, you'll come to the orange-blazed Bull Run

KEY AT-A-GLANCE INFORMATION

LENGTH: 4.9 miles

CONFIGURATION: Out-and-back with 2 loops

DIFFICULTY: Moderate

SCENERY: Soapstone and Santee branches, Patapsco River, forest

EXPOSURE: More shade than sun

TRAFFIC: Moderate

TRAIL SURFACE: Packed dirt

HIKING TIME: 1.5–2 hours

ACCESS: 9 a.m.–sunset

MAPS: USGS Relay; map of PVSP trail system available at the park or online at www.easycart.net/ MarylandDepartmentofNatural Resources/Central_Maryland_Trail _Guides.html.

WHEELCHAIR ACCESS: No

FACILITIES: Restrooms, water, pavilions, and playground at the paved area at 0.8 miles of this hike

SPECIAL COMMENTS: The official park entrance can be reached by taking I-95 to Exit 47 (BWI Airport) and traveling east on I-195. Take Exit 3 to Elkridge. Turn right on US 1, heading south, and take the next right onto South Street. The park entrance is immediately on the left.

Directions

Take I-195 west toward Catonsville / Park and Ride; continue toward the Park and Ride to where I-195 ends at Rolling Road. Turn left and continue on Rolling Road; after it turns into Selford Road, immediately look for the gravel parking area on the shoulder of Selford Road across from the Park and Ride lot. The trail starts just off the parking area.

GPS Trailhead Coordinates

UTM Zone (WGS84) 18S

Easting 351634

Northing 4345360

Latitude N 39° 14.692662'

Longitude W 76° 43.157194'

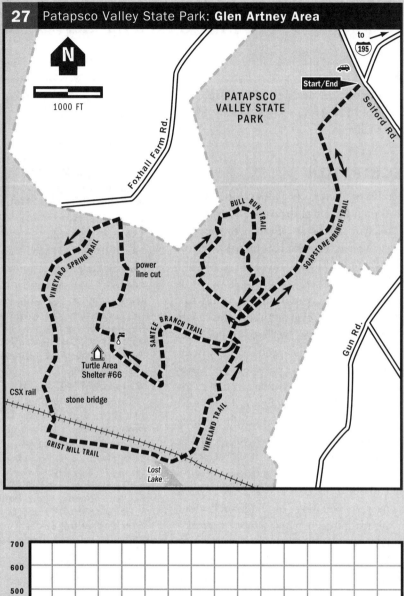

27 Patapsco Valley State Park: **Glen Artney Area**

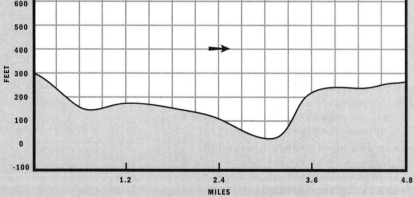

Old growth

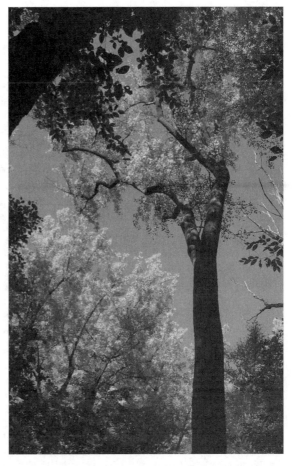

Trail; take note that this trail will be part of your return route. For now, stay on Soapstone Trail. Immediately after the Bull Run Trail cut, you'll come to the longest crossing over Soapstone Branch; the large rocks here make this easy, too. On the other side, you'll come to a little parking area that has a pavilion and bathrooms, as well as a playground.

From the parking area, head diagonally up the hill to the right to stay on the Soapstone Trail. On the right at 0.9 miles, you'll see Santee Branch Trail at the top of the hill. Abandon the Soapstone Trail (it heads back down the hill to the left and ends in a section where you will be later), and take Santee Branch Trail to a road and parking area. Walk along the road to continue the hike. Since this is a park road, it's narrow, doesn't have a lot of traffic, and is bordered by thick woods on one side, making it actually quite pleasant. At the split in the road, head right and go past the DO NOT ENTER (for car traffic) sign.

At the wooden posts to the right at 1.25 miles, pick up the trail (barely discernible, but among spread-out trees and easy to navigate) and then go left up the hill. You'll come to the Turtle Area Shelter, #66. Turn right, back onto the asphalt. You'll find a water fountain here next to the parking area on the right; expect these parking areas to be largely empty during the week. Across from the parking area, you'll see a little dirt trail heading into the woods, at just under 1.5 miles; take the trail and you'll soon see white blazes on the trees.

The topography changes drastically. Before, it was soaring old-growth; here it's short, with nubbly trees and lots of underbrush. Obviously people used this area as an open field sometime in the last 20 or 30 years, but vegetation is now filling it in nicely. You'll cross through a power line cut with its nice views of the forest on the right, and then pass a circular brick structure to the left;

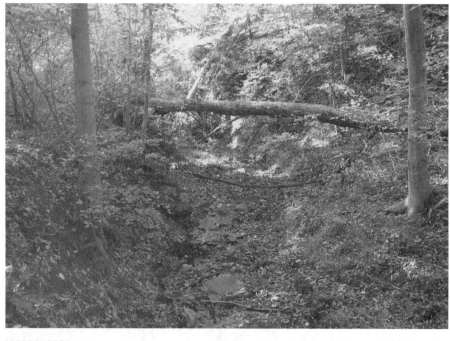

Stream bed

this section feels eerily isolated and exposed. You will come to a trail intersection at about 1.6 miles; go straight and link with the red-blazed Vineyard Spring Trail. Be sure to stay on the red-blazed trail; if you head to the right here, you'll come to the park boundary and eventually join Santee Branch Trail, which heads northward to the Hilton Area of the state park (see page 142). You'll be rewarded with another beautiful area, dominated by tall, thin tulip poplar. This spot attracts many kinds of birds, and during fall and spring migrations, you may see bluebirds, scarlet tanagers, and Baltimore orioles. The trail here has numerous rocks and exposed roots, and it also has lots of underbrush, midlevel shorter trees and hanging vines, and soaring older ones.

At 1.8 miles, you'll see a cut to the right, which will also take you to the Santee Branch Trail. Pass that cut and head steadily down into a valley, where a trickle of water flows on the left. At just over 2 miles to the left, you'll come to the loop cut for the Vineyard Trail; continue straight (taking the left cut would lead you back to the white-blazed trail where you were before). At 2.1 miles, you'll pass, on the right, the concrete slabs and foundation of some long-gone building, now covered in moss.

At 2.25 miles, go under a stone bridge on a boardwalk (above you is the CSX rail line); you'll emerge at the paved, wheelchair-accessible Grist Mill Trail. Go left on this trail, which is popular with walkers, bikers, and Rollerbladers. It's something of a shock to land here after the isolation of the trails from which you've just come, but that's not to say that the Grist Mill Trail isn't nice. It's quite scenic, with nice shade trees to the right fronting the Patapsco River as well as the rising hill to the left where the trains run infrequently.

At a little over 2.5 miles, you'll come to a parking area with bathrooms fronting Lost Lake, an interesting fishing lake reserved only for people who are 61 years of age or older, are under 16, or have disabilities. As soon as you pass the lake, head left under the stone bridge and railroad tracks at the sign that points toward Glen Artney and Lower Glen Artney. On the other side of the bridge, look for the crossing over Soapstone Branch. Since there are no large rocks in the water here, you will not be able to cross in high water; if you can't cross, head straight to get back to the road and ultimately reach the same place as you would crossing Soapstone Branch. Clearly, the more pleasant option is to take the narrow trail on the other side of Soapstone Branch if water levels allow. Once you cross the branch, head left on the purple-blazed Vineland Trail.

At 3 miles, the trail runs right into Soapstone Branch. You'll have to cross here, but big rocks make it easy. Head up the hill and go right; you'll soon emerge at the parking area you came across at 0.8 miles. Backtrack from where you came before, crossing Soapstone Branch again, but this time head left up the hill on the orange-blazed Bull Run Trail. (If you're short on time, you can go straight; your car is just 0.8 miles ahead.)

The Bull Run Trail splits immediately. In fact, it will split several times. It's a loop, so you can go either way; I took the leftward choice each time to make the longest loop possible, which totals not much more than a mile. The trail goes quickly and steeply uphill among mostly tulip poplar. At the top of the hill, you'll come to a power line cut; follow the tree line for a while and cut back into the woods when the trail ends at the power tower. Now the path becomes pebble and rock. You'll come to another split here; again I took the left, onto the dirt trail. This upland forest consists of mostly beech and oak, with poplar still popping up here and there. Some of the enormous trees here are at least second-growth, if not old-growth.

At 3.9 miles, the trail turns rock and pebble again. When it does so, take a right and soon after (about 1,000 feet) take a left onto the packed dirt trail down the hill. You'll come to a little switchback; when the trail splits again, head left. Now the trail runs through a deep-rutted gulley as it continues down the hill; you'll soon come to the other side of Soapstone Branch from where you began the hike. When the trail ends at 4.2 miles, cross Soapstone Branch for the last time and head left; you'll be back on the way to your car.

NEARBY ACTIVITIES

You might enjoy hiking through the nearby Orange Grove and Hilton areas of Patapsco Valley State Park; for hike descriptions and directions, see pages 284 and 142. I-195 runs from the Park and Ride at the Glen Artney trailhead to BWI Airport at the other end. If you can't fly off to paradise, check out the BWI Trail (see page 16).

28 PATAPSCO VALLEY STATE PARK: HILTON AREA

(i) KEY AT-A-GLANCE INFORMATION

LENGTH: 4.1 miles

CONFIGURATION: 2 jagged loops

DIFFICULTY: Moderate–strenuous

SCENERY: Buzzards Rock, Ilchester Rocks, Santee and Sawmill Branch, upland forest, Patapsco River, historical structures

EXPOSURE: Mostly shade

TRAFFIC: Light–moderate

TRAIL SURFACE: Packed dirt; short sections of crushed rock, gravel, and asphalt

HIKING TIME: 2 hours

ACCESS: 9 a.m.–sunset

MAPS: USGS Relay, Savage, Ellicott City, Baltimore West; map of PVSP trail system available at the park or online at www.easycart.net/ MarylandDepartmentofNatural Resources/Central_Maryland_Trail _Guides.html.

WHEELCHAIR ACCESS: On paved Grist Mill Trail only

FACILITIES: Phone, restrooms, camp-sites, pavilions, and playgrounds can all be reached at the park entrance from the Forest Glen Trail.

SPECIAL COMMENTS: There is a $2 day-use fee if you undertake the hike from the official Hilton entrance.

GPS Trailhead
Coordinates
UTM Zone (WGS84) 18S
Easting 349083
Northing 4345288
Latitude N 39° 14.627352'
Longitude W 76° 44.929140'

IN BRIEF

Two of PVSP's more popular overlooks, plus enough elevation changes for a great workout.

DESCRIPTION

The initial trail is the yellow-blazed Buzzards Rock Trail. But its first stop isn't Buzzards Rock. Instead, it's the popular rock-climbing area at Ilchester Rocks. You'll reach it by passing the first trail split at 0.1 mile. Then, just before 0.2 miles, go downhill to the right over the log steps. This little section is blazed in green. You'll reach this popular and beautiful overlook in a tenth of a mile.

Facing the valley, go left; the path almost immediately reconnects with the Buzzards Rock Trail. Take a right. There's a quick split—go straight and stay on the ridge. Heading downhill, you'll reach the paved Grist Mill Trail at 0.5 miles. Head left. At 0.6 miles, look for the little trail heading down

---

Directions ————————→

To hike trailhead: Take I-695 to Exit 13, Frederick Road west. From Frederick Road, take a left on Hilltop Place (0.7 miles beyond Hillcrest Elementary). Go 1 mile. As the road makes a big rightward curve, you'll see the parking area on the left and straight ahead. Take the trail beyond the PVSP sign, to the right of the power line cut.

To the main Hilton entrance: Take I-695 to Exit 13, Frederick Road west. After 2 miles, turn left onto South Rolling Road. At the first intersection, bear right on Hilton Avenue. Continue 1.5 miles until you reach the park; turn right and follow the park road around to a parking area, about 0.2 miles. A sign on the right marks the Forest Glen Trail.

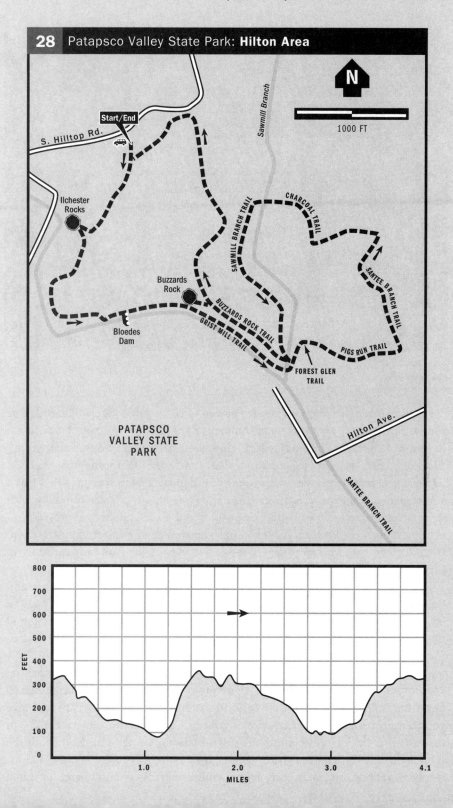

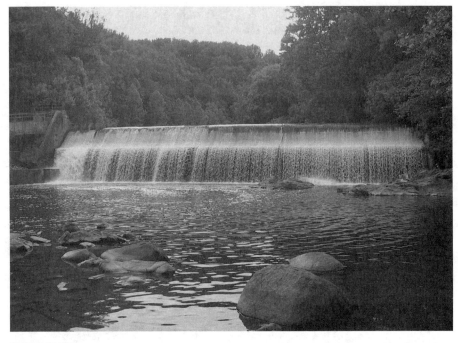

Bloede's Dam

the hill to the right when you hear the sound of rushing water. (There is one yellow blaze there.) This takes you to Bloede's Dam. Now listed on the National Register of Historic Places, the 100-hundred-year-old dam housed the world's first submerged electrical generating plant inside the dam's concrete shell. In addition to its history, the area around the dam is a beautiful spot to sit and contemplate. It also provides great fishing, as the area is stocked annually with rainbow and brown trout. Belted kingfishers and great blue herons provide colorful additions to the scene. It looks like the trail dead ends at a concrete and fence barrier, but you can walk around it and even make your way carefully to the river.

To continue the hike, go back uphill to the Grist Mill Trail and take a right. Follow the Grist Mail Trail for half a mile until you reach the leftward cut at a big stone bridge at 1.3 miles for both the yellow-blazed Buzzards Rock Trail and the blue-blazed Forest Glen Trail. You'll also see the red-blazed Sawmill Branch Trail to the left, but skip it for now.

Cross the water and take the Forest Glen Trail. Parallel Santee Branch on your left as it joins Sawmill Branch. At 1.5 miles, you'll come to the purple-blazed Pigs Run Trail. (Going right here to continue on the Forest Glen Trail will take you to the official Hilton Area park entrance—see Facilities on page 142—in 0.3 miles.) A thick, full upland forest surrounds you on the Pigs Run Trail; the trees are primarily oak, but you'll also see tulip poplar, beech, dogwood, maple, sassafras, redbud, and sycamore. Many wildflowers also abound here, including

Buzzards Rock Trail

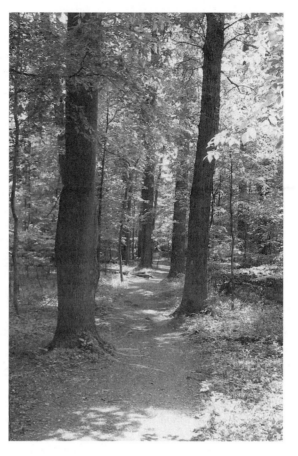

lady's slipper, jack-in-the-pulpit, mayapple, bloodroot, mountain laurel, goldenrod, black-eyed Susan, and Indian pipe. You'll cross a wooden footbridge and then pass through a power line cut before reaching the white-blazed Santee Branch Trail on the left at 1.8 miles. Take the Santee Branch Trail to its namesake waterway. At 2.1 miles, cross the Santee Branch. It's not very deep, but the rocks are spread out, which requires a bit of a well-coordinated leap. Once across Santee Branch, take a left on the orange-blazed Charcoal Trail. The Hilton camping area sits just within the woods to your right.

On the Charcoal Trail, parallel and then cross the power line cut as you reach the red-blazed Sawmill Branch Trail at 2.4 miles. Take it to the left. Follow the Sawmill Branch trail for 0.4 miles as it winds through upland forest dominated by American Beech, tulip poplar, and oak, with mountain laurel, dogwood, witch hazel, spicebush and other shrubs in the understory.

At 2.8 miles, when you reach the Sawmill Branch at the stone bridge where you came in earlier from the Grist Mill Trail (you'll see the CSX rail line to the right), this time take a right uphill on the yellow-blazed Buzzards Rock Trail. Be warned: Buzzards Rock Trail in this section involves a very steep climb over rocks and tree branches; you'll gain about 200 feet in elevation in less than two-tenths of a mile.

As you climb, you'll rise higher and higher above the train tracks; the Patapsco River and Grist Mail Trail where you were earlier, lie just on the other side of the tracks. At 3.2 miles, the trail levels out a bit, providing a reprieve from climbing. On the left at 3.4 miles is Buzzards Rock, named for the birds that used to congregate there. It's easy to see why they did—the spot commands a sweeping view, making it easy to spot prey.

The Buzzards Rock Trail continues to the right of the rock. You'll come to a power line cut at 3.7 miles. Go through the open area and pick up the trail on the other side at the edge of the woods. The trail becomes crushed rock and gravel and looks like an old fire road. Pass the Sawmill Branch Trail to the right. Soon, the Buzzards Rock Trail comes close to South Hilltop Road and parallels it back to the parking area, which you'll reach at 4.1 miles.

NEARBY ACTIVITIES

You might enjoy hiking through the nearby Orange Grove and Glen Artney sections of Patapsco Valley State Park; for hike descriptions and directions, see pages 287 and 137. Also nearby is historic Ellicott City; the former mill town, founded in 1772, has been immaculately preserved, and you will find shops and restaurants on the main street (**www.ellicottcity.net**). To reach Ellicott City from the Hilton Area, reverse the directions given above to Frederick Road and head west (instead of east back to I-695); Frederick Road turns into Main Street in Ellicott City.

PATAPSCO VALLEY STATE PARK: McKELDIN AREA 29

IN BRIEF

Walk to Liberty Dam on unmaintained trails, which take you to the developed, popular McKeldin Area of Patapsco Valley State Park.

DESCRIPTION

Starting at the trailhead, you'll walk on a rocky, packed dirt trail that parallels the North Branch of the Patapsco River. After about 300 feet, much of the rock spreads across the trail and into the water. You'll see massive ferns and mountain laurel on both sides of the trail.

At 0.3 miles, you'll see the first sign of the great contrasts this area offers: while you will walk much of this hike through upland forest, here you are in riverine wetland. A low-lying marsh and boggy area sits to the left, while the trail rises and crosses over a few feeder streams and brooks. Head up the hill to the right at 0.4 miles, and soon after cross a stream in a pine forest. A cut path to the right goes to the top of Liberty Dam; head straight and you'll come to the bottom of the dam, where the trail ends. Liberty Reservoir sits on the other side. When you've reached the dam, turn around and go right toward the river; at a little over 0.7 miles you'll come to a spit of rock and sand that allows you to cross in one jump.

On the other side, you have some options. You can take a right turn that leads to the

KEY AT-A-GLANCE INFORMATION

LENGTH: 6.3 miles

CONFIGURATION: Combination

DIFFICULTY: Moderate–strenuous

SCENERY: Patapsco River, Liberty Dam, McKeldin Rapids

EXPOSURE: Shade

TRAFFIC: Light–moderate

TRAIL SURFACE: Dirt, asphalt

HIKING TIME: 2.5 hours

ACCESS: Open Memorial Day–Labor Day 8 a.m.–sunset and 9 a.m.–sunset the rest of the year

MAPS: USGS Sykesville, Finksburg; a map of the McKeldin Area and/or entire PVSP trail system is available at the park or online at www .easycart.net/MarylandDepartment ofNaturalResources/Central _Maryland_Trail _Guides.html.

WHEELCHAIR ACCESS: No

FACILITIES: Restrooms and water at maintained area; also youth camping, picnic facilities, and disc golf

SPECIAL COMMENTS: To go directly to the official McKeldin entrance, follow the directions below but stay on Marriotsville Road another 0.4 miles from the gravel road; the entrance will be on the left. There is a $2 day-use fee for vehicles.

Directions

Take I-695 to Exit 18, Liberty Road west, toward Randallstown. Go 4.5 miles and turn left onto Marriotsville Road. Go 3.9 miles and turn right onto a little gravel road just before the Patapsco River; go straight to the little parking area. The trail starts just beyond the parking area at the edge of the woods.

GPS Trailhead Coordinates

UTM Zone (WGS84) 18S

Easting 337574

Northing 4359214

Latitude N 39° 22.027702'

Longitude W 76° 53.128989'

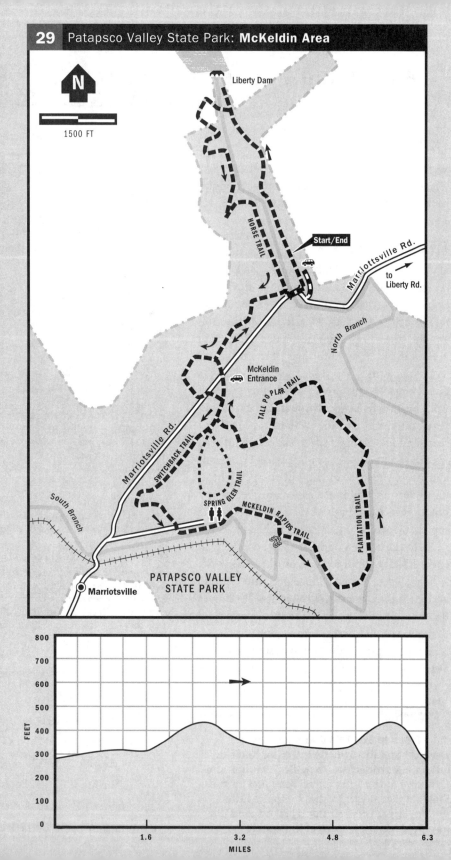

N

1500 FT

Liberty Dam

HORSE TRAIL

Start/End

Marriottsville Rd.

to
Liberty Rd.

North Branch

McKeldin
Entrance

TALL POPLAR TRAIL

Marriottsville Rd.

SWITCHBACK TRAIL

SPRING GLEN TRAIL

McKELDIN RAPIDS TRAIL

PLANTATION TRAIL

South Branch

PATAPSCO VALLEY
STATE PARK

Marriotsville

FEET

800

700

600

500

400

300

200

100

0

1.6   3.2   4.8   6.3
MILES

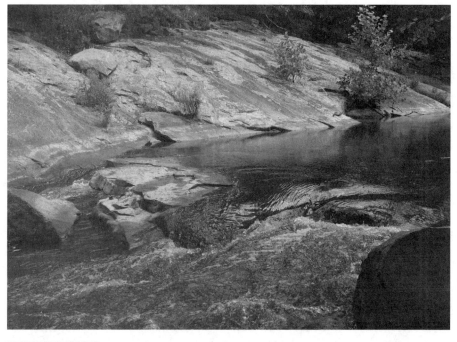

McKeldin Rapids

dam. You can also take a rocky path up the hill; if you stay on this path when it heads left, it will lead you along horse paths toward the official McKeldin Area entrance. Or you can take the more interesting option that lets you walk astride the river along unmaintained trails. Be aware that these unmaintained trails become easy to lose and require more strenuous hiking than the horse trails, but they offer nicer scenery and will link to the horse trail in half a mile. To take the river trail, head left down the hill on a barely discernible groove in the grass and dirt; if you lose the trail, follow the deer paths, which are easily detectable.

You'll be above the river walking away from the dam. You'll have to skirt your way around a big gulley until you find a good place to cross and then follow a narrow stream to the left, which you'll cross at 1.2 miles. Next, head up the hill to the right where the path stops at the river. Go around another little stream full of moss-covered rocks, and cross at 1.4 miles. Once you're across the stream, the trail becomes very discernible. This is the horse trail that you skipped earlier. Take a left, passing a series of hillside mini-waterfalls. For the next 0.8 miles, this trail can be muddy and ground-up because of equestrian use.

When you see the bridge over Marriotsville Road at 1.8 miles, the trail splits. Head right to stay off the road and in the woods. This area is marked by low-level growth: spicebush, greenbrier, and bloodroot. At 2.2 miles, things open up at a power line cut, and a fire road heads to the left up the hill and swings around to Marriotsville Road at the McKeldin Area entrance. Don't take the fire road now—you'll be on it coming back; for now, head left through the woods and cross Marriotsville Road a few hundred feet west of the entrance. This will take you into the pine plantation, a beautiful area with towering pines planted in neat rows. Looking straight on, it seems almost impenetrable, but turn 90 degrees and you'll see order. Take the path here right toward the entrance road for the McKeldin Area and then turn left up the hill; this is the maintained area, and if you've driven here, go to the tollgate and pay the entrance fee of $2.

On foot, you'll have two options when you reach the McKeldin Area entrance: the purple-blazed Tall Poplar Trail and the white-blazed Switchback Trail. Take the Switchback Trail; despite the presence of people in this area, the wildlife seems undeterred; rabbits, gray squirrels, woodchucks, and white-tailed deer run about. You may even spot a shy red fox.

Though you bypassed the Tall Poplar Trail, the Switchback Trail also winds among tall poplars; taking the Switchback Trail simply yields a much larger hiking loop. At 2.9 miles, the trail runs very close to Marriotsville Road, but fortunately it soon turns away toward the river. When you come to a bulletin board and trail split, take a left; you'll pass the other side of the Tall Poplar Trail at 3.1 miles. At 3.2 miles, at a big bamboo grove where mallards congregate, the trail splits again; stay on the white-blazed trail (to the right) up the hill, giving you a great view of the river. You'll come to a paved park road at 3.4 miles, and you'll see a restroom on the right.

Cross the park road and pick up the white-blazed trail again; just 0.1 mile later, down the hill, you'll see a sign for the orange-blazed McKeldin Rapids Trail. According to the Maryland Department of Natural Resources, "The trail's name hints at its destination . . . a cascading rapid on the Patapsco River that flows into a large, deep pool of water." True enough—it's a beautiful spot. Though swimming is prohibited due to strong undercurrents, fishing is very popular, and the park service stocks the river each spring and fall with adult rainbow and brown trout. Smallmouth and largemouth bass, bluegill, redbreast sunfish, and rock bass reproduce in the river.

Turning to the left away from the rapids, you'll cross great rock formations. At one point, the trail itself is a huge rock slab. Be aware that these exposed rocks are favored spots for snakes, including the copperhead, one of only two venomous snakes in Maryland. If you see a snake and it has an hourglass-shaped head, give it wide berth.

At 3.8 miles, you'll reconnect with Switchback Trail, and you'll be standing at a point of interest: while the hike began in Baltimore County, it moved into Carroll County at the first river crossing at Liberty Dam and is now right across the river from Howard County. This is the only place in Patapsco Valley State Park where the three counties converge, the confluence of the north and south branches of the Patapsco River.

Go left at the split and follow the river. When you reach the red-blazed Plantation Trail, take it as it heads gradually up the hill into upland forest. (You could have continued to hug the river on the white-blazed trail. Both options will eventually take you to the same place, but taking the red varies the scenery.) The forest here is primarily oak, but you'll also see tulip poplar, beech, dogwood, maple, sassafras, redbud, and sycamore. Many wildflowers also abound here including lady's slipper, jack-in-the-pulpit, mayapple, bloodroot, mountain laurel, goldenrod, black-eyed Susan, and Indian pipe.

When you reach the top of the hill and a cleared area, you'll see the southern edge of the pine plantation; hawks like to congregate on this tree line. Head left toward the paved park roads, past a basketball court on the left and restrooms on the right. Cross the park road and pick up the purple-blazed Tall Poplar Trail at 4.8 miles. When you see a chalet-style shelter straight ahead and the trail goes in two directions, head right. At another split at 4.9 miles, continue right.

You will see holly trees on the left and the tollgate and contact station on the right, and you'll reach the paved park entrance road at about 5 miles. (You've now completed the outermost loop of the McKeldin Area, but if you still want more, there's a 0.7-mile blue-blazed Spring Glen Trail loop to the left.) This time, follow the entrance road straight across Marriotsville Road and pick up the fire road; follow it down the hill along the power line cut to where you were earlier. (If you hear gunshots, you might feel unnerved, but don't fear; the shots are coming from a nearby firing range.) At 6.1 miles, take a right toward Marriotsville Road and you'll see a river crossing in the shadow of the bridge. Cross the river and head left; your car will be just ahead.

NEARBY ACTIVITIES

You can enjoy more great hiking (as well as fishing) at nearby at Liberty Reservoir, just to the north; please see pages 190 and 195.

30 PATAPSCO VALLEY STATE PARK: PICKALL AND HOLLOFIELD AREA

KEY AT-A-GLANCE INFORMATION

LENGTH: 7.9 miles

CONFIGURATION: Out-and-back with loops

DIFFICULTY: Moderate–strenuous

SCENERY: Piedmont forest, Patapsco River

EXPOSURE: Mostly shaded

TRAFFIC: Light–moderate

TRAIL SURFACE: Packed dirt

HIKING TIME: 3 hours

ACCESS: 10 a.m.–sunset; year-round

MAPS: USGS Ellicott City; maps of the entire PVSP trail system can be purchased at the park headquarters (see Directions) or online at www .easycart.net/MarylandDepart mentofNaturalResources/Central_ Maryland_Trail_Guides.html.

WHEELCHAIR ACCESS: No

FACILITIES: Bathrooms, playgrounds, water, vending machines in Pickall picnic area

SPECIAL COMMENTS: If you don't want to do the whole hike, you can loop down to the water and back by parking in a different spot (see Description for details).

GPS Trailhead Coordinates

UTM Zone (WGS84) 18S

Easting 345387

Northing 4353294

Latitude N39° 18.914666'

Longitude W76° 47.608016'

IN BRIEF

River valleys and deep forest, with a sprinkling of historic structures. This is a prototypical Patapsco Valley hike.

DESCRIPTION

From the parking area, walk down Hollofield Road toward the river and steel bridge. (On the other side, in Howard County, is the former site of Ellicott's Upper Mills [1775], where the Ellicotts lived in Fountaindale, the family manse.) But stay on the Baltimore County side and head toward the Pickall Area entrance.

Walk up the paved park road, above a little stream to the left, and at 0.4 miles cross over I-70. Pass a power-line cut and swing up to the left. When you get to the parking area on the right and pavilion #702, take a right and pick up the footpath in the woods to the right of the pavilion. The footpath arcs around the picnic and playground areas, winding through a forest of oak, pine, poplar, and dogwood. A footbridge gives way to a mowed section of field rising between the woods. Approach I-70 again at 1.3 miles, but take a right at the power-line cut before you reach the interstate. In about 500 feet, you'll be at the park boundary, so take a right back into the woods on the very narrow foot trail. White-tailed deer populate the area, feasting on backyard gardens at night.

Directions

Take I-695 to Exit 17, Security Blvd west. Take Security past the mall and follow signs to Johnnycake Road. Follow Johnnycake to the river and take a right onto Hollofield Road. Take a left onto Dogwood Road and then an immediate left to the parking area off Alberton Road.

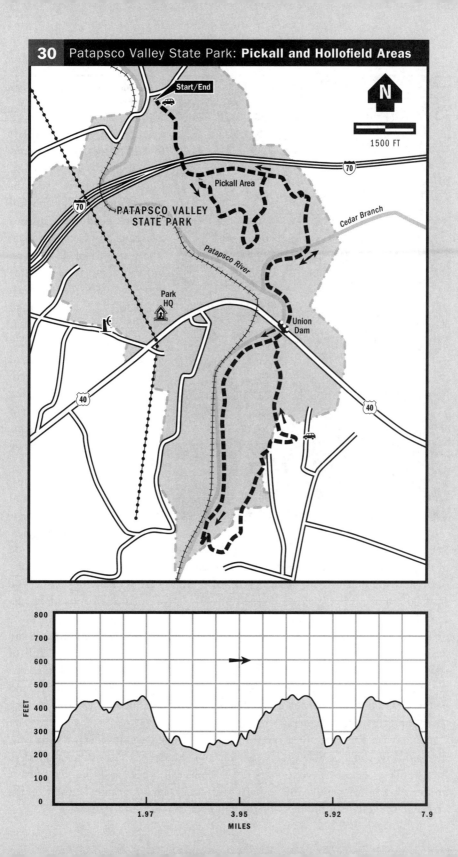

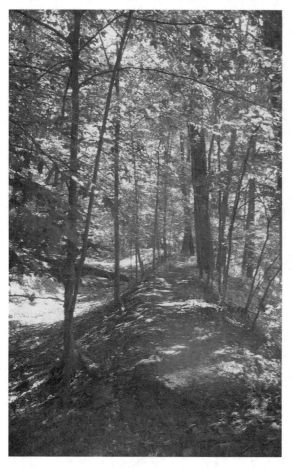

Retaining dam for a water diversion channel

As the trail heads left toward houses, go right onto the barely discernible path. Make your way straight toward the crest of the hill and then head down toward a stream, the Cedar Branch. The trail sort of disappears, but the going is easy. Once you've crossed Cedar Branch at 2.1 miles, a wide fire road runs parallel to the water. You'll see a few sporadic blue blazes. Follow the fire road until it eventually narrows to a foot trail. At 2.6 miles, the Cedar Branch empties into the Patapsco River; at this point, take a left, heading downstream.

Here, the trail is initially very narrow and lightly used, running over rocks and fallen trees. Follow it to the MD 40 bridge and go under, picking up the trail on the other side of the bridge at the remains of the Union Dam, at 2.8 miles. Here now is one of my favorite places in all of Patapsco Valley State Park. For the next mile, the trail (look for a raised section marked initially by wooden slats) runs along the top of an old retaining dam for a water-diversion channel, created for a now-defunct mill downstream. It's a lovely section of trail, with the channel to the left, framed by sloping hills rising above. To the right is the Patapsco, full of rapids in this section. The combination is fantastic. This is also a great place to see the varied river birds, such as great blue and little green herons, killdeer, and belted kingfishers, plus a multitude of geese and ducks making their nests among the sycamores and box elders.

This raised section of trail continues for 1.1 miles, and it's lovely all the way. Occasionally, you'll be able to see stones from the dam where the dirt has eroded. At 3.8 miles, come to a section where the dam wall breaks and then heads back up the other side. Roughly 500 feet after this break, look for and take the wooden bridge to the left—continuing straight will take you out of the park.

This new path is fairly wild, full of broadleaf plants and surrounded by much undergrowth, such as dogwood, mountain laurel, witch hazel, redbud, serviceberry, and spicebush. There are soaring trees as well—oak, hickory, beech, and poplar mostly. You'll see many rightward cuts, but continue on the main path uphill. At the split at 4.7 miles, continue uphill to the right. You'll eventually see a small old stone wall topping the ridge to the right. Cross the wall and you'll come to a wide trail on the left. This is actually Rock Haven Avenue, a road no longer used for vehicle traffic and in the process of being successfully reclaimed by the forest floor. Follow Rock Haven until you see the incongruous 25 MPH speed-limit sign at 5.3 miles. Look for the dirt path heading downhill to the left; if you miss it, you'll soon come to the little parking area on St. Johnsbury Road (see Directions below).

Taking this trail down the hill, you'll reach the river after some dicey progress down the rocky and eroded hill. When you reach the river and Union Dam, head right to backtrack to your car. Only one change on the return route: when you get to the area where the Cedar Branch empties into the Patapsco, stay on the fire road all the way until you reach the power-line cut near I-70. Go left and follow the cut until you reach the portion of the trail where you already were just before crossing over the highway. (This eliminates 0.4 miles—you've earned the shortcut after this difficult but rewarding hike.)

Note: If you only have time for a short hike and/or you just wanted to concentrate on the nicest part of the hike described here (in the Hollofield Area), you can make a nice loop down to the water and back by parking at the following location: Take I-695 to Exit 13, Frederick Road, toward Catonsville. Go 3 miles and turn right onto Oella Avenue. Go 0.7 miles to a right on Westchester Avenue. Go 0.8 miles to a left on St. Johnsbury Road. Park at the end of St. Johnsbury before it hits Rock Haven Avenue. From here, follow the hike as described previously.

NEARBY ACTIVITIES

There's a beautiful public golf course, Diamond Ridge, just a couple of miles from the parking area at Johnnycake and Alberton roads. Go north on Hollofield Road (upriver) and take the first right on Dogwood Road. Take a left on Ridge Road and then the first right into Western Area Park. For more information, call (410) 887-1349 or visit **www2.cybergolf.com/sites/courses/view**. From the parking area at St. Johnsbury Road and Rock Haven Avenue, it's a quick and easy trip to the Benjamin Banneker Historical Park and Museum (see page 14 for a hike here). Follow St. Johnsbury 0.8 miles, then turn right onto Westchester Avenue. Go 0.7 miles and turn left onto Oella Avenue. Look for the park on the right, just before Frederick Road.

31 PRETTYBOY RESERVOIR: CCC TRAIL

IN BRIEF

Enjoy a solitary stroll through a pine forest on an old fire road. The out loop will tease you with water views, and the return loop will lead you to the water's edge.

DESCRIPTION

Beginning at the trailhead, you'll enter the forest on a very wide path, cut by the Civilian Conservation Corps (CCC), the Depression-era jobs program. The dirt and gravel trail here has two clearly discernible tire tracks with higher grass in the middle. Deep woods flank the trail, but the width of the path gives you open walking space.

You'll pass through areas with very tall pines and dense underbrush on either side of the trail. Even though you've just left the road, you probably won't hear any traffic at all; this section of Baltimore County is still very rural. At 0.2 miles, the woods open up a bit, exposing the trail even more. You'll begin to see cuts and side trails on the left and right, but stay straight for now; you'll take one of the cuts on the return trip. At 0.3 miles, an interesting phenomenon occurs that's easy to miss. On the right, the forest is almost entirely pine, but on the left, oaks, hickories, and maples dominate with very few pines at all.

GPS Trailhead Coordinates

UTM Zone (WGS84) 18S

Easting 351076

Northing 4387054

Latitude N 39° 37.218118'

Longitude W 76° 44.102519'

Directions

Take I-83 to Exit 27, Mt. Carmel Road west. Go 3.6 miles and take a right on Prettyboy Dam Road. Go 1 mile and take a left onto Tracey's Store Road. Go 1.1 miles where the road turns sharply to the left; you'll see a small parking area on the right where the road bends. Wooden posts strung with an orange cable mark the trailhead.

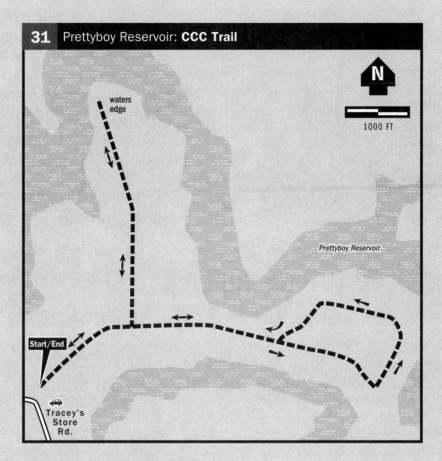

31 Prettyboy Reservoir: **CCC Trail**

waters edge

N

1000 FT

Prettyboy Reservoir

Start/End

Tracey's Store Rd.

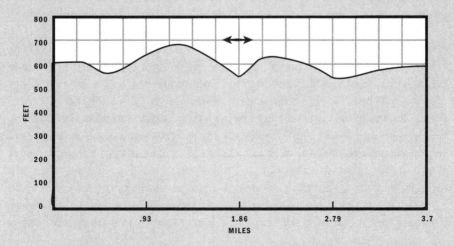

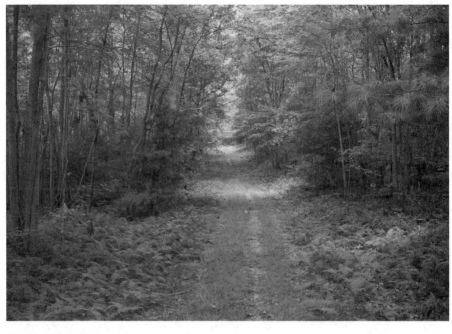

Reservoir fire road

Though it almost defeats the purpose of a hike to keep your eyes on the ground, if you're hiking the CCC Trail in summer, you may want to keep a lookout for a legion of tiny frogs congregating in the grooves of the path. On hikes here in July and early August, I scattered thousands of tiny frogs, and I had to go slowly to avoid crushing dozens at a time. They are especially prominent in areas when the trail is exposed, such as the section between 0.4 and 0.6 miles.

Beyond this point, oaks and hickories overtake the previously dominant pines, and while this results in something of a barren view in the winter, the payoff comes in autumn when the trees explode in vibrant colors. You'll begin to see the reservoir through the woods on the left, even though the water is pretty far away and it's difficult to get a good view.

By 0.6 miles, the tire tracks fade away, but the trail remains wide. The loop begins here; you can go in either direction since you'll come back to this same spot regardless. When I walked this part of the trail, a young white-tailed deer was eyeing me warily off to the left, so I decided to head right. In that direction, the trail rises gradually, and a hill drops off to the right. At just under 1 mile, the trail splits; you want to head left to complete the loop. The reservoir is down below you to the right, but it's something of a tease here as you'll never get a great view through the woods; you can head toward the water on the return trip.

The grass grows much higher here on the path, signaling a lack of use. Continue heading around the loop; you'll complete it by rejoining the trail at

1.4 miles. Walk another half a mile, and then take the wide trail to the right. The scenery is essentially the same as the trail you've been on, but this time you'll reach the water's edge after 0.6 miles. This area won't afford any sweeping views of the reservoir, but it's a nice little spot where you can dip your toes into the water. You might see someone fishing here. When you've had your fill, head back and turn right on the main trail to walk back to your car.

NEARBY ACTIVITIES

You can sample Maryland wines and tour the facilities where they're made at two area wineries. You can reach Basignani Winery at 15722 Falls Road in Sparks by taking Exit 20B off I-83; (410) 472-0703 or **www.basignani.com** for more information. Take Exit 27 off I-83 to reach Woodhall Winery at 17912 York Road in Parkton; (410) 357-8644 or **www.woodhallwinecellars.com** for more information. If you want to do more hiking, opportunities abound at Prettyboy Reservoir (see pages 156–167).

32 PRETTYBOY RESERVOIR: GUNPOWDER RIVER

(i) KEY AT-A-GLANCE INFORMATION

LENGTH: 3.8 miles

CONFIGURATION: Loop

DIFFICULTY: Easy with short moderate–strenuous section

SCENERY: Big Gunpowder River, hemlock groves

EXPOSURE: Mostly shaded

TRAFFIC: Light

TRAIL SURFACE: Packed dirt

HIKING TIME: 1.5 hours

ACCESS: Dawn–dusk

MAPS: USGS Lineboro

WHEELCHAIR ACCESS: No

FACILITIES: None

SPECIAL COMMENTS: Despite its location in the Prettyboy Reservoir watershed, this hike doesn't come into view of the reservoir itself, but rather circles where the Big Gunpowder River begins to enter the northwestern edge of Prettyboy.

IN BRIEF

Feel the temperature drop as you descend from wooded hills to the swift Big Gunpowder River, scrambling through an untamed and isolated section along the way.

DESCRIPTION

Entering the woods, you'll very quickly be in a thick vegetation of oak, pine, black walnut, chestnut, flowering dogwood, maple and poplar above, with several varieties of ferns, raspberry bushes, and honeysuckle below. Resultantly, cardinals, jays, thrushes, woodpeckers, warblers, and vireos avail themselves of this great habitat.

The trail is a very wide fire road, which is good because of the profusion of trailside poison ivy. You'll see a cut to the right at 0.4 miles, but pass it as well as several more cuts to the right coming soon after. These lead to the Big Gunpowder River, where you're headed on a more scenic route. The fire road narrows a bit to a foot trail for about two-tenths of a mile and then widens again along the edge of the watershed boundary—to the left, over a buffer of trees, is a farm field. Mountain

GPS Trailhead Coordinates

UTM Zone (WGS84) 18S

Easting 347529

Northing 4394504

Latitude N 39° 41.206334'

Longitude W 76° 46.683991'

Directions

Take I-83 to exit 31, Middletown road west. Go 4.6 miles to Beckleysville Road and take a left. At 0.2 miles, the road bears left. Stay straight. The road becomes Cotter Road. Cotter turns into Clipper Mill Road at 1.9 miles at a stop sign. Go straight and cross Prettyboy Reservoir on a white bridge. Go 0.4 miles and take a right on Gunpowder Road. After 0.5 miles, pass the Hoffman Cemetery and park at the bottom of the hill to the right. Walk across the road and find the trailhead leading into the woods beyond an orange cable.

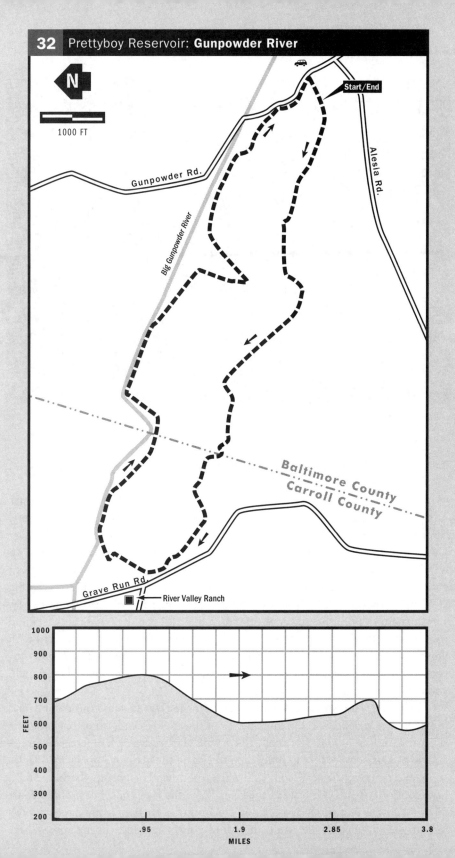

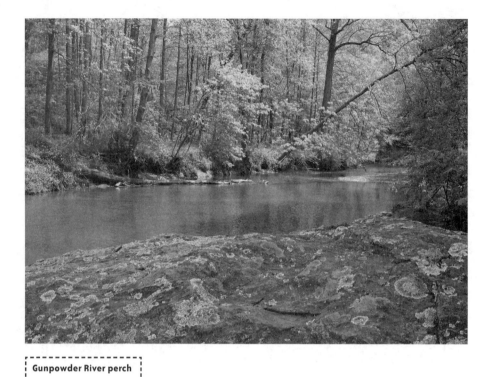

Gunpowder River perch

laurel and blackberry can soon be seen; if it's summer and you didn't fill up on the raspberries earlier, the blackberries are a special treat.

There's a Y at 1.25 miles; continue left. The trail narrows and becomes increasingly rocky as you leave Baltimore County and enter Carroll County. Approach Grave Run Road at 1.6 miles. Just to the right is the entrance to River Valley Ranch, a resort and Christian youth camp founded in 1952 by two Irish immigrants. When you reach the road, turn around and you'll see a different path heading into the woods about ten feet from the one you just left—the Big Gunpowder River will be below you to the left. The river is narrow and twisty, carving banks out of the meadow. Similarly, the trail you're now on is twisty and narrow as well; unlike the fire road coming in, however, this one is spotted with horse manure from the nearby ranch. To the right, moss-covered rock outcroppings dot the hillside. If you look through the trees to the left toward the ranch, you might catch a glimpse of the resident bison.

Below you and about 200 feet to the left, the river widens considerably and provides a nice loud accompaniment. Continue to descend, soon reaching the river and joining a wide fire road, filled with the aroma of hay-scented fern. A jumble of moss-covered rocks and fallen trees give the area an Appalachian feel.

At 2.1 miles, the trail splits. The fire road heads right up the hill, and a little foot trail heads left toward the river. Take the foot trail, but prepare yourself first by pulling up your socks or cinching the cuffs of your pants: there's lots of vegetation over the trail, including poison ivy and thorny rose. There is a reward for the coming work, however: utter isolation comes almost immediately, embodied by a massive rock in the river—a great place to stop and contemplate.

Soon, it looks as if the trail disappears. You have to cross over a little island to the right—there's a tree trunk to help you along. Be aware of nesting Canada geese; it's easy to sneak up on them and get startled by their fleeing—or become a victim of their maternal aggressiveness. Many mallards also make homes here. Make your way along the hillside through the brush along big rocks and wildflowers, mostly wild geranium and jewelweed, or "touch-me-not," the name derived from the popping noise that comes when you touch the plant's mature seed pods. As long as you stay near the river, the trail will reappear, as it never strays too far from the water. The river alternates between roiling over rocks and then settling into deep flat pools. It's very cool in the river valley with an obvious temperature drop after coming off the hill.

Don't be discouraged by all this work during the first quarter-mile, as the trail soon opens up and becomes much more obvious. By 2.4 miles, the trail widens to rejoin the old fire road. You'll still have everything you had before in terms of scenery, just an easier passage now.

Leave the river valley at 2.6 miles and ascend the hill. To the left, you'll begin to see big beautiful hemlocks shading the river. By 2.7 miles, at the top of the hill, there's a trail split. Continue straight, crossing over a stream and then hitting another intersection. Take a left, heading back down in the direction of the river. Pass the stream to the left, crowded with hemlock. By 3.3 miles, the Big Gunpowder River comes back into view through those hemlocks. Descend once again to river level, where things open up. Reach Gunpowder Road at 3.6 miles. Cross and walk along the wide grassy shoulder to the right.

Before you go too far, look to the left. Over the bridge is another parking area. If you want to add a quick but memorable hike, head there for the Hemlock Trail—see Nearby Activities and page 164. Otherwise, continue up Gunpowder Road and reach your car at 3.8 miles.

NEARBY ACTIVITIES

Hike through a hemlock gorge to a spectacular swimming spot on the Hemlock Trail—see page 164. Sample Maryland wines and tour the facilities where they're made at two area wineries. You can reach Basignani Winery at 15722 Falls Road in Sparks by taking Exit 20B off I-83; (410) 472-0703 or **www.basignani.com** for more information. Take Exit 27 off I-83 to reach Woodhall Winery at 17912 York Road in Parkton; (410) 357-8644 or **www.woodhallwinecellars.com** for more information.

33 PRETTYBOY RESERVOIR: HEMLOCK TRAIL

KEY AT-A-GLANCE INFORMATION

LENGTH: 1.25 miles

CONFIGURATION: Approximate out-and-back (see Special Comments)

DIFFICULTY: Moderate to strenuous

SCENERY: Hemlocks, Gunpowder River, swimming hole, rock outcroppings

EXPOSURE: Mostly shaded

TRAFFIC: Light

TRAIL SURFACE: Packed dirt

HIKING TIME: 1 hour (longer with swim)

ACCESS: Dawn–dusk

MAPS: USGS Lineboro

WHEELCHAIR ACCESS: No

FACILITIES: None

SPECIAL COMMENTS: It's difficult to follow precisely the same path out and back. At some points, there seems to be no trail at all, but passage is guaranteed by the open forest floor.

GPS Trailhead Coordinates

UTM Zone (WGS84) 18S

Easting 347285

Northing 4394869

Latitude N 39° 41.400948'

Longitude W 76° 46.859715'

IN BRIEF

Get a taste of Appalachia within a grove of centuries-old hemlocks. After a hike that can be strenuous at times, cool off with a refreshing dip in the icy Gunpowder River.

DESCRIPTION

The trail goes downhill toward the water and almost immediately, you will see the graffiti-covered underside of the bridge you just crossed in your car. When you see this, head left on the little dirt path following the river downstream. The trail is packed dirt and can be very close and narrow, especially in summer. Hike up the socks if you don't want poison ivy. The river to the right is swift and loud ,and occasionally you'll see it through the thick underbrush. Over the river as well as up the hill to your left, you'll see tall trees, but this part of the path is pretty exposed.

Directions ⟶

Take I-83 to exit 31, Middletown road west. Go 4.6 miles to Beckleysville Road and take a left. At 0.2 miles, the road bears left. Stay straight. The road becomes Cotter Road. Cotter turns into Clipper Mill Road at 1.9 miles at a stop sign. Go straight and cross Prettyboy Reservoir on a white bridge. Go 0.4 miles and take a right on Gunpowder Road. After 0.7 miles, you'll come to a bridge. Park on the shoulder on the left as soon as you cross the bridge. Once you've parked, you'll see a guardrail on the other side of the road 100 feet or so from the bridge. There's a sign telling you not to swim, wade, camp, etc. The trail begins just behind that sign. (Be aware: there's another, wider path to the left strung with an orange cable. Though a nice little walk, it does not lead to the one described here.)

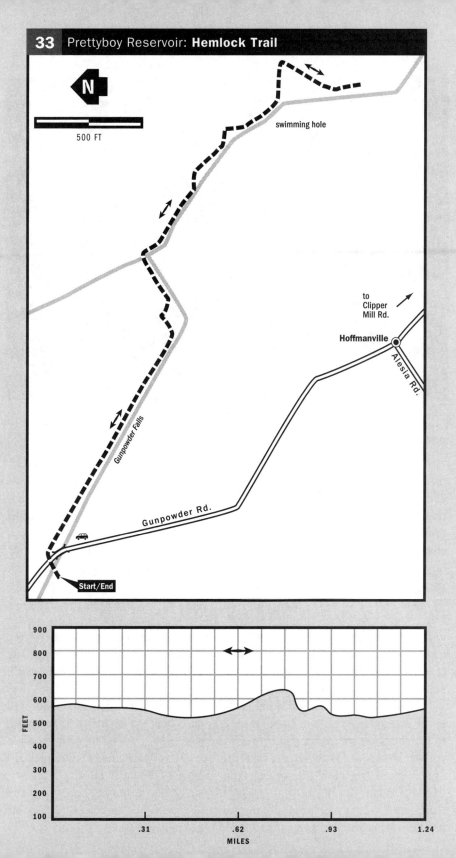

N

500 FT

swimming hole

to
Clipper
Mill Rd.

Hoffmanville

Alesia Rd.

Gunpowder Falls

Gunpowder Rd.

Start/End

900
800
700
600
500
400
300
200
100

FEET

.31   .62   .93   1.24
MILES

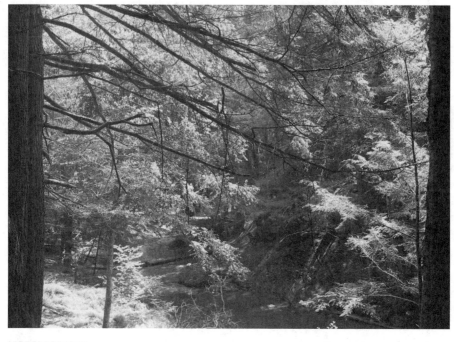

Hemlock shade

At 0.1 mile, the trail opens up a bit, and soon you'll begin to see some beautiful rock formations on the hill to the left. The trail becomes rocky, and moss abounds. The still well-defined trail heads right to the river at 0.2 miles, but then heads away from the river soon after, going up the hill. At a quarter-mile, cross over a stream. A large fallen tree spans the stream to help you along. You'll emerge into a hemlock forest as these beautiful old trees begin to completely dominate the landscape. It's a beautiful spot, but now things begin to get a bit tricky.

The trail becomes very hard to follow. Because of the nature of these thick trees, they crowd out sunlight and little to no underbrush grows. This creates wide alleys between the trees that can look very much like a trail. Due to the trail's inexplicable underuse, you can find yourself at a loss as to exactly where to go. That said, so long as you keep the river within view on your right, you'll be fine. In fact, this confusion is half the fun.

When it seems that you should head to the water, the path gets swallowed up by an eroded bank or a stand of vegetation. Then you decide to head uphill, to clamber over the rocks and through the hemlocks. Depending on how often you decide upon this route, the hike can become very strenuous very quickly. I only had one free hand (the other taken up by my GPS unit) and the going was very difficult at times; this is not to say it wasn't a blast, though. Every now and then, you'll find a nice level middle ground between hill and river. Here, pine needles carpet the soft soil. In this middle ground, you'll have the swift, clean river to your right and lots of rock outcroppings covered in moss to the left, all the while traversing the many hemlocks all around you. All this zigzagging will take you to the hike's end point all the same.

That end point appears at half a mile. You'll come to a deep pool and swimming area surrounded by big rocks. It's the perfect destination on a hot summer day. Beware—because of the swiftness of the river, the water is downright icy and is only for the brave or numb. The trail essentially ends after another couple of hundred feet in a tangle of vegetation and underbrush.

NEARBY ACTIVITIES

Sample Maryland wines and tour the facilities where they're made at two area wineries. You can reach Basignani Winery at 15722 Falls Road in Sparks by taking Exit 20B off I-83; (410) 472-0703 or **www.basignani.com** for more information. Take Exit 27 off I-83 to reach Woodhall Winery at 17912 York Road in Parkton; (410) 357-8644 or **www.woodhallwinecellars.com** for more information. If more hiking is your goal, an easy trek is just beyond the orange cable you passed when you first came in. It heads up through the woods and leads to the Hoffman family cemetery. The Hoffmans owned a paper mill used for making the first paper currency in the United States. Many of the headstones date to the 1700s.

34 ROBERT E. LEE PARK: LAKE ROLAND

 KEY AT-A-GLANCE INFORMATION

LENGTH: 5.6 miles

CONFIGURATION: Out-and-back with a loop

DIFFICULTY: Moderate

SCENERY: Jones Falls, Lake Roland, upland forest

EXPOSURE: Mostly shade

TRAFFIC: Light–moderate on the trail; moderate–heavy at the lake

TRAIL SURFACE: Packed dirt, short stretch of asphalt

HIKING TIME: 2–2.5 hours

ACCESS: Dawn–dusk; you can reach the park from the Falls Road Light Rail stop and walking east on Copper Hill Road; this will take you to Lake Roland.

MAPS: USGS Cockeysville

WHEELCHAIR ACCESS: No

FACILITIES: Water fountain at the lake

SPECIAL COMMENTS: The bridge in front of Lake Roland Dam was closed for repairs in July 2008, with the reopen date unclear. For alternate route, see Description. If you are afraid of dogs, be aware that the section of Robert E. Lee Park near Lake Roland just over the light rail tracks is a favorite for dog owners who blatantly disregard leash laws.

- -

GPS Trailhead
Coordinates
UTM Zone (WGS84) 18S
Easting 356778
Northing 4362073
Latitude N 39° 23.776639'
Longitude W 76° 39.795792'

IN BRIEF

Follow an old rail bed along the Jones Falls to Lake Roland and back.

DESCRIPTION

Climb over the guardrail and head right. Unless there are drought conditions, it's more than likely this beginning section will be full of mud. If it's really bad, a parallel trail heads uphill to the left and eventually rejoins the trail in approximately a quarter-mile when it rises above the low-lying area.

Once above the floodplain, the trail runs along the rail bed of the now-defunct Baltimore and Susquehanna Railroad. You will parallel the Jones Falls downriver on the right, and on the left you'll see rock outcroppings with clinging tree roots. At 0.3 miles, you'll notice the first of many old railroad ties still in the trail. Oak and maple trees dominate this section, offering wonderful, colorful foliage in autumn and abundant shade on hot days. At 0.4 miles, you'll come to a big dip in the trail. The bog on the left provides home to a multitude of bullfrogs. Pass by the cut paths heading up the hill on the left, as they lead to private land.

At just under 0.7 miles, the trail rises above a precipitous drop on the right; lots of hanging grapevines weigh down some of the smaller trees below. Just beyond you'll see an

- -

Directions ⟶

Take I-695 to Exit 23, Falls Road. Follow to the first light at Joppa Road and make a left back onto Falls heading south. Cross Old Court Road and go another 0.3 miles. Park on the left shoulder where the road sweeps to the right. The trail starts just beyond the guardrail.

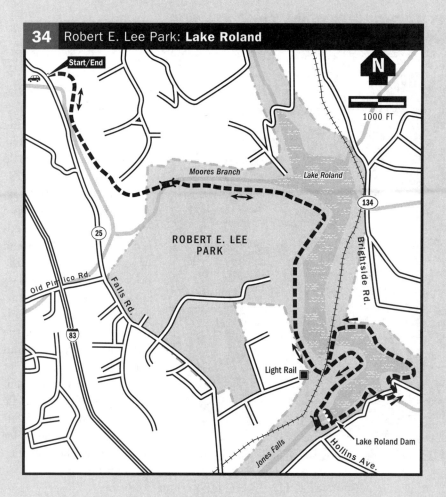

34 Robert E. Lee Park: **Lake Roland**

Start/End

N

1000 FT

Moores Branch

Lake Roland

134

ROBERT E. LEE
PARK

25

Old Pimlico Rd.

Falls Rd.

83

Brightside Rd.

Light Rail

Jones Falls

Hollins Ave.

Lake Roland Dam

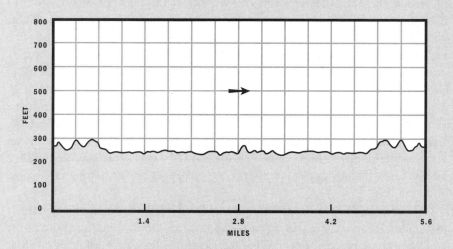

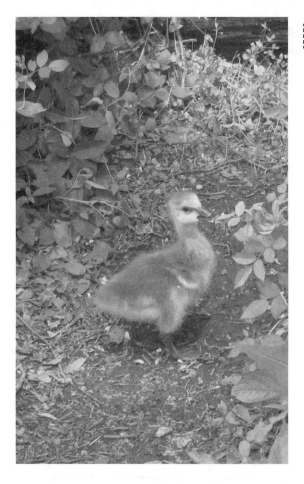

old steel bridge over the stream. This is a favorite spot for dog owners; expect to see a few frolicking canines in the water. The path on the left runs a little more than a mile along the edge of Lake Roland and follows Roland Run before it dead-ends in a residential neighborhood. Instead of taking that, cross the bridge and you'll soon pass some man-made berms built by bikers. At the railroad ties, you can see the indentations from the rail bed heading straight, but as a hiking path, it eventually gets lost in a tangle of vegetation; so head left instead, keeping the water on your left. The trail runs through tall, mature oaks. You will see periodic white blazes here, but nothing consistent.

Soon, you'll see well-worn paths going down the big gullies on the right; bikers use these. In addition, you will see lots of little cut paths spread out in both directions; bikers also use these single-track paths. Keep going straight; you'll have no problem recognizing the main trail—it's wide and well-trod. The biggest problem you'll encounter along the trail is mud puddles, made worse by erosion-causing mountain bikes (I'm guilty of contributing to this myself, so I shouldn't complain).

At 1.2 miles, the Jones Falls comes into better view through tall thin trees. Here, it empties into Lake Roland. Check out the path down to the water; the river runs nice and clean here. Go back up and rejoin the trail, which heads up and down a bit before opening to a clearing at the edge of the lake. You will see a bird feeder sticking out of the marshy area; keep an eye out for ducks, herons, and even ibis.

The trail suddenly drops downhill and rejoins the rail bed on the left. At just under 1.5 miles you will come to my favorite spot to look for those birds; you'll see some railroad ties heading left down to the water—you can go sit at

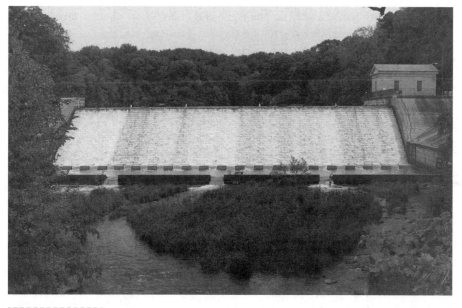

Lake Roland Dam

the lake's edge and watch the birds, turtles, and snakes (and though less romantic, I've seen nutria here, too). Invariably, you'll also see a light rail train gliding by on the tracks on the other side of the lake.

Back on the trail, you'll soon see the defunct railroad tracks, now covered with plants; you will follow them for a while. You can either stay on this wide path or take the smaller one that parallels it about ten feet to the left, closer to the water. Either way, the two trails connect at 2.1 miles.

At this point, you'll come to the light rail tracks. Of course, use caution when crossing, even though this section sits in the middle of a long straightaway, making it impossible for a train to surprise you.

Once you cross the tracks, head uphill. This portion of the trail is badly eroded, and you'll have to clamber over some roots and rocks, but you'll see daylight ahead to the right. Once you reach the top of the hill, you'll see a pavilion and picnic tables. Now you're on a cracked asphalt path; take a left and follow it around the water. Although this is a nice spot to sit waterside and contemplate the lake, I recommend that you keep moving—your chances for solitude here are next to none. It's nearly impossible to escape this section of the park without hearing the screeching tussle of a couple of canines that have been allowed to roam free (see Special Comments). So head around on the asphalt path—you'll have the opportunity for good views and solitude on the other side of the lake. Pass the caretaker's house on the left and head down the very steep hill toward the bridge; you will see Lake Roland dam on the left, at 2.5 miles. The Jones Falls behind you rolls toward the Inner Harbor. As indicated in Special Comments, the bridge may be closed. You can head down a little footpath to the water on the right and cross where there are rocks; wet feet are a possibility, however.

Once across, take the road to the left; you'll see a lovely spot to sit next to the marble building that reads LAKE ROLAND 1861, a reminder of the lake's prior use as a city reservoir. Fishermen frequent the pier on the left of the little cul-de-sac. Take the dirt path at the end of the cul-de-sac and head uphill over the rocky path. At the top of the hill, where there's asphalt again, take a left onto the wide dirt path and head uphill again. As the path turns right, you'll have a glorious view of the lake. Usually, the underbrush is cut down; the view is spectacular and offers wonder in all seasons—spring blooms, summer green, fall foliage, and winter barrenness.

From the overlook, head right about 50 feet or so, and then left down the hill, picking your way through the little trail. When you get to the water's edge, follow it on your left until you cross a little feeder stream. Rain levels will determine how messy this will be, but it shouldn't ever be difficult.

The trail becomes wide on the other side. Follow it to a rock grotto at 3.2 miles, another great lookout point over the lake. Continue on toward the Light Rail tracks. Tread quietly here—invariably you'll see many turtles sunning themselves on half-submerged tree branches. Reach the Light Rail tracks at 3.5. There is a little path to walk to the left of the tracks; this will keep you clear of any trains. In a tenth of a mile, you'll reach the trail you used before. Take a right and backtrack to your car, reaching it at 5.6 miles.

NEARBY ACTIVITIES

You might be interested in visiting two nearby sites that have great historical significance. You can walk from the trailhead to Rockland Historic District, listed on the National Register of Historic Places, at the corner of Falls Road (north of the trailhead), Ruxton Road (to the east), and Old Court Road (to the west). The buildings in Rockland, Baltimore County's first permanent settlement dating back to 1706, remain and have been lovingly maintained, while the mill now houses businesses and shops. From Rockland, you will have a short drive to the Colored Methodist Protestant St. Johns' Chapel of Baltimore County. Built for free blacks in 1833, it has held services continually since 1886. To get there, head north on Falls Road and take the first right onto Ruxton Road; when it ends at a stop sign, go right onto Bellona Avenue, and you will see the church 0.3 miles ahead on the right.

ROBERT E. LEE PARK: SERPENTINE-BARE HILLS

IN BRIEF

Follow an old rail bed along the Jones Falls to an upland forest containing rare serpentine landscape.

DESCRIPTION

The first 0.75 miles of this hike follows the same route as the previous hike in this book, Robert E. Lee Park: Lake Roland. For a more specific description of the beginning of this hike, see that hike profile. For now, climb the guardrail and follow the trail 0.75 miles to the steel bridge spanning the Jones Falls.

Cross the bridge and look for two path offshoots—both to the right, one leading downhill and one leading uphill; pass both of these and take the next path you see to the right, which is easy to spot. This trail is very rocky and rooty; you'll see a blue blaze or two, but these will die out. At just over 0.8 miles, the trail suddenly opens up, and you'll be in an entirely new landscape in an area that's part of Bare Hills. You'll see prairie grass and smell the short, stubby pines as you walk over the rocky topsoil. The sharp rocks you see about you are serpentine, or serpentinite, a mineral that produces extremely nutrient-poor soil. According to the Maryland Geologic Society, serpentine landscapes are "stony, unfertile, and sparsely vegetated—hence the term "serpentine barren." Typically

KEY AT-A-GLANCE INFORMATION

LENGTH: 3.7 miles

CONFIGURATION: Out-and-back with a loop

DIFFICULTY: Easy–moderate

SCENERY: Jones Falls, serpentine ecosystem, upland forest

EXPOSURE: Mostly shade

TRAFFIC: Light–moderate

TRAIL SURFACE: Packed dirt, serpentinite

HIKING TIME: 2 hours

ACCESS: Dawn–dusk

MAPS: USGS Cockeysville

WHEELCHAIR ACCESS: No

FACILITIES: None

SPECIAL COMMENTS: Because of their differing natures, the two Robert E. Lee Park hikes described in this book are treated separately; however, because they share the same trailhead, they can be easily combined for one long hike. See the previous hike in this book for details.

Directions

Take I-695 to Exit 23, Falls Road. Follow to the first light at Joppa Road and make a left back onto Falls. Cross Old Court Road and go another 0.3 miles. Park on the left shoulder where the road sweeps to the right. The trail starts just beyond the guardrail.

GPS Trailhead Coordinates

UTM Zone (WGS84) 18S

Easting 356781

Northing 4362069

Latitude N 39° 23.774507'

Longitude W 76° 39.793646'

35 Robert E. Lee Park: **Serpentine–Bare Hills**

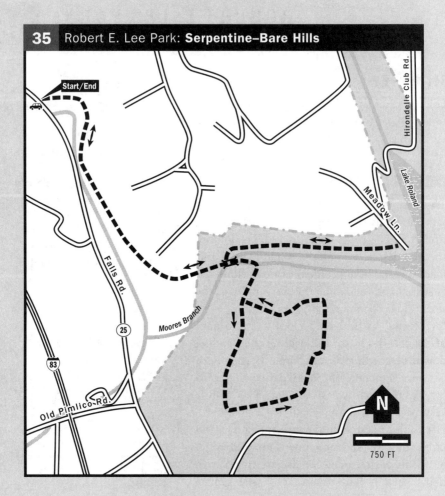

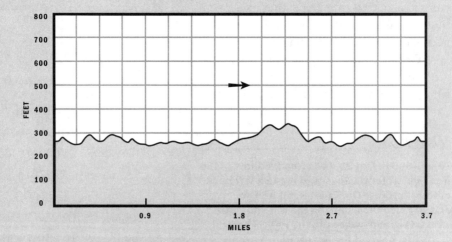

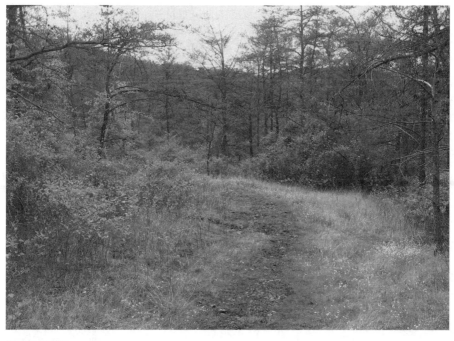

Bare Hills

a serpentine barren contains scrub oak and pine, cedar, grasses, and some unique and rare wildflowers." It also produces chromium, or chromite, the raw ingredient for chrome. This extremely rare ecosystem exists in only a few places in Maryland. (For a heavy dose of serpentine, take the hike at Soldiers Delight Natural Environmental Area, described on page 177. Between Bare Hills and Soldiers Delight, almost all the chrome in the world was mined and produced in the early to mid-19th century.)

The landscape here is a new world from the forest you just left. After turning uphill, follow the trail 500 feet to a clearing. Here, the trail splits; go left. The foliage is dominated by short, stubby pines, crisscrossed by loads of deer trails. There are also many little trail offshoots. Take the main trail, which is recognizable as the widest. It's full of rocks and heads uphill. But do note all these little paths; they offer plenty of opportunities to explore, as they form a spiderweb of trails across the hillside. The hike described here simply follows the main trail, but feel free to veer off and explore.

This is a beautiful place, and one that can be a real revelation to those living in the Baltimore area who have never seen a serpentine landscape before. With its many rocks and minimal vegetation, it looks little like the typical hardwood and piedmont forests of the region. At a little over 1 mile, you'll see the remnants of a pit mine to the left. Don't expect a massive open pit, but rather a filled depression about three feet by three feet across. There's a tiny and very pretty stream that you'll jump over soon after. The rightward path here eventually goes to a private road.

After another couple of hundred feet, where the trail opens onto another clearing, head right up the hill. In spring, this area is dotted with little white wildflowers. At 1.2 miles, the foliage begins to change again, to the more recognizable forests of the area. At the next fork, head left back into woods. There's a trail intersection soon after. Head left. Then, a few hundred feet later, go left again onto a wider trail, near a gorge to the right. This trail meets the main one you used coming in. Take a left to head back to the bridge. (Another trail heads to the left up the hill soon after, so if you want to do more exploring in the serpentine area, take it).

This time, when you cross the bridge, head immediately downhill to the right. This little trail follows the Moores Branch of the Jones Falls for a 1-mile out-and-back, toward where Roland Run enters Lake Roland. Along the way, look for the foundations and existing brick structures of some old ruins to the left, 0.1 mile from the steel bridge. You'll have to leave the trail and head up the hill; there's no established path. Do tread considerately—just up the hill from these structures is a private home.

You will reach the steel bridge on your return at 2.9 miles. Backtrack to your car.

NEARBY ACTIVITIES

See the previous hike in this book, Robert E. Lee Park: Lake Roland (page 168), for two nearby historical sites. If you're hungry, there are great coffee shops and bakeries along Falls Road heading south. Continuing on Falls Road south, you'll come to Mount Washington in just a few miles, containing shops, markets, and one of the nicest business districts anywhere around. Take a right over the Kelly Avenue Bridge to reach Mount Washington.

SOLDIERS DELIGHT NATURAL ENVIRONMENTAL AREA

IN BRIEF

Take a quick trip to a look-alike Midwest prairie, where the serpentine landscape provides a rare environment. Then head to the "other side" of Soldiers Delight—more typical of the mid-Atlantic.

DESCRIPTION:

Many mistakenly assume that the Soldiers Delight Serpentine Trail is thus named because of its shape. In fact, the name refers to the type of soil. Serpentine, or serpentinite, is a mineral that produces extremely nutrient-poor soil, making plant growth a difficult prospect. Exceptions include the serpentine grasslands found in Soldiers Delight. Many of these grasses are not only atypical in Maryland, but are rare all over the planet.

Before European settlement, much of Baltimore County was covered by serpentine grassland, cultivated by Native American fire hunting. Natives used to set extensive fires to drive deer toward the open areas; the fires also had the effect of creating the grasslands that fed the deer. According to the Maryland Department of Natural Resources, even though what serpentine grassland remains in

KEY AT-A-GLANCE INFORMATION

LENGTH: 6.3 miles

CONFIGURATION: 2 jagged intersecting loops

DIFFICULTY: Moderate

SCENERY: Rare prairie, Chimney Branch, abandoned mines

EXPOSURE: Half and half

TRAFFIC: Moderate

TRAIL SURFACE: Packed dirt, serpentine rock

HIKING TIME: 2.5 hours

ACCESS: Sunrise–sunset; Visitor Center open Wednesday–Friday 9 a.m.–4 p.m., Saturday and Sunday 10 a.m.–4 p.m. (info: [410] 922-3044; www.dnr.state.md.us/public lands/central/soldiers.html)

MAPS: USGS Reisterstown, trail maps at bulletin board outside visitor center. Excellent maps can be purchased online www.easycart .net/MarylandDepartmentof NaturalResources/Central Mary land Trail Guides.html.

WHEELCHAIR ACCESS: No

FACILITIES: Restrooms, water, vending machines in visitor center

SPECIAL COMMENTS: Wear sturdy hiking boots or trail shoes— serpentine rock is very sharp.

Directions

Take I-695 to Exit 18, Route 26 west. Go 4.5 miles and take a right on Deer Park Road. The park entrance is 1.9 miles to the left. Park in front of the visitor center. The trailhead parallels the parking lot next to the bulletin board.

Alternate directions: Take I-695 to I-795 west to Owings Mills Blvd. Follow to Owings Mills Center and then pass the mall and turn right on Lyons Mill Road. Take Lyons Mill to a right on Deer Park Road.

GPS Trailhead
Coordinates
UTM Zone (WGS84) 18S
Easting 341930
Northing 4363785
Latitude N 39° 24.546211'
Longitude W 76° 50.161257'

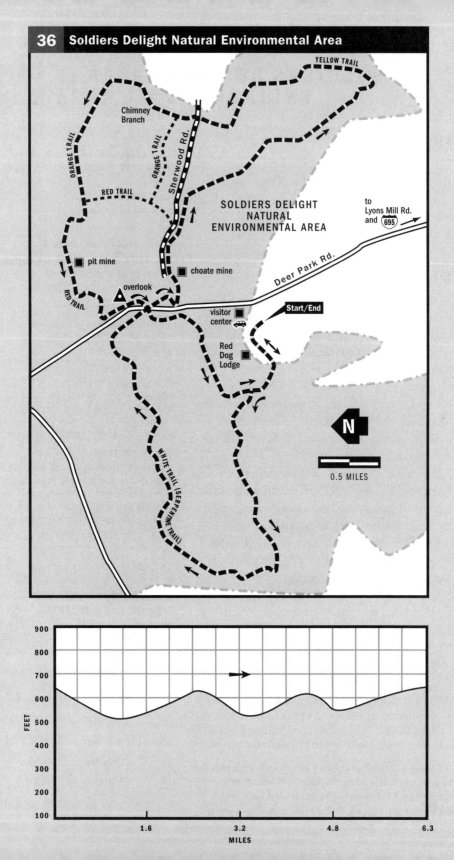

YELLOW TRAIL

ORANGE TRAIL

Chimney Branch

ORANGE TRAIL

Sherwood Rd.

RED TRAIL

SOLDIERS DELIGHT
NATURAL
ENVIRONMENTAL AREA

to
Lyons Mill Rd.
and 695

pit mine

RED TRAIL

choate mine

Deer Park Rd.

overlook

visitor
center

Start/End

Red
Dog
Lodge

N

0.5 MILES

WHITE TRAIL (SERPENTINE TRAIL)

FEET

900
800
700
600
500
400
300
200
100

1.6   3.2   4.8   6.3
MILES

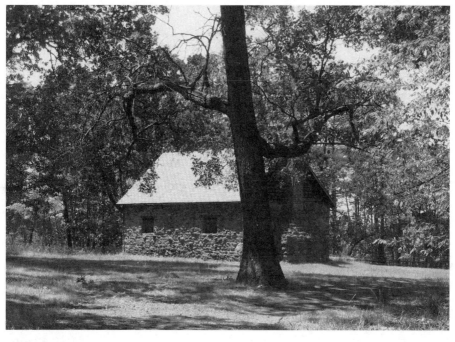

Red Dog Lodge

Maryland amounts to less than 5 percent of the original, it harbors no fewer than 39 rare and endangered plant species. Those found in Soldiers Delight include papillose nut rush, serpentine aster, whorled milkweed, grooved flax, and fringed gentian. Other rare plants include bluestem, three-awn, turkey foot, broomsedge, and beardgrass. Not surprisingly, the rare grasses also host rare insects, including Edward's hairstreak, an unnamed leafhopper, and a black pear-shaped beetle, usually found only in deserts. Soldiers Delight remains the largest remaining serpentine area in the eastern United States and is among the most species-rich in the world.

Begin the hike by heading left on the white-blazed trail. Very soon, you'll come to the Red Dog Lodge, an old defunct hunting lodge built in 1912. Pass it and emerge onto an open area created by a power line cut. Inevitably, along the way, you're bound to hear a sudden shuffle and then see the bounding hops of white-tailed deer. They are abundant in Soldiers Delight.

Walk through a pine forest, a welcome spot of shade on a hot day. As you turn north, come to a creek, where an odd sight greets you. To the left sits an old rusted automobile, the make of which is no longer distinguishable. It belongs to nature now, with grasses growing through the trunk and hood. It doesn't seem to have much of an effect on nearby stream life, if the thousands of darting minnows, skimmers, and dragonflies are any indication.

Continue your walk up a fairly steep hill. The trail here is entirely loose rocks; this is the serpentinite. If you were barefooted, you'd get an unwelcome

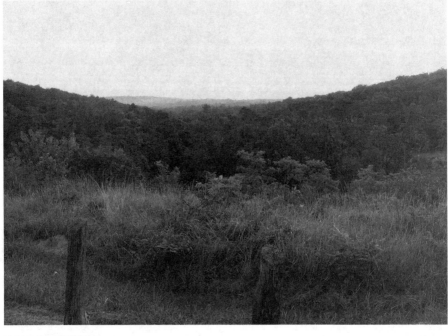

Deer Park overlook

understanding of how sharp the edges of this mineral can be. As the trail takes you back into a pine forest at the top of the hill, turn around. The view before you is astounding: prairie sweeping in all directions. You'll be surrounded by red and yellow-tipped grasses swaying in the breeze. Depending on the season, you might see yellow from the gray goldenrod and grooved flax, white from the serpentine aster and whorled milkweed, and purple from grass-leaved blazing star and fringed gentian.

The prairie is dotted here and there with the stubs of culled pines. This is no act of arson, but rather an ongoing attempt to restore the grasslands, free of the invasive and non-native pines. Head back into the woods, and come to another section of the power line cut you crossed earlier.

After the power line cut, things are still pretty stubbly, but some small, drought-resistant trees offer shade, mostly blackjack oak, post oak, and Virginia pine. Trees that are native are left to grow as best they can in the soil. Approach Deer Park Road; it can be a bit noisy. Come to an overlook on Deer Park at 2.1 miles. A historical marker here tells you that chrome was first discovered in Baltimore County in 1808. Chromite mines existed at Soldiers Delight from 1828 to 1850, and they produced almost all the world's chromium.

Cross Deer Park and head right to continue hiking on the east side, a series of three trails blazed in red, orange, and yellow, which run across landscape far more typical of the Baltimore metro region.

Begin on the rocky red-blazed trail. Initially, the landscape looks much as it does in the serpentine section. But as there is far less serpentine grassland on this side of Soldiers Delight, many mature Virginia pines line both sides of the trail, with wildflowers to the right. Very soon, at 2.3 miles, you'll notice a wooden post pointing to the yellow trail and the choate mine to the right. The abandoned mine sits within a wooden fenced area, but if you circle around the fence, you can walk within and as close as the opening. You'll have to stop there, as the mine is now filled with water. The mine was part of the big operation that thrived in the area in the early to mid-1800s, digging for chromite, talc, asbestos, magnesite, and soapstone, among other minerals.

Moving on, the trail becomes very rocky; often the entire trail itself is one large slab of rock spreading across. The area is nicely shaded and has flourishing greenbrier underbrush, which gives the first indication of the difference between these trails and the Serpentine. As I walked, I was accompanied by the hoot of an owl, but was unable to spot it within the thick canopy of pine, poplar, and oak. At just under 2.7 miles, the trail opens up. You can head left to make a quick loop of the red trail (1 mile total), diagonally left to head to the orange trail (2 miles), or keep going straight onto the yellow trail to make the complete 3-mile circuit. Initially, there is still a lot of serpentine rock strewn about on the yellow trail. The right side of the trail is completely full of green underbrush, but prairie grass grows to the left. In both cases, the dominant pine and Eastern red cedar shades either side. Also, many deer scurry about in the forest cover.

At 3 miles, cross a small stream and head uphill to the right. At 3.3 miles, come to and cross Chimney Branch, which flows into Liberty Reservoir. Just beyond is an area where lots of pines are being eliminated. Head to the right on the other side of the stream; the trail is extremely rocky again.

Cross through another open serpentine area before plunging back into the woods at 3.5 miles. The soil is good here, with lots of underbrush. The trees are still mostly conifers, but much taller than elsewhere. The soil also supports oak, beech, sycamore, and maple. Amazingly (and testament to the varied nature of Soldiers Delight), there's even enough moisture in this section to allow ferns and mosses.

At 3.7 miles, cross Sherwood Road, a narrow lane that leads to a private home. The trail picks up in a field on the other side, among very tall prairie grasses. When you enter the woods again, head left. There's a path straight ahead to private homes. It's confusing because there are no signs pointing you in the correct direction, and the path ahead is wider than the one to the left, but you should head left anyway. Once you do, the blazes return. Unfortunately, the trail skirts the edge of the park boundary, and lots of backyards appear to the right among the mixed hardwood.

You'll hit the orange trail by going straight at 3.9 miles. The trail begins to head left away from the houses and over a nice sweeping hill to the right. The next 0.3 miles is pretty hilly—the contrast between here and the Serpentine section of Soldiers Delight is very stark, aided in part by the appearance of a small stream to the right. But then, at 4.3 miles, emerge into a serpentine barren, with its attendant cut pines. The stream still runs to the right and gives off a pleasing sound created by its rocky bed.

Soon after, come to a post: red trail to the left, yellow to the right. Take a right, walking past a thick stand of grass-leaved blazing star with its purple blossoms. Cross over a tiny stream and enter an open area as you head gradually uphill. At 5.1 miles, there's a fenced area to the right; within is a pit mine. It's closed off, but still quite dangerous. Peer in the hole, but don't climb the fence. (Incidentally, on the trail map, when it says "pit mine," it's not unreasonable to expect a massive open pit, but it's actually quite small.) Reach the road at 5.6 miles. Cross and head to the left to make your way back to the visitor center on the only section of trail in Soldiers Delight that you haven't yet hiked.

NEARBY ACTIVITIES

Just down the road from Soldiers Delight is the family-friendly Northwest Regional Park, home to many ball fields, paved paths, and wheelchair-accessible gardening plots. From the Deer Park Overlook, head back toward Route 26. The park entrance is approximately 3 miles to the left, just before Lyons Mill Road. For additional information on Northwest Regional Park, contact the park office at (410) 887-1558.

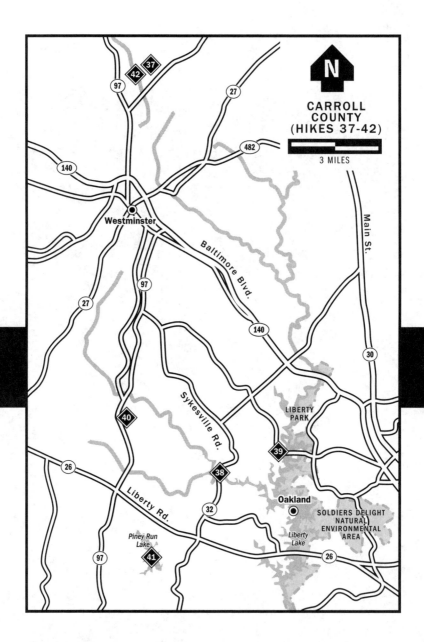

CARROLL COUNTY

37 HASHAWHA ENVIRONMENTAL APPRECIATION AREA
AT BEAR BRANCH NATURE CENTER

KEY AT-A-GLANCE INFORMATION

LENGTH: 2.5 miles

CONFIGURATION: Loop with short spur

DIFFICULTY: Moderate

SCENERY: Wildflower meadows, Bear Branch, raptors

EXPOSURE: More sun than shade

TRAFFIC: Moderate

TRAIL SURFACE: Dirt, rock, asphalt

HIKING TIME: 1–1.5 hours

ACCESS: Dawn–dusk on trails; Bear Branch Nature Center open Wednesday–Saturday 10 a.m.– 5 p.m. and Sunday noon–5 p.m.; info: (410) 848-2517

MAPS: USGS Manchester; trail maps also available in Bear Branch Nature Center or online at ccgovern ment.carr.org/ccg/mapserver4/ gis/webpage/trails.html.

WHEELCHAIR ACCESS: At Bear Branch Nature Center

FACILITIES: Water and restrooms at Bear Branch Nature Center

SPECIAL COMMENTS: The Hashawha Residential Camp is closed to the public; please respect the no-entry areas, which designate the private rental area. Trails to the north of this hike are largely covered under Union Mills (see page 209).

GPS Trailhead
Coordinates

UTM Zone (WGS84) 18S

Easting 329583

Northing 4390472

Latitude N 39' 38.824339"

Longitude W 76' 59.171677"

IN BRIEF

Start at Bear Branch Nature Center and stroll through ten different examples of environmentally friendly land usages.

DESCRIPTION

Enter the trailhead and follow the sign to the pavilion. The wooden fence flanking the crushed rock trail zigzags to the bottom of the hill. When you see the pavilion on the left, head right through the open field and then left at the sign pointing to the blue-blazed Vista Trail. Almost immediately you will come to a three-way intersection; take a left up the hill.

You'll be on a wide dirt path surrounded mostly by short oaks and dogwoods. The trail quickly heads up and then down as it circles the pavilion you passed at the top of the trail. Head up the hill at 0.4 miles in a grove of pines; you'll see the surrounding farmland beyond the pines. Walk through a nice buffer of thick vegetation and emerge at a raptor pen at about 0.6 miles. There are a number of birds being rehabilitated here, including hawks, eagles, and vultures.

Directions ———————————→

Take I-695 to Exit 19, I-795 west; continue until I-795 ends at MD 140 (Baltimore Boulevard) north to Westminster. Continue on MD 140 for 12 miles and turn right onto MD 97 north to Union Mills and Gettysburg. Continue on MD 97 (it becomes Littlestown Pike) 2.8 miles and then turn right onto John Owings Road. After 1 mile, you'll see a WELCOME TO HASHAWHA AND BEAR BRANCH NATURE CENTER sign on the left; turn here and then take a right at the sign for the nature center. The trail begins on the blue-blazed Vista Trail just to the left of the nature center.

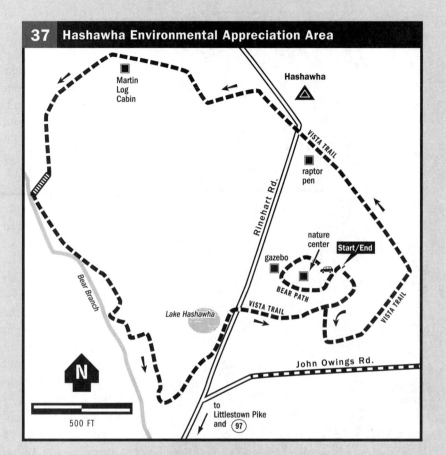

37 Hashawha Environmental Appreciation Area

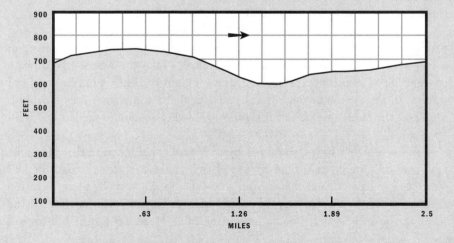

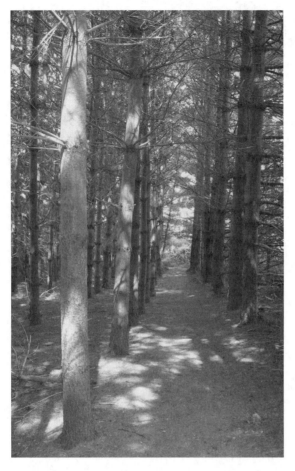

Pine grove

Continue the hike by heading to the right, away from the cages; you'll come to a gravel road and then an asphalt road. In about 100 feet, you'll see yellow (Wilderness Trail) and green (Stream Trail) arrows pointing to the right, and straight ahead lies the restricted area of the Residential Hashawha Camp, a camp for Carroll County sixth-graders. Go right, back into the woods, and then turn right at the exercise course at just under 0.8 miles. You'll pass the restored Martin Log Cabin at 1 mile. Trails heading north here head toward Saw Mill Road and are covered in the Union Mills hike (see page 209).

Parallel a wildflower meadow on the right, filled with goldenrod and cacophonous crickets and grasshoppers in summer. You'll reach a boardwalk at about 1.25 miles. Take a right over the boardwalk and then a left on the other side through another wildflower meadow.

At 1.5 miles, you'll be paralleling Bear Branch, and you'll come to a beautiful open area where a tremendous old maple shades a picnic bench sitting in a crook of the semicircular sweep of the creek. Take the wooden boardwalk straight ahead over the creek; you'll pass a clump of beech trees as you head up the hill. At the top of the hill, take a right; the trail quickly heads downhill. You'll see the creek again on your right as you swing around to the left and head back uphill.

At just under 2 miles, you'll see a gravel road heading left to the camp area and a paved asphalt road heading to the right; take the asphalt road for 500 feet, passing Lake Hashawha on your left. Pick up the Vista Trail again to the right across the road. Pass a marsh on the right, and you'll soon be back at the pavilion you passed at the beginning of the hike. Head left up the hill toward your car; this time, however, take a brief detour by heading left when you come to the parking area. You'll come to an informational sign on "forest edging" and a paved concrete path beyond. Take a left; this is the Bear Path, which winds around the nature center and ends at a gazebo from which you can view examples of land usage that maintain the ten healthy environments in the Hashawha Environmental Appreciation Area: wildlife habitat, field strip cropping, grass waterway, contour strip cropping, grass diversion, lined outlet (rip-rap), pond, woodland, field border, and nontidal wetland. You can take a mowed-grass path from the gazebo to the nature center, which has exhibits on hundreds of butterflies, as well as live box turtles, and stuffed mink, deer, raccoon, and beaver; you can also learn about the interesting changes in the habitat in this area all the way back to the Paleozoic period.

NEARBY ACTIVITIES

Hashawha Environmental Appreciation Area sits within the Union Mills environmental area, which contains approximately 8 miles of hiking trails; please see page 209 for hiking suggestions in Union Mills. For sustenance after a hike at Hashawha, head south on MD 97 into downtown Westminster. Full of restaurants, antiques shops, and museums, Westminster offers many diverse activities. The Maryland Wine Festival takes place each September at the Carroll County Farm Museum grounds in Westminster; for information: (410) 386-3880, (800) 654-4645, or **www.marylandwine .com/mdwinefest**. For the museum: **ccgovernment.carr.org/ccg/farmmus**.

LIBERTY RESERVOIR:
38 LIBERTY WEST-MORGAN RUN

 KEY AT-A-GLANCE INFORMATION

LENGTH: 6.7 miles

CONFIGURATION: Loop

DIFFICULTY: Easy–moderate

SCENERY: Liberty Reservoir, Morgan Run, Little Morgan Run, white pine plantations

EXPOSURE: Shade

TRAFFIC: Light

TRAIL SURFACE: Packed dirt

HIKING TIME: 2.5 hours

ACCESS: Sunrise–sunset

MAPS: USGS Finksburg

WHEELCHAIR ACCESS: No

FACILITIES: None

SPECIAL COMMENTS: This hike includes a difficult river crossing at Little Morgan Run; expect wet feet in all but the lowest water levels.

IN BRIEF

A taste of Loch Raven Reservoir, but with fewer people.

DESCRIPTION

You may not think that starting a hike on a fire road with busy Route 32 just above you is very pleasant, but you'll quickly move away from civilization. About 900 feet down the fire road, you'll see another fire road heading downhill on your left. Take the road down the hill, and at a quarter-mile, you'll reach the reservoir; you'll see a thick forest of white pine on the right.

Although you might still be able to hear the traffic on Route 32, when I was here the quacking and wing-beating of ducks, the pounding of a woodpecker, and the whispering glide of a gray heron effectively drowned it out. Moving on, the trail more or less follows the contours of the reservoir. As you walk along, notice the edge of the reservoir as you parallel it; heavy rainfall raises the water level and submerges the trunks of the trees, giving the area a look reminiscent of cypress swamp. Ravens and red-winged blackbirds frequent this area.

Unlike the trails at Loch Raven Reservoir, which often run right alongside the water, the trails here at Liberty Reservoir run

GPS Trailhead
Coordinates
UTM Zone (WGS84) 18S
Easting 333270
Northing 4367091
Latitude N 39' 26.234715"
Longitude W 76' 56.242855"

Directions

Take I-695 to I-70 west, and continue to MD 32 north; go 10 miles to Liberty Reservoir Bridge. Cross the bridge and immediately look for the gravel parking area to the right; park your car, walk across MD 32, and go over the guardrail. The trail starts on the fire road at the bottom of the hill.

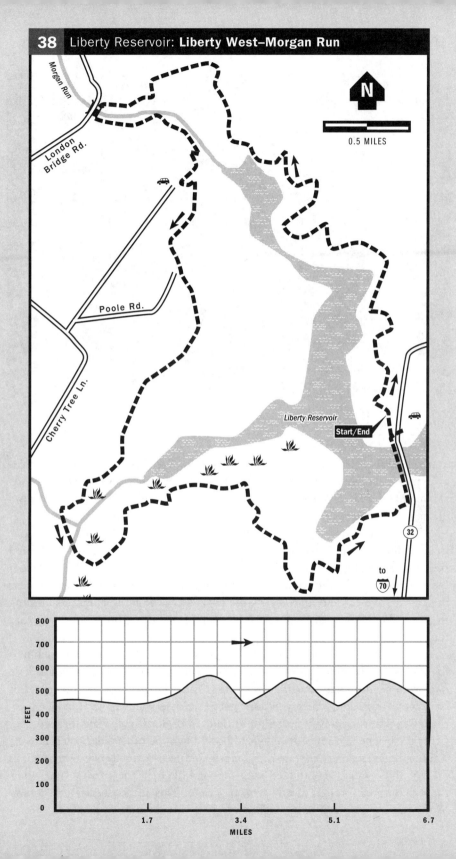

N

0.5 MILES

Morgan Run

London Bridge Rd.

Poole Rd.

Cherry Tree Ln.

Liberty Reservoir

Start/End

32

to
70

FEET				
800				
700				
600				
500				
400				
300				
200				
100				
0				

1.7   3.4   5.1   6.7

MILES

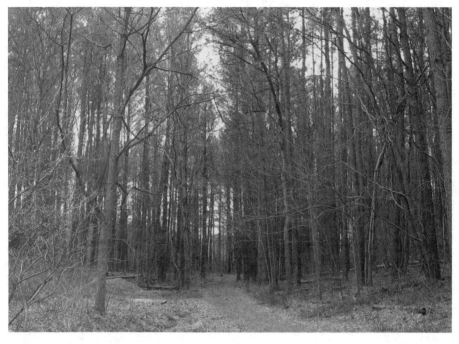

Liberty fire road

up the hill, away from the water a bit. This is because these trails have remained primarily fire roads, as opposed to cut single-track for bikes. Since the fire roads run about a hundred or so feet above the water, you will have many good views of the reservoir spreading out in several directions.

By 0.7 miles, once again the trail runs through the pine forest and will continue so for a while. Cross a stream at 1.1 miles; look for a bog and milkweed swaying in the breeze at 1.5 miles. Here you'll head up a steep hill, away from the reservoir; you'll come to a power line cut at the top of the hill. You can hear the crackle of electricity in the air—the buzz is a bit unnerving, but it's nothing to worry about. The trail here takes the form of two tire grooves directly under the power lines.

At 1.9 miles, the path veers away from the power lines and heads back into the woods; you'll cross a little stream and soon after come to Morgan Run, a wide river with small rapids coursing over rocks. You'll hear the wonderful sound of swiftly moving water, which you don't get at the reservoir. The trail, now a footpath, follows Morgan Run upstream to London Bridge Road, a small rural road. Cross the bridge and immediately head back down the other side; you'll now be walking downstream. On your right, moss- and fern-covered rock outcroppings line the hills, which are studded with mountain laurel. The narrow trail winds through an area forested mostly with oak trees. This section bears little resemblance to the previous 2 miles, highlighting the varied nature of this hike.

You'll probably see some horseshoe impressions in the dirt path here. At a grouping of fir trees at 2.6 miles, you'll pass a marsh on the left; if you're walking in late spring or summer, the chorus of frogs will be almost deafening. The trail soon splits, and you can either go to the left along the reservoir or straight ahead to rejoin the fire road; take the fire road. You'll soon come to Poole Road, marked by a set of orange cables with a small parking area beyond. Make a U-turn and look for another orange cable; head in that direction. The trail takes you into an incredibly beautiful white pine plantation; you'll find it easy to get lost in contemplation here as you walk along a little stream on the left with the pines to the right.

At 3 miles, unfortunately, civilization comes into view, and you'll see a few houses on the right beyond the pine forest. Over the next half mile or so, you'll pass a bunch of trails leading off to the left—these all dead-end at the reservoir. At 3.3 miles, you'll see a wide fire road to the left, the end of a residential road to the right, and a set of orange posts straight ahead. Follow the orange posts, continuing straight alongside the narrow paved road to the right. Though it's a bit disappointing to be passing backyards, if you look only left, it's all pines as far as you can see—and you'll probably hear the hammering of a woodpecker or two. Keep an eye out for red foxes as well.

The trail will take you to a stream valley and across a little stream. Immediately after, you'll come to Little Morgan Run. As mentioned in the Special Comments section, you might have difficulty crossing here without getting wet. If the water level is low, however, you should be able to cross relatively easily and stay dry.

On the other side of Little Morgan Run, the trail parallels a twisty little stream that empties into a marsh and then bleeds into the edge of the reservoir. You'll come to a trail split at 4.9 miles; take the leftward cut to stay in the woods. Over the next half mile or so, you'll go up and down a series of hills, skirting the edge of the forested reservoir boundary; houses will reappear through the woods on the right. The trail swings around toward the reservoir, giving you a great view of the water, which here splits off into four directions. It's a lovely spot.

At 5.9 miles, you'll come to a T-intersection; go left and you'll quickly come to the edge of the reservoir. It offers a nice view, but unfortunately you'll probably also see trash; debris seems to float this way and accumulate here. Head uphill to the right, keeping the reservoir on your left; mountain laurel lines the path here. When you reach the fire road at the top of the hill, go left. You'll start to hear the traffic on Route 32 again; take the narrow footpath through the woods. You will come to Route 32 at 6.4 miles; walk carefully along the shoulder of the highway, taking extra care when you cross the Liberty Reservoir Bridge, as the shoulder narrows considerably. You'll find your car on the right on the other side of the bridge.

NEARBY ACTIVITIES

In addition to the other trails in the Liberty Reservoir watershed, this area offers an abundance of hiking opportunities. To the south, check out the Hugg-Thomas Wildlife Management Area of Patapsco Valley State Park; it is open to hikers on Sundays from mid-February through August (open to hunters only the rest of the year); take MD 32 south to the first right over the Patapsco River and turn left onto Main Street and then right onto Forsythe Road. Also visit Morgan Run Natural Environmental Area to the west (see page 199); take MD 32 south to MD 26 west and continue to MD 97 north. You also have the option of hiking, boating, or fishing in Piney Run Park (see page 204); take MD 26 west and turn left onto Martz Road into the park.

LIBERTY RESERVOIR: MIDDLE RUN TRAIL 39

IN BRIEF

An anomaly: despite this hike's location at Liberty Reservoir, it rarely offers views of the reservoir itself. Nevertheless, it's arguably the prettiest and most diverse hike in the Liberty Reservoir watershed—it's also my favorite.

DESCRIPTION

The trail splits almost immediately; a fisherman's path to the right heads downhill toward the water, and the main trail, a wide fire road, continues straight. If you want to spend a little while by the water, take the cut down to the edge of the reservoir. To continue this hike, go straight.

Pine dominates the landscape here, evidenced by the smell and innumerable needles underfoot. You'll also see some hardy holly trees that are managing to eke some living space despite the crowding pines. At a quarter -mile, you'll come to a four-way crossroads; turn right and move away from the pines into a forest of oak, poplar, mountain laurel, and redbud, filled with birdsong.

On the left at 0.4 miles, you'll pass a great rock outcropping rippling down the hill like a dinosaur's spine. When the trees are bare, the tip of the ridge offers a great view of the river valley. Mountain laurel lines both sides

KEY AT-A-GLANCE INFORMATION

LENGTH: 3.7 miles
CONFIGURATION: Out-and-back with a loop
DIFFICULTY: Moderate
SCENERY: Middle Run, pine plantations, mixed hardwoods
EXPOSURE: Mostly shade
TRAFFIC: Light
TRAIL SURFACE: Packed dirt
HIKING TIME: 1.5 hours–2 hours
ACCESS: Sunrise–sunset daily
MAPS: USGS Finksburg
WHEELCHAIR ACCESS: No
FACILITIES: None
SPECIAL COMMENTS: This hike requires crossing Middle Run four times; although the water is never too wide nor too deep, expect wet feet and legs, perhaps up to your knees.

Directions

Take I-695 to Exit 19, I-795 west. Take Exit 7, Franklin Boulevard, but head west to Nicodemus Road just before you get to Franklin Boulevard. Nicodemus Road turns into Deer Park Road after Ivy Mill Road. Cross Liberty Reservoir bridge and continue 1 mile to the big turn to the right; look for the gravel parking area on the left. Walk into the woods behind the parking area and look for the footpath.

GPS Trailhead Coordinates

UTM Zone (WGS84) 18S
Easting 336810
Northing 4368285
Latitude N 39' 26.920545"
Longitude W 76' 53.793583"

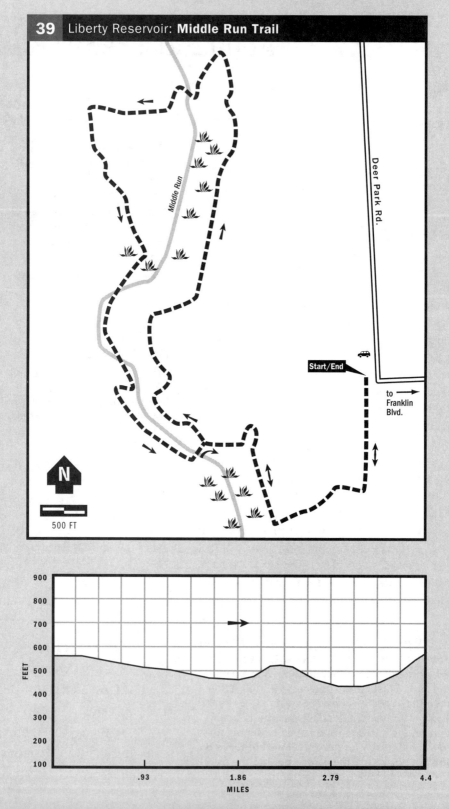

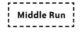

Middle Run

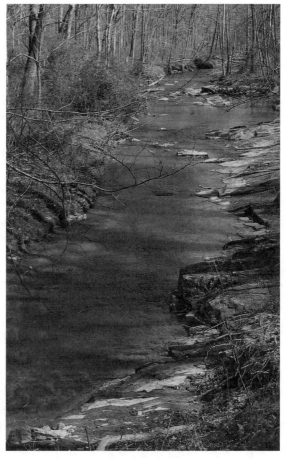

of the trail. Down the hill on the left, you'll see the edge of the reservoir, complete with a marshy buffer area between the reservoir's end and the trail; continue along the edge of the reservoir until the trail splits at a jumble of rocks on the right at 0.7 miles. You'll see Middle Run on the left, where you'll end up in a few miles.

Go to the right at the split; you'll head gradually uphill, passing through a pine and spruce forest that supports a plentiful white-tailed deer population, at 1 mile. You'll cross a modest stream at 1.2 miles—a little warm-up for what's ahead. At 1.3 miles, you'll come to another little stream with a towering cathedral of pine on the other side. You'd be hard-pressed to see dirt here—a carpet of pine needles covers the trail. At 1.5 miles, you'll see a power line cut straight ahead; turn left (turning right leads to another parking area at Deer Park Road, north of where you parked).

Middle Run appears soon after. This decent-size crossing requires removing your shoes; take time to look in both directions, upstream and down, while you're crossing. The beautiful, meandering stream runs clean and clear. On the other side, the trail splits; keep going straight ahead, moving gradually uphill through more pines. The pine plantation ends abruptly and gives way to oak and poplar, with a few flowering dogwoods here and there.

The trail splits again at 1.8 miles; this time head left. Mountain laurel dominates this section of the trail, and if you're lucky to catch it during spring bloom, you're in for a treat of white clustered flowers. You'll cross Middle Run a second time at 2.3 miles; use the fallen tree approximately 50 feet to the right of the trail to help you across. It's not easy, but it's certainly doable if you want to avoid taking off your shoes again; if you do remove your shoes, don't lace them back up when you reach the other side—you'll be crossing the water again in a tenth of a mile.

After you cross Middle Run the third time, you'll see blue blazes on some of the trees, but they promptly disappear. Pass the trail cut going straight up the hill on the right, and stay on the trail parallel to the stream. At 2.8 miles, you'll notice some nice smooth flat stones leading down to the water; checkered with green moss, they make a perfect place to stand and take in the beauty of the stream valley.

At 3 miles, the main trail continues straight ahead, and a cut to the left leads back to the water; follow the cut and cross Middle Run for the fourth and final time. If you've somehow managed to make it this far without removing your shoes, you'll have to do it before crossing here, where the stream is wide. Take extra caution walking over the rocks, which can be quite slick. Once across, backtrack to the parking area, remembering to take a left at the four-way crossing at 3.6 miles.

NEARBY ACTIVITIES

If you're looking for more hiking, Morgan Run Natural Environmental Area is nearby to the west (see page 199). From Liberty Reservoir, continue on Deer Park and turn left onto Gamber Road; turn right onto Nicodemus Road, and then turn left onto MD 97 south. Look for Morgan Run on the left. If you're interested in antiques or a meal in a cozy restaurant, go to historic Reisterstown, which dates back to the mid-18th century; backtrack toward I-795, take a left onto Ivy Mill Road, and then turn right onto Westminster Pike, which turns into Main Street.

MORGAN RUN NATURAL ENVIRONMENTAL AREA 40

IN BRIEF

Morgan Run Natural Environmental Area includes approximately 1,400 acres of wonderful hiking and equestrian trails. The entire area has been blissfully left alone, with well-maintained trails but no unnecessary "improvements," making it a perfect place to get away from it all.

DESCRIPTION

The first thing you'll notice at Morgan Run is birds: songbirds flit about, shuttling from the tall trees to the regenerating fields and bird-houses; within the woods, woodpeckers and owls make their incessant noises; hawks and turkey vultures wheel above; and startlingly massive wild turkeys waddle over the trails. Because this hike frequently leads from woods to the edge of fields, you'll constantly hear branches cracking and leaves crunching as the creatures move about, but you'll have a hard time spotting them. Abundant life and energy surround you here.

At your first trail split option, head left into the woods; be on the alert for manure, evidence of the trail's equestrian traffic. Also

KEY AT-A-GLANCE INFORMATION

LENGTH: 5.7 miles

CONFIGURATION: 2 jagged loops

DIFFICULTY: Easy–moderate

SCENERY: Mixed hardwoods, regenerating fields, stream valleys

EXPOSURE: Half shade and half sun

TRAFFIC: Light

TRAIL SURFACE: Packed dirt, grass

HIKING TIME: 2 hours

ACCESS: 7 a.m.–sunset daily

MAPS: USGS Finksburg, Winfield; maps also available online at ccgovernment.carr.org/ccg/mapserver4/gis/webpage/trails.html.

WHEELCHAIR ACCESS: No

FACILITIES: None

SPECIAL COMMENTS: Numerous trails at Morgan Run, many of which are connector trails, provide many different possibilities and configurations for hiking—to make the longest hike, keep heading left whenever you come to intersecting trails. The online maps above can help you make better sense of the trails that head out in many directions.

Directions

Take I-695 to I-70 west to Exit 76, MD 97 north to Westminster. After you cross MD 26, turn right onto Bartholow Road and then make an immediate left onto Jim Bowers Road and an even more immediate left onto Ben Rose Lane. Continue straight to the end of the large gravel parking area at the end of the road. At the far left end of the parking area, you will see two picnic benches; the trail begins straight beyond the picnic tables. In about 200 feet you will be able to discern the trail's worn groove in the grass.

GPS Trailhead Coordinates

UTM Zone (WGS84) 18S

Easting 327861

Northing 4370386

Latitude N 39' 27.951214"

Longitude W 77' 0.062821"

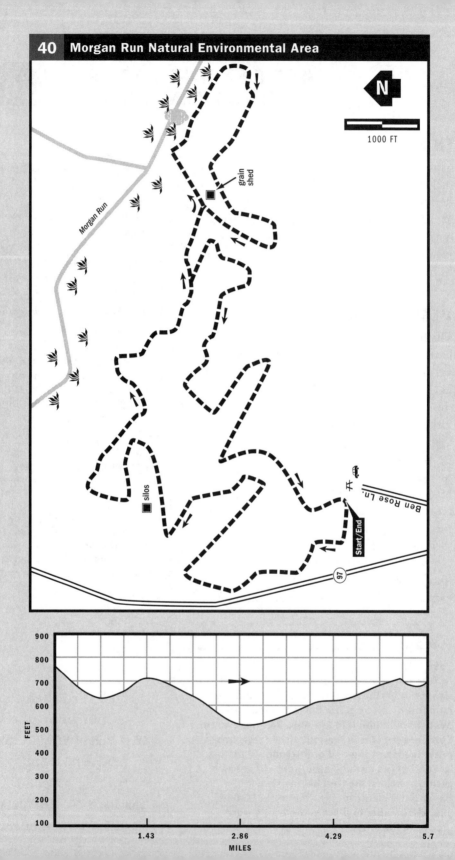

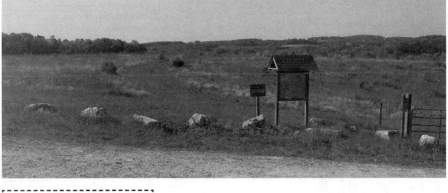

View from trailhead parking lot

be alert for ticks, which lurk in the tall grasses in the tree-line buffer, and take extra time looking for and removing ticks from your clothing and body at the end of the hike. I hiked Morgan Run in the summer and picked off no fewer than two dozen ticks.

After a quarter-mile, you'll be able to hear the traffic on MD 97 on the left, but a thick buffer of poplar, oak, maple, sassafras, ash, and dogwood prevents you from seeing it. Unfortunately, the trail continues toward MD 97, coming as close as ten feet before heading away at a branch of Morgan Run, which at this point is not much more than a trickle. You'll see an overgrown foot trail heading toward the water, but go right instead on the obvious and wide trail that leads up the hill. As you head away from MD 97, the sounds of civilization fade away and isolation returns.

Be on the lookout for some old stone foundations on the right at 0.6 miles. At 0.8 miles, emerge into an opening where you have several options; again, head left. Deer favor this habitat, and you'll probably see a few of them. Clumps of isolated vegetation pock the land, and the field on the right, once cleared, is growing back. Unfortunately, autumn olive, an invasive species, has found a home; if you're hiking in the spring, you'll smell a pleasant scent reminiscent of lilac from its white flowers. The autumn olives provide habitat for songbirds and other wildlife, and the trees also serve as a windbreak for the area's big pockets of deforested land; on the negative side, the dominating autumn olives do a superb job of crowding out native species, something you'll notice as you continue your hike. When I revisited Morgan Run to update this book, I noticed that the autumn olive wasn't quite as dominant as it once was, but it's still there.

You'll see some old abandoned silos on the left at 1.3 miles; continue around and swing back into the woods at 1.4 miles. When you emerge at the next clearing, head right to stay away from MD 97 (going straight will lead you to the same place but add a tenth of a mile to the hike). Just before you reenter the woods, turn around for a great view of a wooded valley—a farm on the right

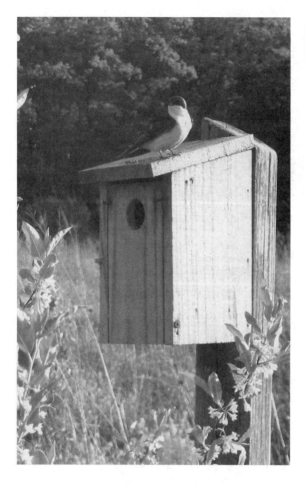

One of many Morgan Run avian denizens

is the only indication that people live in this area.

When you reemerge to the open field, take a left. Swing around where the hill levels a bit, and take a left back into the woods; you'll see oak, maple, and dogwood trees on your left, and pines on your right. Take another leftward cut after another 900 feet. You'll very quickly come to a rightward cut; pass it and take the next rightward cut instead. The path becomes a well-worn groove in the grass and merges with the more obvious trail and links to the other end of a loop you earlier skipped. (Again, this can get confusing with the profusion of paths, so taking along the map is a good idea. On the other hand, a good sense of direction should be sufficient to get you where you want to go.) You'll come to another wide path immediately after; take a left, but notice the cut to the right at 2.5 miles—you'll be taking it on the way back.

At 2.6 miles, you'll see an old decrepit garage stable and a newer one closer to the trail. Swing around to the left to continue the hike, and you'll see a corn bin just ahead. Cross a branch of Morgan Run on some logs; once across, you can head right to go back to the parking area, or go straight to extend the hike. Be sure to look left to see a beautiful pond in a grove of towering beech trees; you would have a difficult time finding a more peaceful place.

Ultimately, you'll be taking a right, and you have three chances to do so: a path at 3 miles, one just beyond that, and then a third path that will take you to the farthest edge of the trail. I recommend taking the third path because it leads you through thick forest with no sign of humanity even though the park boundary means nearby suburban backyards. You will reenter the woods at 3.3 miles; take a left at 3.4 miles and head deeper into the woods. Parallel a branch of Morgan Run as you walk upstream. Cross the branch at 3.6 miles. It soon joins the wider Morgan Run, which operates as a catch-and-release trout stream; cross the water again. After asking this, you might have some trouble spotting the trail; look for it about ten feet to the right of where you've crossed.

Go uphill and turn right onto the wider path that runs along a hillside covered with ferns and honeysuckle. You'll gradually rise above the stream valley on the right and emerge from the woods at 3.8 miles at the shed you passed earlier. Take a left; you will backtrack a little bit before heading left again, at the cut you noted earlier at 2.5 miles. At a little over 4 miles, come to a T-intersection; go left. You'll begin passing cuts to the right at about 4.5 miles; all of these cuts head back to the parking area, but pass them to make the hike longer.

For some variation, turn right at the connector trail at 5.1 miles (otherwise you'll continue to the parking area along the tree line, adding a half mile to the hike) and then turn left at the central field trail. It will lead you straight to the parking area, affording some nice views of the entire area on the way. Again, remember to check for ticks when you finish hiking this section.

NEARBY ACTIVITIES

In the mood for some fishing? Nearby 300-acre Piney Lake is often lauded as one of the best fisheries in the state. Head back to MD 26 and take a left. Then take a right onto White Rock Road and follow the signs. For a description of Piney Run's hiking trails and nature center, see page 204.

41 PINEY RUN PARK

KEY AT-A-GLANCE INFORMATION

LENGTH: 4.7 miles

CONFIGURATION: Loop

DIFFICULTY: Easy

SCENERY: Piney Run Lake, pine forests, mixed hardwoods

EXPOSURE: More shade than sun

TRAFFIC: Moderate on trails; heavy at boat ramp

TRAIL SURFACE: Packed dirt with small sections of asphalt

HIKING TIME: 1.5 hours

ACCESS: Sunrise–sunset daily

MAPS: USGS Finksburg; some You ARE HERE maps along trails; maps also available online at ccgovern ment.carr.org/ccg/mapserver4/gis/webpage/trails.html.

WHEELCHAIR ACCESS: No

FACILITIES: Boat launch, pavilions, boat rental, restrooms and water at nature center; food at boat launch

SPECIAL COMMENTS: The park charges a vehicle fee April 1–October 31: $4 for Carroll County residents, $6 for nonresidents. The nature center is open April 1–October 31, Tuesday–Friday 10 a.m.–5 p.m and Saturday and Sunday 1–5 p.m.; it is open the rest of the year from 10 a.m.–4 p.m.

- -

GPS Trailhead
Coordinates

UTM Zone (WGS84) 18S

Easting 329152

Northing 4362338

Latitude N 39' 23.618181"

Longitude W 76' 59.039454"

IN BRIEF

Leave the boating and fishing crowds behind as you explore the forests around popular Piney Lake.

DESCRIPTION

Before you start your hike, stop in the nature center, which features live reptiles and knowledgeable naturalists. The nature center hosts an astounding 300 programs a year, ranging from presentations for toddlers to ones for senior citizens. Make sure you check out the outside hummingbird garden and aviary. The birds you might see include black vultures, turkey vultures, barred owls, great horned owls (the largest resident owl in Maryland), red-shouldered hawks, and red-tailed hawks.

Beginning on the Lake Trail behind the nature center, you'll be in thick woods that obscure 300-acre Piney Lake, which many believe to be the best fishery in the state. According to the Maryland Department of Natural Resources (DNR), fish species found in the lake include "pumpkinseed sunfish, redbreast sunfish, brown bullhead, smallmouth bass, white sucker, spotfin shiner, bluntnose minnow, banded killifish, golden shiner, creek chub, and tessellated darter." These are in addition to the more common largemouth bass, bluegill, yellow perch, channel catfish,

- -

Directions

Take I-70 to MD 97 north; turn right on Streaker Road and continue until it ends at White Rock Road. Turn right and go 0.4 miles; turn left onto Martz Road and follow the signs to Piney Run Park. Take the first right to the parking area for the nature center; the trail starts 100 feet behind the nature center.

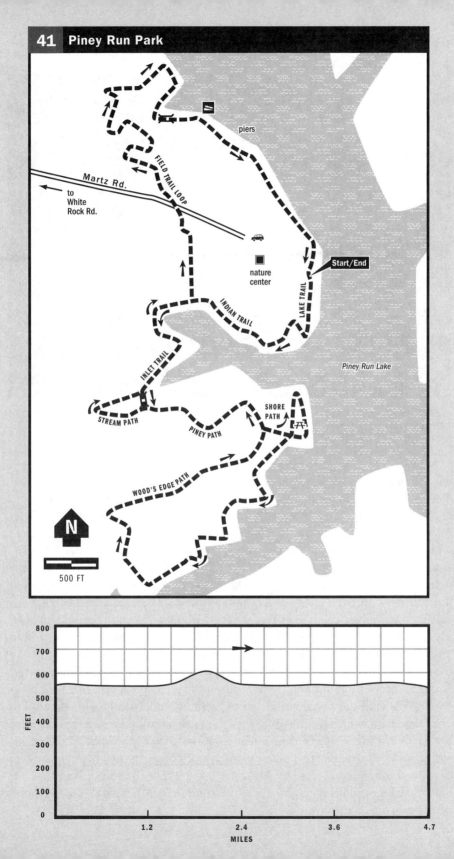

piers

FIELD TRAIL LOOP

Martz Rd.

to
White
Rock Rd.

nature
center

Start/End

LAKE TRAIL

INDIAN TRAIL

INLET TRAIL

Piney Run Lake

SHORE
PATH

STREAM PATH

PINEY PATH

WOOD'S EDGE PATH

N

500 FT

800
700
600
500
400
300
200
100
0

FEET

1.2   2.4   3.6   4.7
MILES

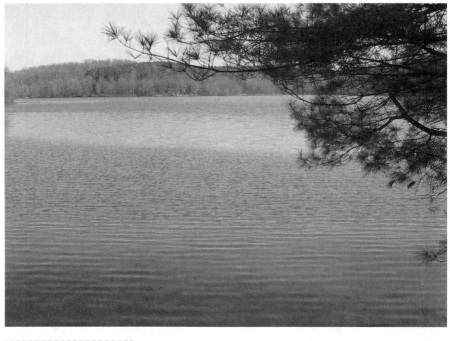

Piney Lake: fishing heaven

black crappie, striped bass, and redear sunfish. In addition, the DNR introduced tiger muskie to the lake in 1996 and stocks it annually with rainbow trout.

If you haven't brought your fishing pole, stick to the blue-blazed Lake Trail as it heads right and circles the aviary. After 250 feet, pick up the red-blazed Indian Trail continuing in the same direction. When the trail splits, at 0.2 miles, take the yellow-blazed Inlet Trail to the left, and follow the contours of the lake. You'll soon come to an open field on the right buffered by pine trees and forsythia; an overwhelming smell of pine fills the air here, a sample of what's to come. At 0.5 miles, you'll see a YOU ARE HERE trail map facing a footbridge; cross the bridge. The trail splits on the other side of the small stream; take the trail to the left now—you'll take the one to the right on your way back.

The trail gradually rises above the lake through an oak and poplar forest with lots of moss, and the trail blazes turn orange as you approach a pine plantation. The trail splits again at 0.7 miles; again, head left and follow the trail to the Shore Path, which dead-ends to the left in just a few hundred feet. Take it for a nice view and an area of contemplation at the edge of the lake, where ducks, geese, and fish congregate. Several gnawed tree trunks in the area indicate that beavers live here, too. Heading back, go to the left to the spit of land that juts into the lake. Studded with pines, it's an extraordinarily beautiful spot that boaters often use as a picnic area.

Continuing your hike back on the trail, pass the cut heading to the right that leads to Piney Path and continue along the lake. You'll walk on a short exposed section of the trail before you plunge again into a pine forest with a very high canopy that offers blissful shade on a hot day. Despite the glorious smell and sight, however, the high canopy blocks so much of the sunlight that ground-level growth is very limited and the forest floor is fairly barren.

You'll see spruce, fir, and the occasional redbud trees along the edge of the woods before you reach a farm field at 1.6 miles. The trail then swings around to the right and reenters the canopy of pines; take the unblazed Wood's Edge Path straight ahead (heading left would connect you with the Piney Trail you passed earlier).

Now, on Wood's Edge Path, you are paralleling Inlet Trail. To your left is entirely pine, while the right is mostly oak. At 2 miles, take a left; pass by Inlet Trail to the right, and take Stream Path straight ahead toward the footbridge. Go past this bridge; continue on the trail and cross a different footbridge over a pretty little rock-strewn stream farther ahead, and emerge onto an open field full of clover. Take the path back to Inlet Trail, but this time at 2.8 miles, go straight (instead of heading right where you came in before), cross the footbridge, and swing to the right at the field onto the gravel. Turn left onto the paved park road.

Cross the paved road and head straight toward Pavilion 4; after you pass the boat launch parking, look for a sign for the Field Trail. The sign is some distance from the actual trailhead; if you are confused, just head right toward the new pavilion, parallel the paved road in the grass, and continue past the second pavilion on the right. Here you'll find the trail sign and the trail soon after, which is blazed white.

Red cedar dominates here, and cardinals, jays, ravens, and blackbirds flit about in the branches, while hawks circle overhead. Continue on the carpet of cedar needles, and at 3.1 miles, you will see a sign pointing in both directions for the Field Trail. Take a few minutes to sit on the bench straight ahead and enjoy the great views over the lake. Moving on, go to the right, following the signs to Field Trail Loop. At 3.6 miles, cross a footbridge and go left toward the boathouse at the popular fishing and picnic area. Pick up the asphalt path as it heads past the boat launch, where you can rent a canoe or kayak. Traffic is heavy with people and boaters, but a prohibition on gasoline motors helps ensure that at least it's quiet.

You'll pass a series of wooden piers on your left; continue straight ahead on the paved road until you see a sign for Lake Trail, marked by a series of two-by-fours heading up the hill. This section of Lake Trail takes the form of a very pleasant footpath that winds along the lake. Eventually it heads up the hill and rejoins the wider, more established Lake Trail, but it's easy to miss because fishermen have extended the footpath all along the lake's edge. If you find yourself still on the footpath along the lake, but you can see the nature center through the woods, find a path and take it up the hill.

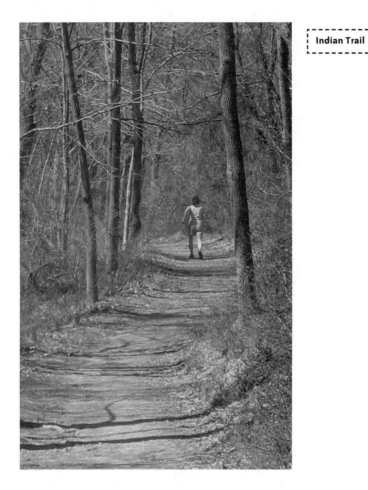

Indian Trail

NEARBY ACTIVITIES

You can find much more hiking at nearby Morgan Run Natural Environmental Area to the north (see page 199), Liberty Reservoir to the east (see page 195), and Patapsco Valley State Park's northern sections to the south (see page 284). If you're looking for a perfect antique for your home, visit the shops in New Market, "Maryland's Antique Capital," just 10 miles down I-70 west in Frederick County.

UNION MILLS

IN BRIEF

Take a rugged hike through rural northern Carroll County, slogging over creeks, through steep switchbacks, and along pleasant rolling fields.

DESCRIPTION

Once past the trailhead, you'll soon see a sign that reads BOULEVARD TRAIL. The trail, which is dirt and crushed rock, plunges into a grove of pines. Then it runs along a ridge with a slight rise on the left and a steep plunge on the right. At the top of the hill, it opens up, which gives you a nice vista of woods and fields loaded with goldenrod.

As the trail winds up and down the hills, you'll see a BOULEVARD TRAIL sign every 0.3 miles or so. At 1.4 miles, Big Pipe Creek comes into view, and you'll soon see a CROSSOVER TRAIL sign on the right. Take this trail across the creek; there's no natural crossing over the creek, but it often has only two inches of water in its shallowest section. Expect your feet to get wet and also muddy; this section is pretty wild, and equestrian use ensures that the creek banks remain soft and muddy. Since you have just begun the hike, take off your shoes and put them back on once across the creek.

KEY AT-A-GLANCE INFORMATION

LENGTH: 6.2 miles

CONFIGURATION: Out-and-back with large loops

DIFFICULTY: Moderate–strenuous

SCENERY: Forest, streams, bogs

EXPOSURE: Half and half

TRAFFIC: Light

TRAIL SURFACE: Dirt, crushed rock

HIKING TIME: 3.5 hours

ACCESS: Trails are open seven days a week, sunrise–sunset, February 16–August 31; they are closed Monday, Wednesday, Friday, and Saturday September 1–February 15 for the Cooperative Hunting Program, and they are completely closed for 2 weeks beginning the Saturday after Thanksgiving.

MAPS: USGS Manchester; maps also available online at ccgovernment .carr.org/ccg/mapserver4/gis/web page/trails.html.

WHEELCHAIR ACCESS: No

FACILITIES: None

SPECIAL COMMENTS: The hike described here attempts to pull together the diverse opportunities presented by the numerous trails, offshoots, and connectors. Take along a map.

Directions

Take I-695 to Exit 19, I-795 west; continue until it ends at MD 140 (Baltimore Boulevard) north toward Westminster. Go 12 miles and turn right onto MD 97 north to Union Mills and Gettysburg. MD 97 turns into Littlestown Pike; go 2.8 miles and turn right onto John Owings Road. Go another 0.7 miles and turn left at the stables and sign for EQUESTRIAN TRAIL PARKING. The trail starts up the hill behind the stables between the two ponds.

GPS Trailhead Coordinates

UTM Zone (WGS84) 18S

Easting 328875

Northing 4390084

Latitude N 39' 38.606222"

Longitude W 76' 59.660468"

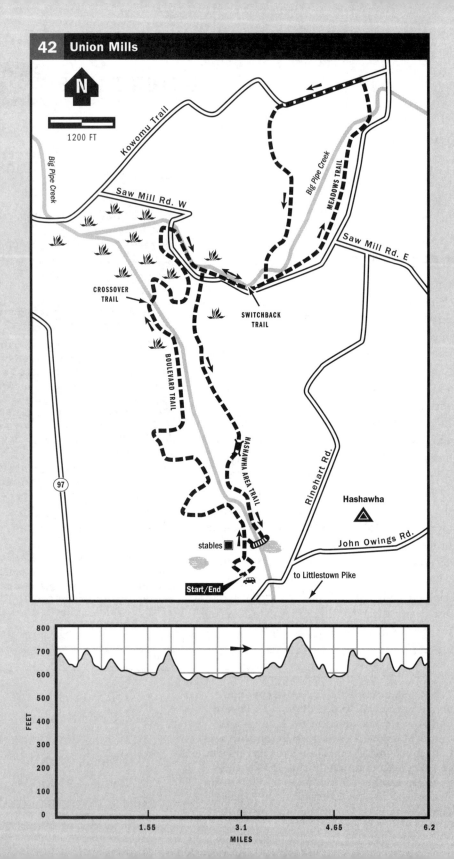

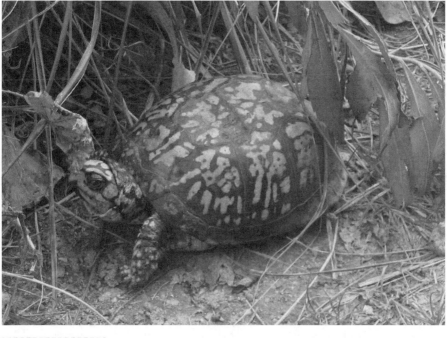

Box turtle along trail

The trail, sporadically marked with white blazes, parallels the stream to the left on the other side. It's more up and down here, with moderate to strenuous switchbacks. At the top of the hill at 1.8 miles, head left and follow the trail toward a sign that reads: LOOP. It runs through an open field and comes to Saw Mill Road at 2.1 miles. The trail then runs parallel to Saw Mill Road, sometimes running on the shoulder itself, before plunging back into the woods. You will find that this is not nearly as unpleasant as it sounds; the shoulder is wide and the woods are thick all around. Take proper caution here, however—the area is rural and not very heavily traveled, but the road has lots of blind curves and folks sometimes take these too quickly.

Just beyond 2.4 miles, you'll see a cut to the right; you can take that trail to begin making the loop back to the trailhead, but to extend your hike, continue along Saw Mill Road trail, named the Switchback Trail in this section. The creek will be down the hill below you to the left. The trail cuts away from the road for good at just under 2.9 miles and crosses the creek—again, expect to get your toes wet. Take the trail up the hill, where a profusion of ferns decorates the hillside. You'll emerge into an open meadow full of goldenrod; you'll be on a wide fire road here. This, understandably, is the Meadows Trail. Take a left and, at 3.2 miles, cross a stream (you won't get wet toes this time—the stream has lots of rocks you can use as stepping-stones). You'll see some beautiful rock formations on your right.

The trail becomes crushed rock before it splits at 3.3 miles. Take a left (going right takes you out to a parking area on Rinehart Road in a little less than half a mile). Follow the trail as it winds parallel to the creek and then heads uphill. You'll reach the Kowomu Trail at 3.7 miles. Take a left, following the rural road. When you begin to head left away from the road, at 4 miles, you'll head precipitously uphill once again; in fact, you're now at the hike's highest elevation, more than 750 feet. You'll begin to make your descent toward Big Pipe Creek and the Meadows Trail / Switchback Trail junction. Cross the creek at 4.4 miles, and then rejoin the trail by going right at 4.5 miles.

At 4.8 miles, you'll reach the trail split you earlier passed to extend the hike. This time, take a left, crossing Saw Mill Road. Take a right at 5.3 miles, and cross a wooden footbridge; the area opens up into a field of wildflowers. Take a left; you're now in the Hashawha Environmental Appreciation Area (see page 186), and you'll see Big Pipe Creek on the right. Paralleling the creek, is a beautiful open area—a tremendous old maple tree shades a picnic bench that's surrounded on all sides by the semicircular sweep of the creek. Take a right on the boardwalk over the creek and up the woods—you'll pass a sign alerting you that you are leaving Hashawha.

Climb a hill that is steep and rocky but relatively short, less than a third of a mile. At the top of the hill, take a left. You're now on a portion of the trail that you took at the beginning of the hike, but this time, take a left at the white blazes at the group of pine trees at 6.1 miles. Follow this short switchback through the pines and emerge at the edge of a pond. Take a right, and you will find your car ahead on the left.

NEARBY ACTIVITIES

The Union Mills hiking area includes the Hashawha Environmental Appreciation Area and Bear Branch Nature Center. See page 186 for a description of hiking opportunities at Hashawha. To reach Bear Branch Nature Center, follow the directions above for Union Mills, but pass the stables and the EQUESTRIAN TRAIL PARKING sign and continue another 0.7 miles until you see the WELCOME TO HASHAWHA AND BEAR BRANCH NATURE CENTER sign. Turn here and then take a right at the sign for the nature center. For sustenance after the tough hike at Union Mills, head south on MD 97 into downtown Westminster, which is full of restaurants, antiques shops, and museums. The Maryland Wine Festival takes place each September at the Carroll County Farm Museum grounds in Westminster; for information: (410) 386-3880, (800) 654-4645, or **www.marylandwine.com/mdwinefest**. For the museum: **www.ccgovernment.carr.org/ccg/farmmus.**

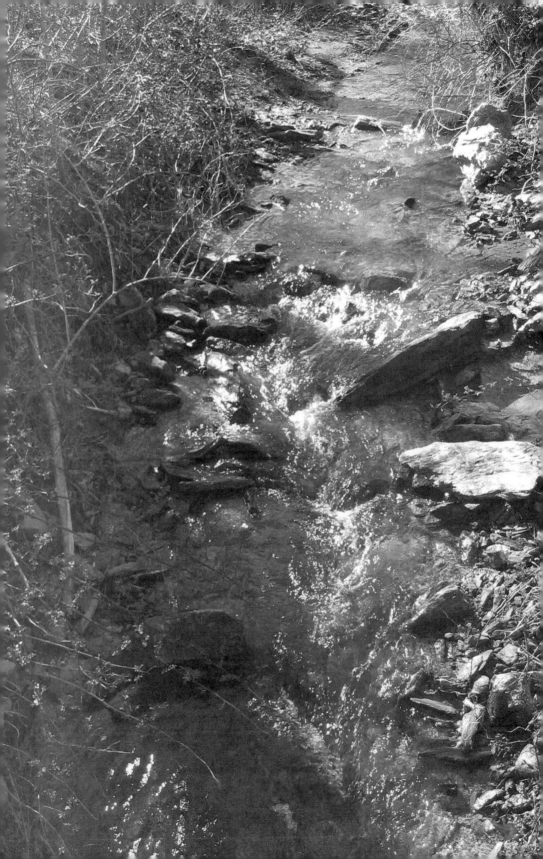

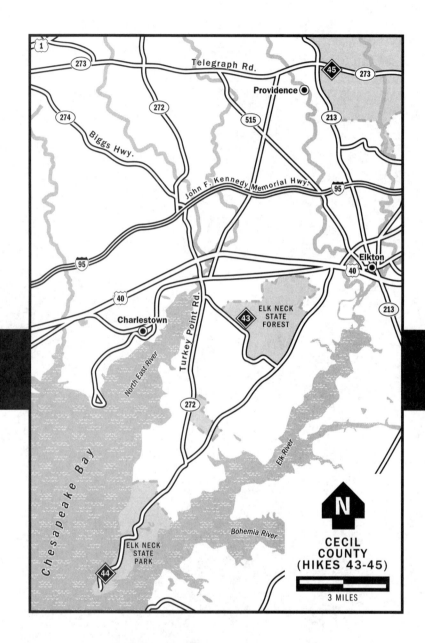

CECIL COUNTY

43 ELK NECK STATE FOREST

KEY AT-A-GLANCE INFORMATION

LENGTH: 6.9 miles

CONFIGURATION: 2 intersecting loops

DIFFICULTY: Moderate–strenuous

SCENERY: Mature forest, marsh, Plum Creek Pond

EXPOSURE: More shade than sun

TRAFFIC: Light

TRAIL SURFACE: Sand/gravel, dirt

HIKING TIME: 2.5–3 hours

ACCESS: Sunrise–sunset

MAPS: USGS North East. A detailed trail map is available at the Elk Neck State Park headquarters and online at www.easycart.net/ MarylandDepartmentofNatural Resources/Central_Maryland _Trail_Guides.html.

WHEELCHAIR ACCESS: No

FACILITIES: Shooting range (bow, handgun, rifle)

SPECIAL COMMENTS: Elk Neck State Forest is popular for hunting. If you hike during hunting season (generally during the autumn months), wear orange or hike on Sundays, when hunting is prohibited. For a hunting schedule, call (410) 260-8540 or (877) 620-8367, or visit www.dnr.state.md.us/ huntersguide.

- -

GPS Trailhead
Coordinates
UTM Zone (WGS84) 18S
Easting 421371
Northing 4381620
Latitude N 39' 34.841452"
Longitude W 75' 54.933958"

IN BRIEF

Hike through diverse wooded flatland, rolling hills, and marshlands in Elk Neck State Park's lesser-known cousin.

DESCRIPTION:

Identified on maps as Trails 1, 2, and 3, the "trails" are actually forest roads. Though wide and offering limited vehicle access, the roads are flanked by thick woods: mixed deciduous trees and evergreens. Initially, things can be a bit unnerving; in addition to the occasional car coming through, you'll hear gunshots from the handgun and rifle shooting range you'll pass at 0.6 miles. Beyond it is a landfill (out of sight of where you are now) that offers good habitat for whippoorwills and a variety of owls. Once beyond the shooting range, things become considerably more pleasant and isolated. Vehicles are prohibited from going farther than this point.

Now that the road is all yours, the encroaching forest of pine, maple, oak, sassafras, ash, hickory, and poplar seems to crowd in even more. At 1.3 miles, to the left, is the blue-blazed Mason-Dixon Trail, a 190-mile trail that runs through Pennsylvania, Delaware, and Maryland. Pass it for now. Come

- -

Directions ─────────────────→

Take I-95 north from Baltimore to Exit 100, MD Route 272 south. Go 2.5 miles through the town of North East, and then take a left on Irishtown Road. The Forest entrance is 1.7 miles to the left. Go 0.4 miles to the parking area to the left in front of the water tower. The sand and gravel road you just turned off is Trail #1. Head left on it. (If it's spring and you're interested in seeing nesting worm-eating and hooded warblers, first walk down the hill behind the tower.)

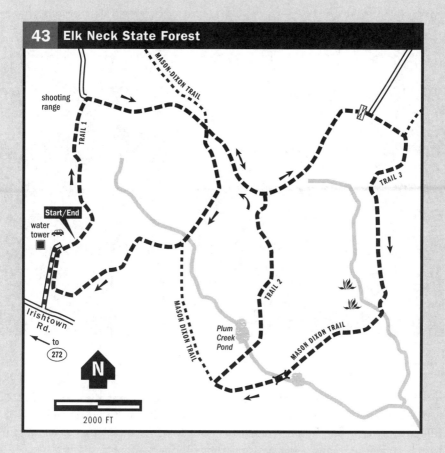

43 Elk Neck State Forest

MASON-DIXON TRAIL

shooting range

TRAIL 1

Start/End

water tower

Irishtown Rd.

to 272

N

2000 FT

MASON-DIXON TRAIL

TRAIL 3

TRAIL 2

MASON DIXON TRAIL

Plum Creek Pond

MASON DIXON TRAIL

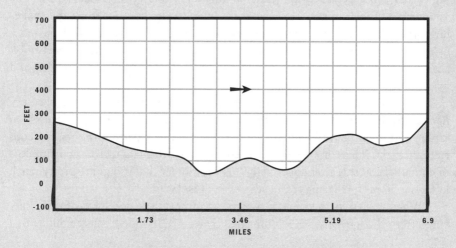

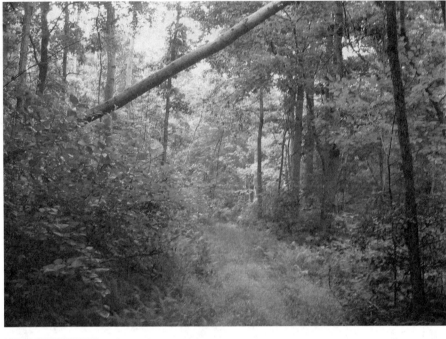

Mason-Dixon Trail

to a Y at 1.6 miles. To the right is Trail #2; continue straight ahead on Trail #1, here identified as Mountain Laurel Lane. The road begins to narrow a bit, soon filled with the strong summertime aroma of cedar. An understory of mountain laurel, azalea, fern, and other native shrubs fill out the forest.

When you reach a gate at 2.1 miles, take a right onto Trail #3 and then another quick right at 2.3 miles into the woods on the narrow, blue-blazed Mason-Dixon Trail. This is a very woodsy and tight, packed dirt trail. At 2.9 miles, tall grass overtakes the trail in summer—hike up the socks. This lasts 100 feet and then returns to packed dirt. Be on the lookout for frogs and snakes lurking in the grass. The trail soon hugs the edge of a big marsh. I passed a great heron rookery here. At the sound of my approach, some dozen birds took flight. Their enormous wingspans and odd guttural calls were both startling and magnificent.

Cross a tiny marsh outlet and then head back into the woods on the very narrow trail. In fact, for a moment, it's barely discernible, but the blazes soon return and then the trail widens again. There are many path offshoots, but continue straight. There are trees over the trail every 100 feet or so, requiring lots of climbing. But this strenuous exercise is a reminder that things are pretty much left alone here, furthering the heady sense of isolation.

When you come to an earthen dam spanning a little pond, look for the tiny cut path to the left—there's a footbridge there. At 2.8 miles, emerge onto Road

Trail #2; take a right. You'll soon come to Plum Creek Pond, a beautiful open spot ringed by aquatic plants. Between the marshy area and the thick forest surrounding, it's the perfect spot for birding. Depending on the season, some of the birds you may see include kinglets, thrushes, nuthatches, woodpeckers, vireos, and the occasional scarlet tanager.

If the collapsed trail bridge spanning the pond feeder has not been repaired enough for easy crossing, you can take a small path before and around the pond. Once you're beyond the pond, take another right and then go around it that way; you'll soon link up to the trail.

Either way you've gotten beyond the pond, continue straight away from it on Trail #2. When you reach the intersection of Trails #1 and #2, where you went straight before, take a left and begin to backtrack. When you soon see the Mason-Dixon Trail you passed earlier (this time on the right), be on the lookout for the Mason-Dixon Trail portion on the left—it comes 0.1 mile later. Take it.

You're now back in deep woods. Cross a stream. Keep going straight at the next split and stay straight until you come to a T, and then take a right. At a little over 6 miles, you'll emerge onto the Road Trail #1 you used to enter the forest in your car. Take a right and your car will be just up ahead to the left.

NEARBY ACTIVITIES

The town of North East is a pleasant place to spend a few hours. Among the attractions is the Upper Bay Museum, two big buildings on the North East River, housing an extensive collection of hunting, boating, and fishing artifacts. Call (410) 287-5909 for information. Heading back to I-95, if you continue past the exit, you can follow the signs to Plumpton Park Zoo in Rising Sun. It is home to a collection of indigenous animals as well as African creatures. Visit **www.plumptonpark zoo.org** or call (410) 658-6850 for information.

44 ELK NECK STATE PARK

KEY AT-A-GLANCE INFORMATION

LENGTH: 13.5 miles total hike/bike/drive

CONFIGURATION: Varies

DIFFICULTY: Easy–moderate

SCENERY: Beach, Elk River and Chesapeake Bay, forests, marshes

EXPOSURE: Varies

TRAFFIC: Light–moderate

TRAIL SURFACE: Packed dirt; some sand and gravel on Green and Orange

HIKING TIME: 1 hour each for Red and Blue; 1.5 hours each for Orange and Green; 0.5 hours for White

ACCESS: Sunrise–sunset; there's no fee for the park, but there is a $5 toll bridge on I-95 crossing into Cecil County.

MAPS: USGS Earleville, Spesutie. A detailed trail map is available at the Elk Neck State Park headquarters and online at www.easycart.net/MarylandDepartmentof NaturalResources/Central_Maryland_Trail_Guides.html.

WHEELCHAIR ACCESS: No

FACILITIES: Picnic pavilions, campsites; playgrounds; boat launch

SPECIAL COMMENTS: None of the trails intersect—bringing a bike makes going from one to another easy and pleasurable.

GPS Trailhead Coordinates

UTM Zone (WGS84) 18S

Easting 413444

Northing 4368265

Latitude N 39' 27.576585"

Longitude W 76' 0.367119"

IN BRIEF

Do it all at Elk Neck State Park in one long day of hiking and biking. If it's summer, leave time for swimming as well.

DESCRIPTION

Head straight away from the parking area on the wide, packed dirt trail. Great views of the Chesapeake Bay are yours by just peering to the right. Eventually, thick woods crowd out the views. At the split at 0.6 miles, go left, where there's a raptor viewing area. Depending on the season, you'll see vultures, eagles, ospreys, buteos, hawks, harriers, kites, kestrels, merlins, and falcons.

Reach the Turkey Point Lighthouse at 0.8 miles. Highest of the Bay's 74 lighthouses, it was built in 1833. (For more information on the Lighthouse, visit **www.caracove.com/tpls.**) Sheer cliffs fall away from the lighthouse ahead, dropping into the bay. Though many signs warn of danger, you can go right to the edge. With the lighthouse behind you, head right and back into the woods onto a narrow trail that eventually comes to water level. Walk along the water for a few hundred feet and then turn back into the woods at a little beach, following the trail back to the parking area.

Back in your car, drive north on Old Elk Neck Road and take a right on Rogues Harbor Road after about a mile (look for signs

----

Directions

Take I-95 north from Baltimore to Exit 100, MD Route 272 south through the town of North East. Follow Route 272 South (Old Elk Neck Road) 12 miles until it ends. This is the trailhead for the Blue Trail.

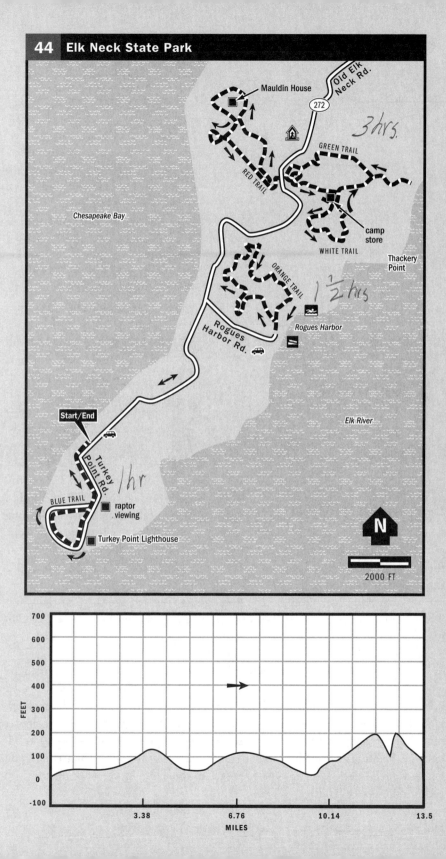

Chesapeake Bay

Mauldin House

Old Elk Neck Rd.

272

3 hrs.

GREEN TRAIL

RED TRAIL

camp store

WHITE TRAIL

Thackery Point

ORANGE TRAIL

1½ hrs

Rogues Harbor Rd.

Rogues Harbor

Elk River

Start/End

Turkey Point Rd.

1 hr

BLUE TRAIL

raptor viewing

Turkey Point Lighthouse

N

2000 FT

700
600
500
400
300
200
100
0
-100

FEET

3.38   6.76   10.14   13.5

MILES

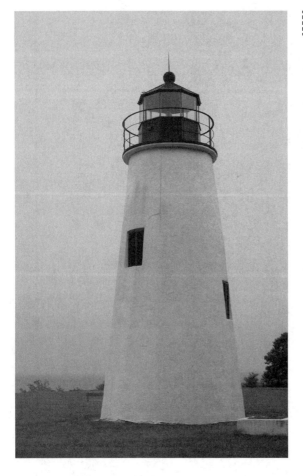

Turkey Point Lighthouse

to the boat launch). Follow it to the parking lot on the left. Go all the way to its farthest end and you'll see the trailhead for the Orange Trail. At the first split soon after starting, go left. Come to the edge of a marsh and look for herons. The Orange is an extraordinarily beautiful trail, wooded with poplar, hickory, and oak and full of wildlife: deer, squirrels, and owls are abundant. It feels quite isolated until it runs near a campground—because of thick woods, you'll rarely see the campground, but it can be noisy during summer. When you reach the beach at 2 miles, take a right and walk along the beach toward the rock jumble in the distance. Climb along the rocks and reenter the woods just before the split you took left coming in. Now go straight ahead to the parking area. It's time to unlock the bike.

Bike back out to Old Elk Neck Road and go right. Take the first right, following signs to the camp store, and go to the registration booth. Purchase an interpretive guide for $1 for the White Trail. Lock up the bike at the camp store and go across the road to the White trailhead.

The White Trail is short and pleasant, with foliage clearly marked by wooden posts. Along the loop, you'll see poplar, three varieties of oak, maple, holly, two types of dogwood, birch, serviceberry, paw paw, beech, hickory, mountain laurel, two types of blueberry, sassafras, gum, witch hazel, sycamore, pine, cherry, and locust. Each is described in the corresponding guide. You'll exit the White Trail on the camp road, but a bit farther east than where you entered. Head back left and when you get to the camp store, walk behind it to pick up the Green Trail.

From behind the camp store, take a left. Don't worry about the lack of blazes—you're actually on a secondary path that connects to the Green Trail.

White Trail

When you reach a split, take a right; otherwise, you'll end up on a park road. You'll soon reach the wide Green Trail; head right on it. After 0.4 mile-sonce you're on the Green Trail, you'll come to a beaver pond, stocked with bass and sunfish. A Maryland Non-tidal Freshwater Fishing license is required to fish. Look for mallards, black ducks, and teal at the pond.

Take a left at the Y at the end of the pond. Follow it to the camp loop and go left until the end of the loop. There's a little path heading to a beach from there. This beach abuts the Elk River, just north of Thackeray Point.

Backtrack and when you reach the pond again, go left. The trail becomes very tight and close. When you come to a T, take a left away from the water and up the hill. You'll quickly come to the back of the camp store. Time to grab the bike for the final trail.

Head back out to Old Elk Neck and take a right. Almost immediately, take a left. The trailhead for the Red Trail is just ahead on the left. Lock the bike to a tree here. The Red Trail follows the contours of the N.E. Beach Access Road until it splits toward a picnic area. The trail loops around the picnic area, passing the Mauldin House near the top of Mauldin Mountain (really a hill, to be more precise), which rises almost 300 feet above the surrounding land.

The Red Trail is listed as "difficult" on the Elk Neck park map because of its ups and downs, but it's nothing too strenuous. However, if this is the last hike of the day after doing all the others above, you'll feel it. Nevertheless, the tall canopy of locust, beech, maple, poplar, hickory, and oak won't fail to inspire. With a thriving understory, including wildflowers (and springtime blooms from dogwoods), the Red Trail is truly beautiful. Among the foliage, look for red-breasted nuthatch, cedar waxwing, and pileated woodpecker. When you reach your bike again, pedal back to the Orange Trail parking lot. Remember that it's at the end of Rogues Harbor Road, at the signs for the boat launch.

NEARBY ACTIVITIES

The town of North East is a pleasant place to spend a few hours. Among the attractions is the Upper Bay Museum, two big buildings on the North East River, housing an extensive collection of hunting, boating, and fishing artifacts. Call (410) 287-5909 for information. Heading back to I-95, if you continue past the exit, you can follow the signs to Plumpton Park Zoo in Rising Sun. It is home to a collection of indigenous animals as well as African creatures. Visit **www.plumptonpark zoo.org** or call (410) 658-6850 for information. For more hiking, visit either Elk Neck State Forest (see page 216) or Fair Hill NRMA (see page 225).

FAIR HILL NATURAL RESOURCE MANAGEMENT AREA 45

IN BRIEF

Almost endless opportunities in this bucolic corner of extreme northeastern Maryland.

DESCRIPTION

With more than 5,600 acres and 75 miles of multiuse trails, Fair Hill has something for everyone. This hike takes in the highlights of the three largest trails—Orange, Green, and Blue—all sitting north of Fair Hill's dividing line, MD 273. As you travel through the diverse landscape, keep an eye out for beavers, coyotes, foxes, raccoons, and white-tailed deer.

From the parking area, walk into the field beyond the collection box toward the wood line. You'll see a groove in the grass and an orange blaze on a post. When you reach a crushed-rock farm road at 0.3 miles, head into the woods, composed of enormous, thick, mature trees, mostly ironwood, beech, oak, and poplar. At the wide trail at 0.4 miles, take a left. Then, after another couple of hundred feet, take a left again into the woods—if you come to a bow hunting parking area, you've gone a bit too far. You'll soon emerge into an open field, one of many in this hike. Follow

KEY AT-A-GLANCE INFORMATION

LENGTH: 13–18 miles (see Special Comments)

CONFIGURATION: Jagged loop

DIFFICULTY: Strenuous

SCENERY: Forest, streams, historical sites

EXPOSURE: More shade than sun

TRAFFIC: Light, but many trails are used for equestrians. Be alert.

TRAIL SURFACE: Sand, gravel, crushed rock, asphalt, packed dirt

HIKING TIME: 6+ hours

ACCESS: Dawn–dusk. Parking $3 for Maryland residents, $4 for others; $5 to cross Millard Tydings Bridge over the Susquehanna eastbound.

MAPS: Stationary maps at parking areas. A complete trail guide can be purchased online at www.easycart .net/MarylandDepartmentofNatural Resources/Central_Maryland_Trail _Guides.html.

WHEELCHAIR ACCESS: No

FACILITIES: Portable toilets at parking areas; water at visitor center

SPECIAL COMMENTS: This hike takes in only the 3 largest blazed trails. The remaining 2 can be added to or substituted for those described.

Directions ——————————>

Take I-695 to I-95 north toward Delaware and Philadelphia. Take exit 100 to MD Rt. 272 north. Go 6 miles to a right on MD Rt. 273. Go 4.8 miles to a left turn into Parking Area #1. The Orange Trail is at the far end of the parking lot, to the left of Rt. 273. To go to the visitor center, pass Parking Area #1 and turn right into entrance #3. Turn left onto Ranger Skinner Road, turn left onto Training Center Road, and cross over Rt. 273. Turn right onto Tawes Drive. The visitor center is on the right.

GPS Trailhead Coordinates

UTM Zone (WGS84) 18S

Easting 426235

Northing 4394797

Latitude N 39' 41.990368"

Longitude W 75' 51.624305"

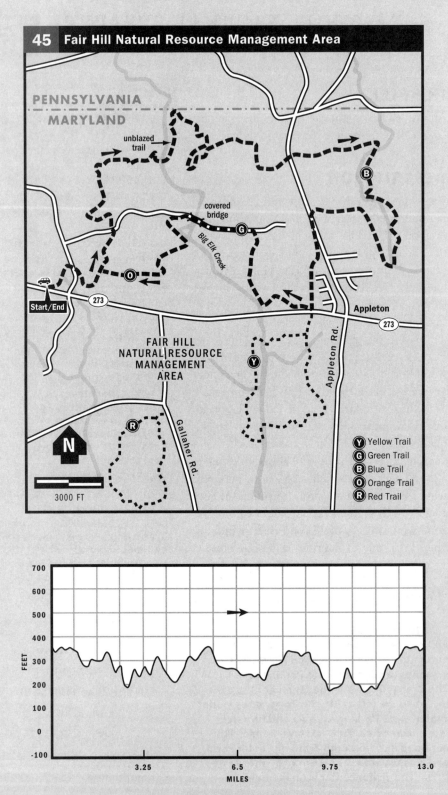

45   Fair Hill Natural Resource Management Area

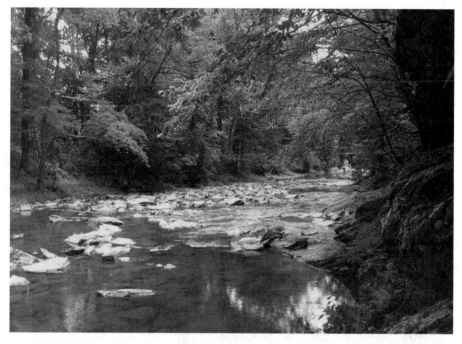

Big Elk Creek

the grooves in the grass (there are still blazes, very prominently marked throughout). When the trail splits, take a left.

At 0.7 miles, cross to the tree line and then to another open field. Take a left into the woods at the NO HORSES sign onto a small, narrow, twisty trail, which is simply gorgeous. You'll find many such hiker–equestrian splits; in each case, taking the hiker trail leads to a path that's too narrow for horses. The trails all wind up in the same place eventually, so take the hiker trails: they're beautiful, not to mention free of manure. At 0.9 miles, cross a little footbridge and emerge into an open field again. Head left and, at just under 1 mile, reach paved Tawes Drive. Take a left and then a quick right back into the woods. At the first split, head right.

At 1.2 miles, cross a little stream and then an unpaved road, which you'll cross yet again at 1.7 miles. Traverse a field at 1.8 miles. On the other side of the field, take a right at the orange blazes. Cross a stream and marshy areas on wooden boardwalks, and follow the trail as it takes in a series of switchbacks. When you reach the wider trail at 2.3 miles, take a left. When you get to the bottom of the hill, go right and continue along Big Elk Creek.

Here things get potentially confusing. You can stay on the Orange Trail all the way to a crossing on the unpaved Black Bridge Road. But the arguably more interesting route is to momentarily walk off the blazed trails and cross Big Elk Creek at 2.8 miles on a solid slab of cement to the left. Big Elk Creek operates

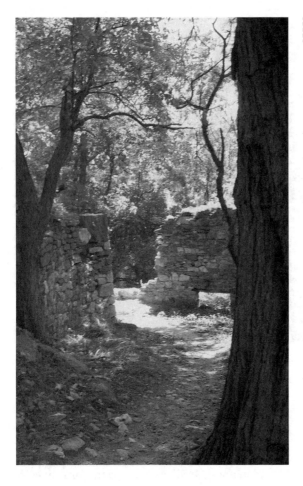

Stone ruins along Orange Trail

as a put-and-take trout stream (stocked with brown and rainbow trout) and is home to smallmouth bass, sunfish, and bluegill. Also be on the lookout for kingfishers and bald eagles. Once on the other side, the trail is prominent and easy to follow, but unblazed. (You might see a sporadic circular blue blaze here and elsewhere along the hike; these blazes are not part of the Blue Trail but indicate the Blue Diamond Trail, an alternative route during muddy or wet conditions that helps fight against erosion on the other trails.) You'll reach Fair Hill's boundary line at 3.3 miles. No sign will tell you this, but the boundary line is actually the Mason-Dixon Line, and stepping a foot beyond puts you in Pennsylvania.

Head right, following the switchbacks to the top of the hill. At the open field at the top of the hill, take a right. Keep an eye out for hawks, owls, and vultures searching for prey here. You'll see a gravel road in front of you and the McCloskey picnic area to the right. Cross the gravel road and you'll soon pass through stone ruins. Go around some deer exclosures in a stunning area. You'll follow the rocky, rooty trail along a farm boundary line, marked by a collapsing fence to the right. A big ridge falls to a valley below you to the left—it's quite beautiful.

At 4 miles, next to Big Elk Creek, you'll emerge onto a wide gravel trail that is blazed green. Go left, then left again immediately at the split. When you reach a field at 4.6 miles, take a right. Take another right at the split at 4.8 miles. Pass more ruins to the right: a silo and stone wall. There's another field at 5.2 miles; down the hill to the right is Parking Area #3. The Blue Trail goes straight. Cross Appleton Road on an elevated bridge, and follow the farm road. Your next spot of shade comes at 5.7 miles.

At 6.1 miles, go right onto a smaller path at a deer exclosure (a wider path goes straight ahead, but turn here to stay on the Blue Trail). You'll quickly come to and cross Christiana Creek at 6.3; unlike every other waterway featured in this book, this creek actually empties into Delaware Bay, not our more familiar Chesapeake. Take a right and follow the blue blazes into the woods, over a little footbridge spanning a vernal pool. The trail leaves the woods, becomes crushed rock, and then crosses the creek. The trail then becomes a farm road splitting the woods. At 7.7 miles, take a left at the split into an open area, following the farm road. This field-and-forest buffer hosts a multitude of birds, including bobolinks, swifts, swallows, bluebirds, flycatchers, thrushes, indigo buntings, and jays.

At 8.1 miles, go left at the blue blaze. Go through the tunnel at Appleton Road, and come to the junction of the Blue and Green trails. Take a left. Following the Green Trail now, you'll be on crushed rock, heading uphill on an exposed farm road. At 9 miles, you'll reach a bridge spanning MD 273. While this bridge is not part of the hike described here, you can use it to reach the Yellow Trail. If you choose to take it, you'll find the trail just up ahead. It's a 3.2-mile loop that heads downhill toward Big Elk Creek and returns via the west side of the creek.

If you're not taking the Yellow Trail, however, don't go all the way to the bridge. Instead, take a right just before the bridge, so that you're paralleling MD 273 on your left. At 9 miles, continue straight; the trail then turns to cement and follows an old abandoned road (there's even a rotting bridge going over it). At 9.5 miles, before you get to the bridge over Big Elk Creek, take a right over the smaller bridge spanning the feeder for Big Elk, turning away from MD 273. You can follow the Green Trail as it heads more or less straight until reaching Old Union School Road at 10 miles; however, it's more pleasant to take a parallel path in the woods. To do so, look for the first rightward cut into the woods, and then go left at the split. Just make sure to go left over the stream at 9.9 miles; otherwise, you'll end up in a maze of little paths east of where you want to be.

Rejoin the Green Trail and go right, reaching unpaved Old Union School Road, where you'll head left. You'll soon pass an old barn and home to the left. Continue straight ahead and pass through the 1860 Foxcatcher Creek Covered Bridge, one of only two left in Cecil County and a Maryland Historic Civil Engineering Landmark. You'll see Parking Area #2 to the right. Take the Orange Trail on the left. You'll immediately come to a marsh and pond on the left. There's a boardwalk and observation deck. Circle around, passing the nature center on the right, at 11.3 miles. (Run by the Fair Hill Environmental Foundation, the center offers nature programs and day camps; call [410] 398-4909 for more information.) You'll soon come to a path marked NATURE TRAIL. CHILDREN LEARNING. Take this trail, which rejoins the Orange Trail after 0.2 miles. At 11.6 miles, in an area of pine and cedar, take a right at the trail split; take another right at the next split and head downhill. At 12 miles cross a wide trail, and at 12.2 miles rejoin a portion of the trail close to where you began the hike. You will see a sign that reads .8 MILES TO PARKING LOT #1. Now backtrack to the parking area.

To hike the last remaining blazed trail at Fair Hill, you can continue by car—take a left out of the parking area, and then go right on Gallagher Road to the first right onto Big Elk Chapel Road. Parking Area #4 is immediately on the left. The Red Trail is a 2.5-mile loop that runs along an old logging road through forest and field. A rather easy hike, it crosses Grammies Run several times.

NEARBY ACTIVITIES

There's plenty to do right here. Fair Winds Stables offers guided trail rides for ages eight and up: **www.fairwindsstables.com,** (410) 620-3883. Fair Hill also hosts the annual Scottish Games: **www.fairhillscottishgames.org,** (302) 453-8998; the Cecil County Fair: **www .cecilcountyfair.org,** (410) 392-3440; and the Fair Hill Horse Race Track: **www.fairhill races.org,** (410) 398-6565.

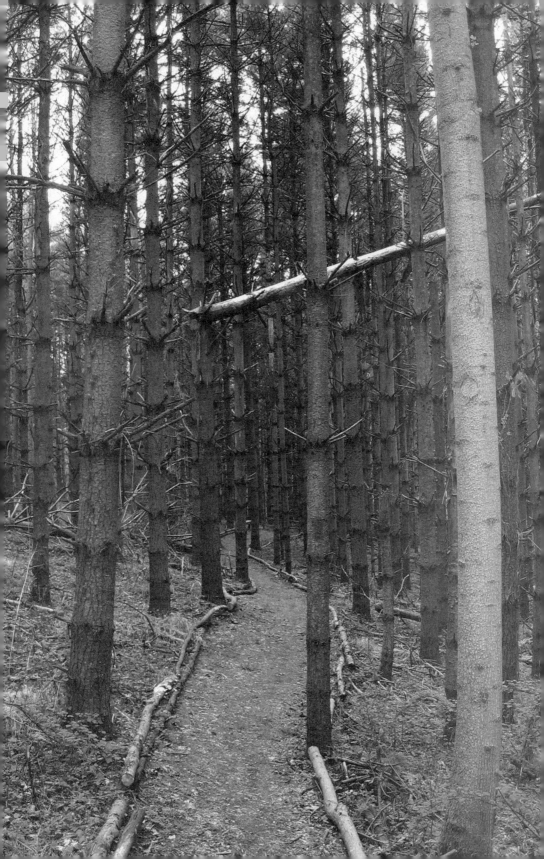

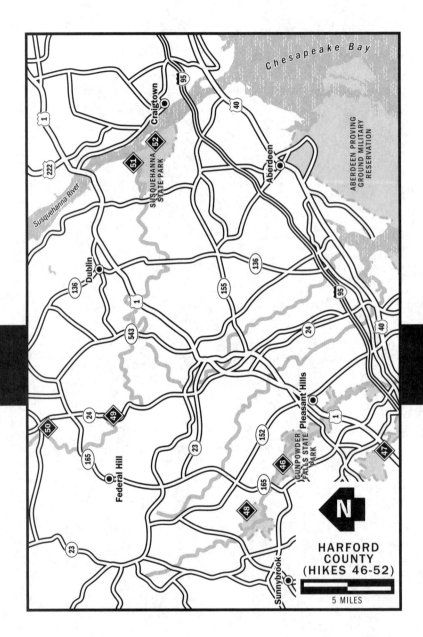

Chesapeake Bay

ABERDEEN PROVING GROUND MILITARY RESERVATION

Susquehanna River

SUSQUEHANNA STATE PARK

Craigtown

Aberdeen

Dublin

GUNPOWDER FALLS STATE PARK

Pleasant Hills

Federal Hill

Sunnybrook

N

HARFORD COUNTY
(HIKES 46-52)

5 MILES

HARFORD COUNTY

46 GUNPOWDER FALLS STATE PARK: PLEASANTVILLE-BOTTOM LOOP

KEY AT-A-GLANCE INFORMATION

LENGTH: 4.5 miles

CONFIGURATION: Loop

DIFFICULTY: Strenuous in summer, moderate otherwise

SCENERY: Riverine and upland forest

EXPOSURE: Shaded

TRAFFIC: Light

TRAIL SURFACE: Packed dirt, rocks

HIKING TIME: 2.5 hours

ACCESS: Dawn–dusk

MAPS: USGS Jarrettsville

WHEELCHAIR ACCESS: No

FACILITIES: None

SPECIAL COMMENTS: You can start this hike on Bottom Road (parking is limited on Pleasantville Road). To get there, take I-695 to Exit 31, Harford Road northwest. Go 8 miles to a left on Fork Road, then go 1.6 miles to a right on Bottom Road. Go 2 miles to the parking spots near the river.

GPS Trailhead
Coordinates

UTM Zone (WGS84) 18S

Easting 374538

Northing 4374092

Latitude N 39' 30.438402"

Longitude W 76' 27.560334"

IN BRIEF

Hike along the Gunpowder River, then ascend to the exceedingly beautiful rail bed of the defunct Maryland and Pennsylvania Railroad.

DESCRIPTION

If you're doing this hike in summer, a word of warning: wear long pants. I didn't, and by the time I was through with the initial section, my legs were a pair of itchy, bloody pulps. There's poison ivy galore, plus sticker bushes, devil's tear thumb, and nettles. I spent a good amount of time cursing, but I'm incredibly glad I didn't turn around—this hike winds up being one of the prettiest anywhere around. (Indeed, even in this first section, there are loads of wild-flowers to temper the irritants.)

Initially heading downstream, make your way through a rather narrow yellow-blazed trail before heading uphill after a few hundred feet. (There's a path heading to the water, but it's used mostly by anglers and often gets eroded.) Uphill now, and away from the blood-inducing foliage, you'll cross a beautiful little horseshoe stream. Many white-tailed deer congregate here. Though you're now well above the water, you'll very quickly descend to water level. When the trail splits, head right toward the Gunpowder River; lots of blazes tell you you're in the right place.

Directions

Take I-695 to Exit 31, Harford Road northwest. Go 8 miles to a left on Fork Road. Go 2.5 miles to a hard right on Pleasantville Road. Go 1 mile and cross the bridge over the Gunpowder to a small parking area immediately on the right. The trail heads downhill toward the river from the parking area.

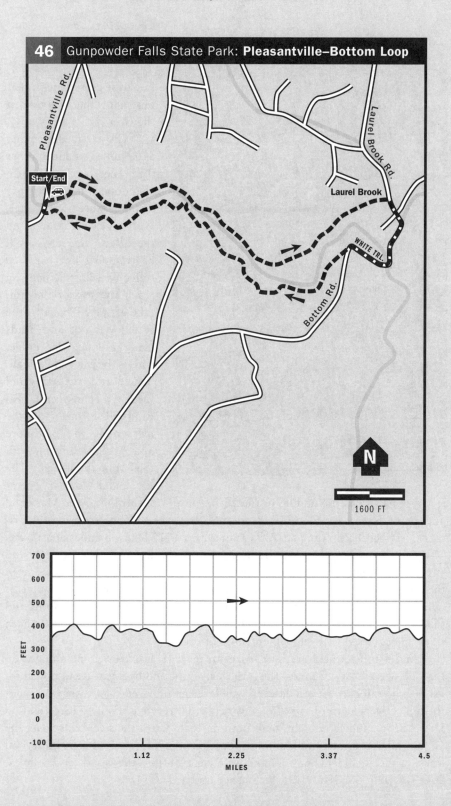

46 Gunpowder Falls State Park: **Pleasantville–Bottom Loop**

Pleasantville Rd.

Laurel Brook Rd.

Start/End

Laurel Brook

WHITE TRL.

Bottom Rd.

N

1600 FT

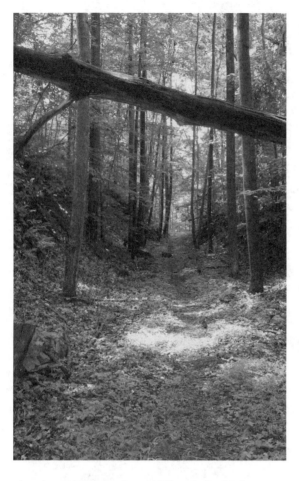

Look for geese, ducks, herons, and kingfishers along the river.

Cross a feeder stream at 0.6 miles, and in another 0.2 miles you'll pass an abandoned stone structure near the water. Soon after, the trail heads straight up the hill to the left; you'll be tramping on shards of reflective schist. When you reach the top of the hill, take a right. Blessedly, the trail levels out and heads along a long, flat grade. This is the Ma and Pa Trail, named after the Maryland (Ma) and Pennsylvania (Pa) Railroad, formed from the merger of the Baltimore and Lehigh Railway with the York Southern. The Ma and Pa was in operation from 1901 to the middle of the 20th century. According to the Maryland and Pennsylvania Railroad Preservation Society, the rail line covering the distance between Baltimore and York, Pennsylvania (45 highway miles apart), was 77 miles, reflecting the meandering nature of the line. But here it's flat and straight—and simply beautiful. For my money, this section of trail is one of the nicest anywhere in the Baltimore metro region. The river flows a couple of hundred feet below to the right, across valleys and hills filled with birdsong and shaded by mature wooded forest. The trail sits on a riser with gorges on both sides, interspersed with sudden uprisings of rock.

At 1.4 miles, there are blue blazes to the left, but keep going straight on the yellow trail. At 1.7 miles, the trail turns right and begins to head downhill, leaving the rail bed. As you descend, you'll see an unpaved road at the bottom of the hill. This is Laurel Brook Road, which you'll reach at 2 miles. Turn right on Laurel Brook and go straight, onto Bottom Road. Cross the steel bridge over the Gunpowder, and then head uphill to the right. Look for white blazes on several trees on the shoulder. Look for the little cut path into the woods at 2.4 miles. Take this white-blazed trail, which heads upstream.

You'll slowly descend to river level. This is very typical Gunpowder: piedmont hills with medium-size, well-spaced forest covered in ferns. At 3.1 miles, when the trail splits, go right down the hill, among the beech trees. Cross a beautiful rivulet at 3.3 miles; notice where the earth has been eroded to rock. The water heads over these little riffles. At 3.5 miles, the trail swings left and heads into a level area. When you get to the other side of this area, head downhill to the right toward the river, among a carpet of ferns. Cross a feeder stream. At 3.7 miles, at the top of the hill, take a right. The trail becomes wide and flat again. This is another great section, running high on a ridge, with the river a couple of hundred feet below to the right. Even though Pleasantville Road isn't too far away, I wouldn't expect any people. In fact, in this section alone I saw three herons, a dozen deer, and no humans.

At 4.3 miles, the trail makes a rightward cut toward the river. You'll no doubt notice that it also continues straight ahead. You can hike there, but the trail is completely overgrown and pretty difficult; take comfort in knowing that you already dealt with that at the hike's beginning (if it's summertime, of course). Assuming you've instead headed downhill, you'll soon hear cars crossing the steel bridge over Pleasantville Road, where you're parked.

NEARBY ACTIVITIES

Boordy Vineyards, Maryland's oldest family-run winery, is a short distance away and offers daily tours at 2 and 3:30 p.m. Head south on Harford Road to a right on Long Green Pike. Follow the signs. For more information, call (410) 592-5015, or visit **www.boordy.com.**

47 GUNPOWDER FALLS STATE PARK: SWEATHOUSE BRANCH WILDLANDS

KEY AT-A-GLANCE INFORMATION

LENGTH: 8.7 miles

CONFIGURATION: Loop and out-and-back with loops

DIFFICULTY: Moderate–strenuous

SCENERY: Gunpowder River and branches, upland forest, ruins

EXPOSURE: Mostly shade

TRAFFIC: Light–moderate on west side of Rt. 1 (Stocksdale, Sweathouse, Wildlands), moderate on east side (Lost Pond, Sawmill)

TRAIL SURFACE: Dirt, rock, sand

HIKING TIME: 4 hours

ACCESS: Dawn–dusk

MAPS: USGS White Marsh; large stationary map on the bulletin board in the parking area

WHEELCHAIR ACCESS: No

FACILITIES: None

SPECIAL COMMENTS: Because the parking area sits in the middle of this hike, you can easily do either just the west (of US 1) trails, or the east. The hike described here does both sides. Bikes are not allowed on the west side Wildland trails. Gunpowder Falls State Park headquarters is located at the Jerusalem Mill; (410) 592-2897.

- -

GPS Trailhead Coordinates

UTM Zone (WGS84) 18S

Easting 375675

Northing 4365230

Latitude N 39' 25.658712"

Longitude W 76' 26.667953"

IN BRIEF

Stroll through the floodplain along Gunpowder River as well as upland forest, taking in an abandoned millpond, sawmill ruins, and swimming holes.

DESCRIPTION

Doing the west side trails first, begin the hike by walking under the US 1 tunnel and entering the Sweathouse Branch Wildlands Area. After 500 feet, go right onto the pink-blazed Wildlands Trail. It initially runs alongside US 1, so it can be a bit loud, but the trail soon heads away through a beautiful area of mature trees, many easily 50 or 60 years old, among them some fantastically large beeches. By 0.75 miles, the sound of US 1 is gone and you're left only in pristine woods filled with birdsong.

At 0.9 miles, the trail gets sandy and crosses a stream soon after; you're likely to scatter a few frogs as you cross. At 1.1 miles, the hill is covered with lichen-stained rocks. At 1.3 miles, come to a big pine plantation straight ahead. Go left here. While these pines do crowd out other tree species, the plantation is really quite beautiful.

At 1.4 miles, take a right onto the blue-blazed Stocksdale Trail, skirting the edge of the pine plantation. Soon you'll see lots of ferns. Take notice of the posts telling hikers to keep left, as there is private land to the right. At 2.1 miles, take a right onto the yellow-blazed

- -

Directions ⟶

Take I-695 to Exit 32, MD 1 north (Belair Road), and go 5.5 miles; look for the parking lot on the right after you cross Gunpowder River. The trails start at the edge of the parking lot behind the bulletin board.

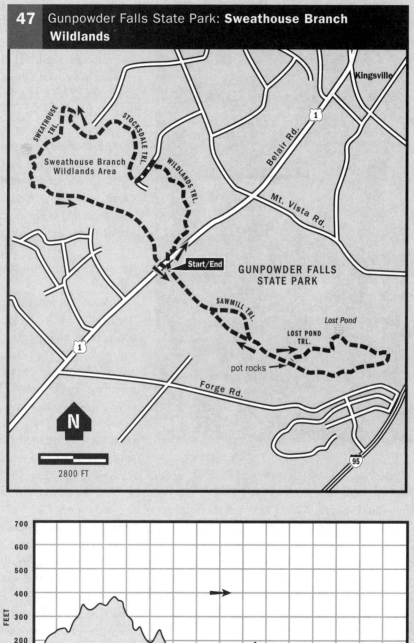

47 Gunpowder Falls State Park: **Sweathouse Branch Wildlands**

Kingsville

SWEATHOUSE TRL.

STOCKSDALE TRL.

WILDLANDS TRL.

Sweathouse Branch Wildlands Area

Belair Rd.

Mt. Vista Rd.

Start/End

GUNPOWDER FALLS STATE PARK

SAWMILL TRL.

Lost Pond

LOST POND TRL.

pot rocks →

Forge Rd.

N

2800 FT

95

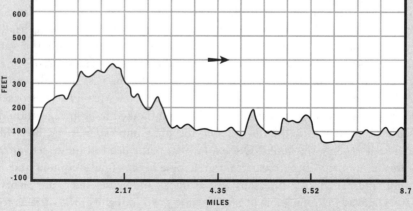

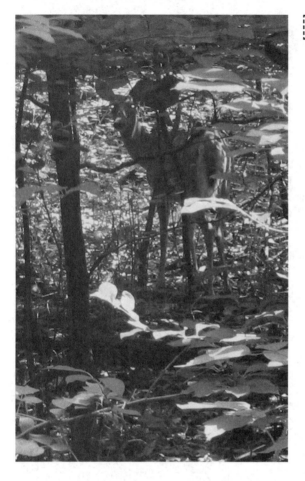

Wary eyes on the Sweathouse Trail

Sweathouse Trail. There's another pine plantation at 2.2 miles. The forest floor here has been affected by the pines crowding out sunlight. But while this spot is not very diverse, it is lovely. In fact, it's quite picturesque, especially in spring and summer, with its carpet of green and wildflowers. Walk along the ridge; the hills fall quite a bit to your left.

Start descending into the valley below; you'll soon hear the gurgle of water. Small rock ledges are piled along the trail to guard against erosion. This is just another example of how lovingly (but unobtrusively) maintained these trails are. At 2.5 miles, reach the Sweathouse Branch and hike alongside it, traveling downstream. At 2.6 miles, look for a knotty old twisted beech on the left; it's a beautiful and unique-looking tree, having suffered the torsions of age and weather.

At 3 miles, cross the stream, its vernal pools teeming with life. There are still yellow blazes on the other side. Once you've crossed, move away from the water and head uphill. Soon after, take a right at the Y-intersection, heading steeply downhill. At 3.2 miles, you'll reach a large pool formed from the waters of Long Green Run where you can swim. When you've had your fill of this charming spot, walk along the trail heading downstream. Pass the rightward cut at 3.4 miles and then cross Sweathouse Branch, a pretty stream full of frogs and fish. The trail becomes a bit more closed in and flanked by lush vegetation, but it's still prominent. You'll be paralleling the Big Gunpowder River. Box elders and sycamores hug the banks. Quite a few cut paths head to the water, providing lots of opportunities to search for great blue herons (multitudinous and easy to spot) and belted kingfishers, as well as ducks and geese. There are plenty of beavers here as well; muskrats live nearby, too. Swimming near the surface, trout and white and yellow perch are easy to spot. Do keep your eyes on the trail occasionally as well, as hordes of tiny frogs leap about underfoot.

At 3.8 miles, you'll see the other end of the Stocksdale Trail to the left. Continue on straight (unless you want to hike the only portion of the trail you didn't do). Many limestone boulders decorate the trail to the left. At 4.4 miles, the other end of the Wildlands Trail is to the left, followed soon by more beautiful rock formations and a little grotto. Reach the US 1 tunnel at 4.6 miles; the parking area is just on the other side.

To continue hiking and take in the Lost Pond and Sawmill trails, go straight, keeping the river to your right. You can either follow the trail along the water's edge or take the official Lost Pond trailhead, which has blue blazes and begins at the edge of the woods up the hill at the end of the parking lot. The two trails closely parallel each other and eventually connect. I took the trail along the water's edge, but be aware that during heavy rains, mud and maybe even a few inches of water may cover it.

Please note that I've reset the mileage here in case you are just hiking one side or the other from the parking area. As you walk along the floodplain, you'll pass a massive sycamore that seems to have long outlived its expected life span. Soon after, you'll see another large sycamore jutting over the water. Someone (for good or ill) has nailed wooden steps into its trunk. The result is that you can climb up to a nice river perch with views of the swiftly running water.

Continuing on, you'll see beech trees with their roots spread over a rock outcropping. Ford a small creek at 0.4 miles, where you will head left to the yellow-blazed Sawmill Trail. Descend and follow Broad Run to the site of the early-19th-century Carroll Sawmill ruins and millrace.

Rejoin the Lost Pond Trail by taking a left; you'll soon see an enormous tulip poplar with a hollowed-out trunk, which would make quite a den for some large rodent or snake. Cross Broad Run on a little footbridge at 0.7 miles; as you continue along the trail, you'll hear the wonderful sound of rapids on the right from the large rocks in the river. Just before you reach the 1-mile mark, head right to the "pot rocks," so called because of the deep potholes created in the bedrock from the river erosion; a wooden signpost points the way. This is an excellent place to sit awhile and take in the sounds of the noisy river.

When you've had your fill, head back up the hill and continue to the right. The trail leads uphill through an upland forest of mature mixed hardwood trees, mostly oaks, poplars, sycamores, and maples. The trail passes the site of the long-gone Long Calm, a fort on the Big Gunpowder used in the late 17th century. The fort was still in use during the Revolutionary War, when Lafayette and his troops camped there. When you get to the top of the hill, you'll begin skirting an open farm on the left through the woods.

Continue walking until you reach the lost pond at 1.8 miles. If you were expecting water, you'll be disappointed. What's left of this abandoned pond is merely the shape and indentation of an oval body of water. Still, it's an interesting

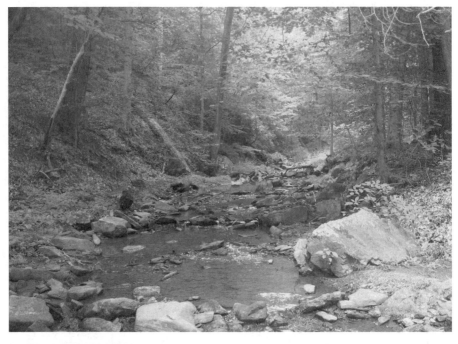

Gunpowder feeder stream

sight since it sits in the middle of the woods and clearly looks out of place in its current incarnation: a grassy marshland surrounded by tall trees.

It gets a bit confusing here; there appears to be a well-maintained trail up the hill to the left of the pond, but that quickly peters out. Instead, head around the pond, keeping it to your right; when you come out on the other side, head away from the pond by going left up the wooded hill. At 2.3 miles, you'll cross a small stream using rocks in the waterway as stepping-stones. Head back to the section of trail where you came in, which you'll reach at 3.1 miles, and follow it back to your car.

NEARBY ACTIVITIES

You'll find several other sections of the noncontiguous Gunpowder Falls State Park close by. The park runs in sections along Gunpowder River, which forms the border between Baltimore and Harford counties. Rocks State Park in Harford County is also close by; to get to the park, continue on MD 1 north, turn left onto MD 24 north, and you will come to the park entrance approximately 5 miles north of Forest Hill. You will find plenty of places to eat in all price ranges in Bel Air, which is off MD 1.

GUNPOWDER FALLS STATE PARK: SWEET AIR AREA 48

IN BRIEF

An amazing amount of variety in a relatively short hike—the scenery changes every mile or so.

DESCRIPTION

It's almost a crime that this exceedingly beautiful 1,250-acre section of Gunpowder Falls State Park is so lightly used. But what a treat that is for hikers seeking solitude. The bulk of traffic in the Sweet Air section is from equestrians.

From the trailhead, follow the path as it merges into a wide farm road. You'll soon pass an open field to the left. There's a cornfield straight ahead where, at 0.1 mile, you'll come to the first split. Head left to stay on the yellow-blazed Barley Pond Loop. Follow the tree line around the cornfield, turning right at a YOU ARE HERE sign at 0.3 miles and reaching the edge of the woods at 0.6 miles. There's a wooden sign here reading, THE WOODS WERE MADE FOR THE HUNTER OF DREAMS. There are many spots along the hike where similar signs have been painted with inspirational, nature-oriented quotations. There's a certain irony

KEY AT-A-GLANCE INFORMATION

LENGTH: 5.1 miles

CONFIGURATION: Jagged loop

DIFFICULTY: Easy–moderate

SCENERY: Upland forest, Little Gunpowder River, Barley Pond, pine plantations

EXPOSURE: Mostly shaded

TRAFFIC: Light

TRAIL SURFACE: Packed dirt, mowed grass

HIKING TIME: 2 hours

ACCESS: Sunrise–sunset

MAPS: USGS Phoenix, Jarrettsville; immovable trails map at the parking area

WHEELCHAIR ACCESS: No

FACILITIES: None

SPECIAL COMMENTS: Alternate directions: Take I-695 to Exit 27 Dulaney Valley Road north. Follow it over the Loch Raven Reservoir bridge and merge left onto Jarretsville Pike (MD Rt. 146 north). Once you cross into Harford County, take the first right onto Hess Road. Follow Hess to a U-turn right onto Park Road and then the first left onto Moores Road. Take a right into the park on Dalton Bevard Road.

Directions

Take I-83 to Exit 20, Shawan Road east until it ends at York Road. Take a right on York and then the first left onto Ashland Road, which becomes Paper Mill Road. Go 6 miles until Paper Mill becomes Sweet Air Road (after crossing Jarrettsville Pike). Go 2.7 miles to a left on Greene Road. Go 1.8 miles to a left on Moores Road and another 0.5 miles to a left on Dalton Bevard Road. The gravel parking area is up to the right. At the leftmost point of the parking area is a sign for the Barley Pond Loop. That is the trailhead for the hike described here.

GPS Trailhead
Coordinates
UTM Zone (WGS84) 18S
Easting 370682
Northing 4377315
Latitude N 39' 32.145967"
Longitude W 76' 30.288184"

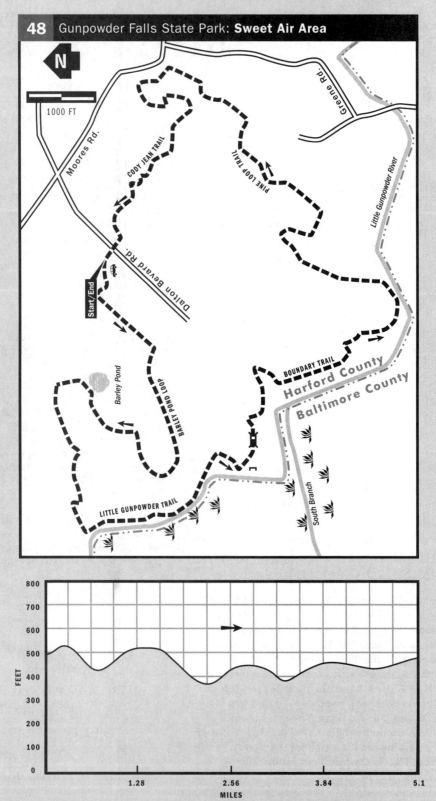

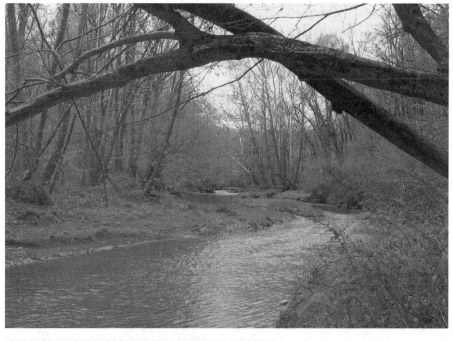

Harford County on the right and Baltimore County on the left

here: though the quotations are nice, this hike is so beautiful that it doesn't require any embellishment.

To the left of the sign is the red-blazed hikers-only trail and to the right is the Barley Pond Trail—continue there. (Red is a good option if there are bikers and horses afoot—it will eventually link up to the hike as described here.) There are several different varieties of ferns covering the ground and mostly oak, maple, and tulip poplar with spicebush and mountain laurel rounding out the midlevel growth.

At 0.75 miles, there's a split; leftward heads to the Gunpowder River, but you'll be there soon—continue straight on the Barley Pond, which soon narrows and zigzags, turning into a foot trail and crossing over a tiny stream with skunk cabbage and lilies. The scenery is very typical of piedmont northeastern Baltimore/Harford County. At 1 mile, at the top of the hill, emerge onto Barley Pond. It's a beautiful spot, and the pond has great visibility. Be on the lookout for red foxes, which inhabit the area.

Head left around the pond—look for water snakes, frogs, and small fish, mostly bluegills. There's another trail split immediately after the pond—head left to stay on the Barley Pond Trail. Just at the top of the hill, look for the massive oak tree that has split at its base into five separate and very tall trees. This process is replicated throughout the woods. Reach the end of the Barley Pond Loop at 1.1 at a T-intersection and take a left to pick up the white-blazed Little Gunpowder Trail.

The Little Gunpowder Trail is twisty and full of green. Little streams wind throughout the landscape amid rolling hills studded with red maple. These riparian streams offer perfect cover for many birds, evidenced by a chorus of song. Another split arrives a quarter-mile later. Left heads to the blue-blazed Boundary Trail, which eventually goes to and through the river. For now, go rightward, where you'll see both blue and white blazes. The trail, soon turning back to only white blazes, winds around gradually and easily, following the contours of the hills, which reach like the fingers of an outstretched hand down to the river.

By 1.5 miles, the landscape is dominated by multiflora rose, which can crowd the trail. Reach the river at 1.6 miles—there's a little wooden resting area with a bench. The hike is entirely in Harford County, but the river is the dividing line between Harford and Baltimore County. Here also is the other end of the red trail you passed at the hike's beginning. Head left along the river. Many long flat rocks extend into the water where you can vie with the snakes and turtles for a spot to sit and sun yourself.

Cross a footbridge and you'll come to the wide blue-blazed Boundary Trail. This is where you can cross the river, but it can be a bit of a challenge—in normal conditions, it's about 30 feet across and can be 3 to 4 feet deep. (If you do cross and walk the Boundary loop, you'll add approximately 2 miles to the total hike.) For now, continue on the white Little Gunpowder, but pause at the bench below the John Muir quotation. In the river is a fallen sycamore, where water eddies into a pool. The sycamore has sprouted five new trees, testament to nature's regenerative power. Many of the trees in this area are covered in moss, with wildflowers strewn about, including asters, bloodroot, boneset, jack-in-the-pulpit, jewelweed, joe-pye weed, and woodland sunflower. Across the river sits a striated rock outcropping supporting some oaks.

As you continue, you'll pass several orange-blazed cuts running vertically along the hills. These are connector paths between the upland and river trails. Pass a grove of beech trees with pristine bark free of graffiti scrawls and when you reach a split, bypass the connector yellow trail, heading instead toward the river and the blue trail.

At 2.8, parallel a cornfield; go through a pine plantation and cross a stream at 2.9 miles. Immediately after, come to an intersection; head left up the hill through mixed hardwood. Along with the trees already named, you'll find some locust and ironwood as well. Emerge onto a big field and head right, as the trail becomes mowed grass. After another tenth of a mile, the trail splits—head right and then back into the woods (you'll see blue blazes again). It emerges from the woods back onto mowed grass after another tenth of a mile, following the park boundary line past a private backyard. As you walk along the fence and trees, look for the trail heading slightly to the left. In early spring or winter, the grass path may be the same height as the field around and can be hard to spot.

Head right at the cornfield where dogwood and pine line the edge. At 3.8 miles, you'll see signs for the Pine Loop Trail both straight and left—go straight.

The trail splits—blue Boundary left, yellow Pine Loop right. Taking the Pine, you'll soon see the reason for the name. Take the discernible cut to the left into the thick of the white pine plantation and pass a footbridge donated by the Chesapeake Trail Riding Club.

At 4.4 miles, you will see a cairn with a hiker icon. Take this green-blazed hikers-only Cody Jean Trail—it moves through the white pines but does so from the top of the hill, giving a nice vantage through the wide spaces between the trees. At a picnic table and another cairn, cross over the Pine Loop to stay on the Cody Jean and follow it as it zigzags through mixed hardwoods, crosses a stream, and heads back into the pines, where it becomes especially aromatic. Emerge onto the opposite side of where you turned right earlier to park and you'll see blue and yellow trailheads to the left. Cross Dalton Bevard, passing the training area for Chesapeake search dogs to the left, and your car is on the other side.

NEARBY ACTIVITIES

The Ladew Topiary Gardens, dubbed the "most outstanding topiary garden in America" by the Garden Club of America, earns its place on the National Register of Historic Places. It's a fascinating and inspiring destination. To reach it from GFSP, reverse the alternate directions under Special Comments to a right on Jarrettsville Pike and follow the signs to Ladew on the right. For info: (410) 557-9466; **www.ladewgardens.com.**

49   ROCKS STATE PARK

KEY AT-A-GLANCE INFORMATION

LENGTH: 3.6 miles

CONFIGURATION: Irregular loop

DIFFICULTY: Moderate–very strenuous

SCENERY: Rural northern Harford County, mature upland forest, rock columns

EXPOSURE: Shade

TRAFFIC: Light on trail, moderate–heavy at King and Queen's Seat

TRAIL SURFACE: Packed dirt, rock

HIKING TIME: 2 hours

ACCESS: 9 a.m.–sunset daily; $2 per person service charge on weekends and holidays at the picnic areas

MAPS: USGS Fawn Grove; trail maps available at park office; downloadable map at www.dnr.state.md.us/publiclands/central/rockmap.html

WHEELCHAIR ACCESS: No

FACILITIES: Restrooms and water at the park office (open Monday–Friday 7 a.m.–3 p.m.); public phone in parking area

SPECIAL COMMENTS: Rock climbing is allowed, but use caution. Regardless of whether you're climbing or merely hiking, wear sturdy boots.

GPS Trailhead Coordinates

UTM Zone (WGS84) 18S

Easting 378777

Northing 4388536

Latitude N 39' 38.281367"

Longitude W 76' 24.761109"

IN BRIEF

Explore 885 acres of dense forest and massive boulders rising above Deer Creek, culminating in the main attraction: King and Queen's Seat, 190-foot rock outcroppings once the ancestral meeting place of the Susquehannock and Mingo Indians.

DESCRIPTION

In 1951, the State of Maryland began purchasing land surrounding the Deer Creek Valley. Originally envisioned as Deer Creek State Park, the name was later changed to the unceremonious but apt Rocks State Park. An amble through the area quickly bears out that decision.

The first thing you will see at the trailhead is the yellow sign that reads: CAUTION: CLIMBERS HAVE BEEN SERIOUSLY INJURED WHILE ATTEMPTING TO FREE CLIMB. This applies to the King and Queen's Seat, which you will visit at the end of the hike. For now, there is enough to occupy you on the steep and rocky approach to the main loop trail. Fallen tree trunks, two-by-fours, and well-placed rocks make the climb a little easier, but it is very strenuous regardless. During the first 900 feet of trail, you will gain 200 feet in elevation.

Directions

Take I-695 to I-95 North. Take Exit 77B, MD 24 north toward Bel Air, and continue through the towns of Bel Air, Rock Spring, and Forest Hill. After 13.4 miles on MD 24, you'll see a sign for Rocks State Park; continue another half mile, and you'll see signs pointing to the park office on the left (you can find trail maps and parking there). Pass this entrance and continue another 0.2 miles to the gravel parking area on the left across from Deer Creek; the trail begins at the edge of the woods in front of the parking area.

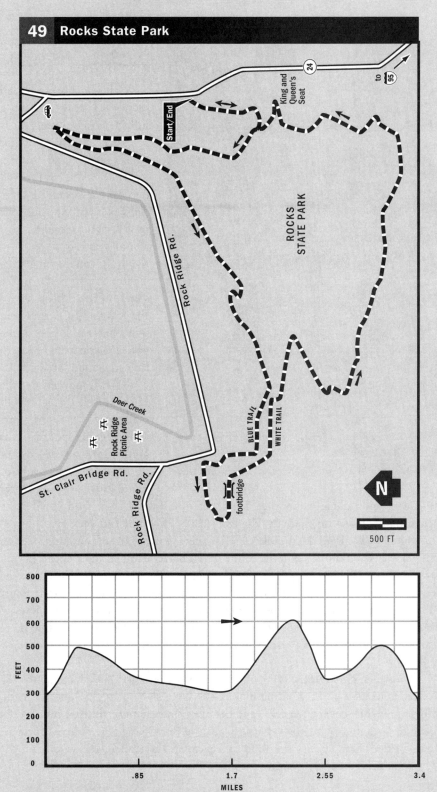

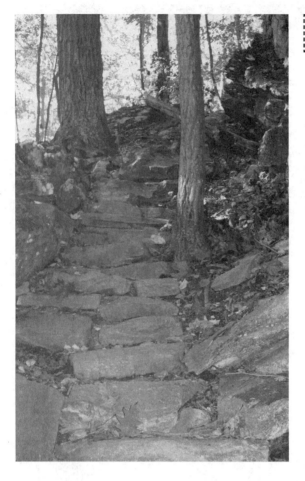

This purple-blazed section of trail leads up a hillside covered with rocks as well as tall, straight oaks, ferns, and sumac. At times, the trail itself becomes a series of large slabs of rock, and massive rock outcroppings surround you. At the top of the hill, you'll come to a T-intersection; if you're short on time, head left to the King and Queen's Seat now, but for a good hike go right and come back to this attraction later.

You'll appreciate the fairly level, wide, well-maintained packed dirt trail surrounded by ferns and sassafras at the top of the hill. The blazes turn to white in this section. After 100 feet, you'll come to another T-intersection. Take a right, and you'll see a bench immediately on the left. The trail heads downhill and then levels out at 0.3 miles. Walk along the middle of a flat ridge, which falls off about 20 feet on both sides. At 0.6 miles, don't take the green-blazed trail straight ahead (it will take you to a parking area on Saint Clair Bridge Road); head left instead. The white blazes return as you gradually head uphill; you'll see lots of nice spongy moss along the trail, and a rock outcropping to the right gives good views of Deer Creek below. (You can tube and swim in the creek, but be aware that there are no lifeguards; you can also fish here if you have a freshwater fishing license and trout stamp.)

Squirrels, chipmunks, wild turkeys, and white-tailed deer accompany you as you continue uphill, winding among the huge slabs of rock along the path. Moss and lichen cover the rocks, and the area is awash in ferns. At 1 mile, you'll come to a small asphalt road that leads to the Rock Ridge Picnic Area from St. Clair Bridge Road. Cross the road and pick up the trail in the woods on the other side at the brown wooden post. At 1.1 miles, look for an oak tree with its trunk growing over a rock; it looks like spilled wax and is absolutely beautiful.

At 1.2 miles, the trail splits; head right onto the blue-blazed trail, which runs a little lower down the hill closer to Deer Creek. The red oaks crowding above provide welcome shade on hot days. You'll continue to see a profusion of rocks covered with moss and spilled tree roots. At the T-intersection at 1.4 miles, take a right through a big grove where ferns carpet the ground. Cross the wooden footbridge here; this area is home to the Scouts Interpretive Trail, and you can pick up trail brochures by heading toward the road, across from the Hills Grove Picnic Area.

Complete the interpretive loop (and return the brochure to recycle). You'll cross over another wooden footbridge at 1.7 miles and another 150 feet farther down the trail. You'll see an open bog just beyond and lots of azalea and mountain laurel on either side of you. There's a wooden post that sits in a big field of ferns with a slight indentation in the ground next to it; you will reach the end of this half-mile loop soon after you see this post. Turn right to head back to the white trail. When the trail splits, you can either go straight or keep to the right to return via a higher elevation than you came and to make another loop so you don't back-track. Either way, you'll reach another trail split at 1.9 miles and rejoin the white trail at 2 miles; take a right, and you'll see white blazes right away.

The trail runs as a switchback, ascending quickly over the ubiquitous rock. A well-placed bench on the left at 2.2 miles provides a welcome resting place. You'll soon reach an intersection with a sign pointing in different directions. If you go right, you'll leave the park; if you go left, you'll come to the picnic area; and if you go straight (actually diagonally right), you'll stay on the white trail. Go straight, and you'll come to another intersection at 2.4 miles. Here you can cut left on the orange trail to head to the picnic area, or stay straight to remain on the white trail, which becomes quite level as it winds through mature upland forest.

At the two wooden posts on the left (they look like ski slaloms), turn left. Go up the hill, which is a moderate climb, and when you reach the top, at 3 miles, take a right; you will soon come to the King and Queen's Seat on the right. Be very careful here—people have fallen off these vertical rock faces, some of which soar 94 feet. Many of these slabs have been carved with graffiti, which at first seems to detract from the sanctity of this place so highly valued by the indigenous Indians. I actually found it sort of nice to see the older scrawls, some of them dating back to the mid-1800s. You might find it interesting that David has been in love with Esther for well more than 100 years now.

The King and Queen's Seat provides a rather stunning vista of the rolling farmlands of northern Harford County sprawling out and Deer Creek running below. In spring and summer, you can see an almost unbroken ribbon of green, and the autumn foliage puts on a spectacular show. In winter months, when you should take extreme caution if you're hiking in snow and ice, the leafless view stretches even farther than it does in summer. In short, it's an amazing spot.

After you've taken it all in, go right off the rocks, and on the right you'll quickly rejoin the purple-blazed trail you used earlier. Remember that this is a very steep section; go slowly since going down can be more difficult and tough on the knees than coming up.

NEARBY ACTIVITIES

Rocks State Park includes two more tracts: the Hidden Valley Natural Area, located 5 miles north at the intersection of Madonna, Telegraph, and Carea roads; and the Falling Branch Area (see the next hike in this book), home to Maryland's second highest vertical waterfall, Kilgore Falls. To reach it from the parking area for this hike, continue north on MD 24 for another 4.2 miles and turn left onto Saint Mary's Road. Go another 0.4 miles and turn right onto Falling Branch Road. Park on the right at the ROCKS FALLING BRANCH AREA sign.

ROCKS STATE PARK: FALLING BRANCH AREA 50

IN BRIEF

Take a short hike with a grand payoff: Kilgore Falls, Maryland's second-highest vertical waterfall.

DESCRIPTION

The relatively small (67 acres) Falling Branch Area of Rocks State Park was once a meeting place for Susquehannock Indians. Local hikers and nature enthusiasts didn't know about it for many years because it sat on private property. Fortunately, in 1993, the state, with the help of many local activists including Harford County public school children, bought the land and turned it over to Rocks State Park officials for administration. It has become one of the most attractive parcels for many miles around.

From the trailhead, you'll wind through a well-exposed section of the trail with thick underbrush of mostly goldenrod and spicebush; a stand of pines provides shade. The path soon runs downhill. You'll see lots of poison sumac on mature red oak trees, as well as an abundance of tulip poplars, beeches, sassafras, hollies, and mountain laurels.

Directions ————————————————→

Take I-695 to I-95 North (Exit 33B). Go 11 miles to Exit 77B, MD 24 north toward Bel Air, and go through the towns of Bel Air, Rock Spring, and Forest Hill. After 13.4 miles on MD 24, you'll see a sign for Rocks State Park. Keep going another half mile; you'll see signs pointing to the park office to the left, but to reach the Falling Branch Area, pass the office sign and proceed another 4.2 miles and turn left onto Saint Mary's Road. Go another 0.4 miles and turn right onto Falling Branch Road; park on the right at the ROCKS FALLING BRANCH AREA sign. The trail starts at the left end of the parking lot.

KEY AT-A-GLANCE INFORMATION

LENGTH: 1.1 miles

CONFIGURATION: Out-and-back with a spur

DIFFICULTY: Easy

SCENERY: Kilgore Falls, hardwoods

EXPOSURE: Shade to the waterfall but mostly sun on the extension along Falling Branch

TRAFFIC: Moderate

TRAIL SURFACE: Packed dirt after an initial small section of crushed rock

HIKING TIME: 15 minutes to the waterfall and 30 minutes adding the extension

ACCESS: 9 a.m.–sunset daily

MAPS: USGS Fawn Grove, trail maps available at the Rocks State Park central office (see Directions)

WHEELCHAIR ACCESS: No

FACILITIES: None on the trail; restrooms and water at the Rocks State Park central office (see Directions)

SPECIAL COMMENTS: A proposed sale of the Falling Branch Area by the Maryland Department of Natural Resources in 2004 roused much public opposition, and fortunately the sale was scrapped. For information on the area, call the Rocks State Park office at (410) 557-7994.

GPS Trailhead
Coordinates

UTM Zone (WGS84) 18S

Easting 377972

Northing 4394346

Latitude N 39' 41.414523"

Longitude W 76' 25.388217"

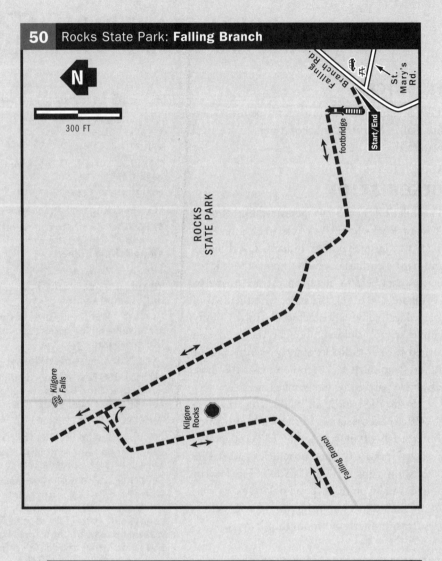

50 Rocks State Park: **Falling Branch**

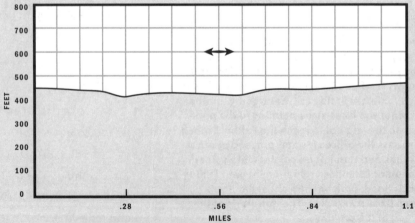

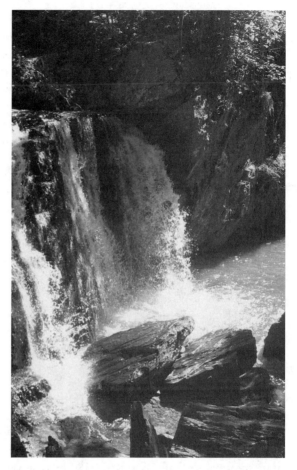

Kilgore Falls, Maryland's second highest vertical waterfall

You'll reach a wooden boardwalk and footbridge at 500 feet. The trail turns to packed dirt on the other side, and red cedars abound as the trail rises above a little valley on the left. This area, as well as the woods on the other side of Falling Branch, provides prime habitat for red fox, white-tailed deer, and a multitude of woodland birds, including wild turkey. You'll soon hear the rumble of Kilgore Falls; Falling Branch comes into view on the left, and you'll parallel it upstream. Also to the left, at 0.2 miles, you can see the remains of an old kiln or stone chimney, as well as the stone foundation of a stagecoach rest stop.

When the trail splits at 0.25 miles, head left toward Falling Branch Stream. (You can also go right, which will take you above the waterfall, but the views of its cascade are largely obstructed from there.) You'll see other trail cuts here and there, but avoid these; with the exception of the trail described here, all of them invariably lead to private property.

Cross over the Falling Branch on the stepping-stones. Be extra careful in winter; the stones are not set very high out of the water, and ice and snow can make them very slippery. Heavy rains will also cover and/or make the stones slippery. In general, though, the water remains pretty shallow. If the water is high and the trail on the other side, which runs just alongside Falling Branch, is covered, you can take another trail higher up the hill.

At 0.3 miles, you'll reach Kilgore Falls, which sits in an absolutely gorgeous spot—a rock amphitheater made up of erosion-resistant Prettyboy schist. The falls, at 19 feet tall, is the second-highest natural vertical waterfall in Maryland. Be sure to sit down and take in the views of the falls. While it certainly can't compare to Niagara or Angel Falls, if you're lucky enough to have it to yourself, you'll find the wildness of the area very inspiring. Over the schist, the water spills into a deep pool, where actress Sissy Spacek swam in the movie Tuck Everlasting. Look closely to the left for the remains of stone steps heading up to the waterfall; it's very possible that the Susquehannock constructed these long ago. You can climb the rock wall to get to the top of the falls; it doesn't require much experience in rock-climbing, but it does necessitate some nimbleness, to be sure.

Before you head back to your car, you can extend the hike by staying on the west side of Falling Branch and going diagonally uphill to the right—you'll come to this portion of the trail just after you pass a bench and just before you reach the Falling Branch crossing. This trail initially follows the old stagecoach route away from the falls; you'll be walking downstream and see lots of ferns, moss-covered rocks, and evergreens decorating the hill on the right. This is also the site of a mill that once stood here.

Continuing on, the trail becomes almost overgrown as it sees relatively little traffic, but it soon opens up into a field of mostly blackberry bushes and goldenrod. Turn around, at 0.5 miles, when you see the ALLIANCE FOR THE CHES-APEAKE BAY sign. Walk back toward Kilgore Falls, cross over the Falling Branch, and head back to your car.

NEARBY ACTIVITIES

In addition to the main section of Rocks State Park (see page 248), you may want to visit nearby Eden Mill Park and Nature Center, at 1617 Eden Mill Road in Pylesville; it offers many short hiking trails perfect for small children as well as picnicking, and canoe launching and fishing on Deer Creek. The nature center, which is housed in a restored gristmill, features a hands-on area for children; for more information, call (410) 836-3050 or visit **www.edenmill.org**.

SUSQUEHANNA STATE PARK: RIVER TRAILS 51

IN BRIEF

Follow the mighty Susquehanna upstream to Conowingo Dam—then return via an obscure wooded foot trail.

DESCRIPTION:

If any area outdoor enthusiasts needs a reminder why he or she is lucky to live in this area, Susquehanna State Park provides it. First, the Susquehanna River's impressive numbers: 444 miles, a 13 million acre drainage basin, the second-largest watershed in the eastern United States. The river begins as an overflow of Otsego Lake in New York and runs through three states before draining into the Chesapeake Bay, just south at Havre de Grace, MD, pouring 19 million gallons of freshwater into the bay every minute.

The Susquehanna was first explored by John Smith in 1608. Of course, the native Susquehannock Indians had already been hunting and fishing in the area for centuries. Smith's assessment of the area is applicable even today: "Heaven and earth seemed never

KEY AT-A-GLANCE INFORMATION

LENGTH: 7.5 miles

CONFIGURATION: Out-and-back with jagged loop

DIFFICULTY: Moderate

SCENERY: Susquehanna River, Deer Creek, historical sites, hardwoods

EXPOSURE: Shaded

TRAFFIC: Moderate–heavy on Lower Susquehanna Heritage Greenways Trail, light on alternate Greenways Route and Woodland Trails

TRAIL SURFACE: Gravel, packed dirt, some asphalt

HIKING TIME: 2.5–3 hours

ACCESS: Sunrise–sunset

MAPS: USGS Conowingo Dam, Aberdeen. Get the *Trail Guide to Susquehanna State Park* at www .easycart.net/MarylandDepart mentofNaturalResources/Central_ Maryland_Trail_Guides.html.

WHEELCHAIR ACCESS: No

FACILITIES: Restrooms, water, campground, Steppingstone Museum, picnic area, boat launch, phone

SPECIAL COMMENTS: Tours of Conowingo Dam were unavailable as of early 2009. Call (410) 457-5011 for updates.

Directions

Take I-95 to Exit 89, MD Route 155 west. Go 2.5 miles to a right on MD Route 161. Go 0.3 miles to a right on Rock Run Road, and follow Rock Run into the park. Follow signs to camping area. At the intersection of Craigs Corner and Wilkinson, take a right. Take a left on Craigs Corner just before the campground gate. Pass a private road to the left and look for parking on either side of Craigs Corner just before you reach the Stafford Road Bridge over Deer Creek to the left. Walk across Stafford Bridge and take a right to reach the trailhead of the Lower Susquehanna Heritage Greenways Trail.

GPS Trailhead Coordinates

UTM Zone (WGS84) 18S

Easting 400126

Northing 4386571

Latitude N 39' 37.384808"

Longitude W 76' 9.818938"

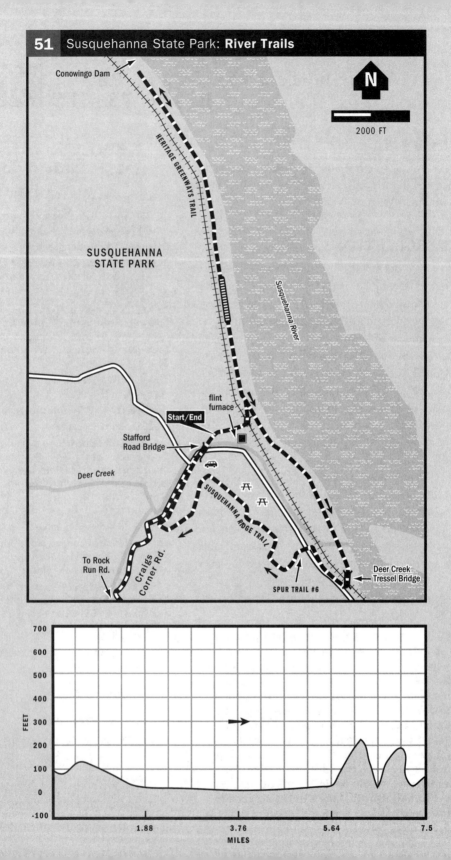

Conowingo Dam

N

2000 FT

HERITAGE GREENWAYS TRAIL

SUSQUEHANNA
STATE PARK

Susquehanna River

flint
furnace

Start/End

Stafford
Road Bridge

Deer Creek

SUSQUEHANNA RIDGE TRAIL

To Rock
Run Rd.

Craigs Corner Rd.

SPUR TRAIL #6

Deer Creek
Tressel Bridge

FEET

700
600
500
400
300
200
100
0
-100

1.88   3.76   5.64   7.5
MILES

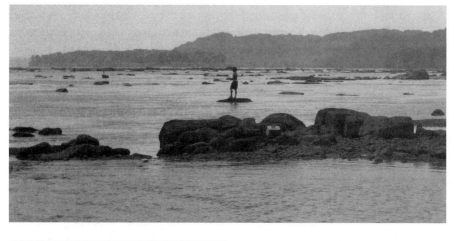

Susquehanna River, near the Chesapeake Bay

to have agreed better to frame a place for man's . . . delightful habitation." European establishments on the river date to 1622 as successful trading posts. By 1658, the settlement that would become Havre de Grace had been established.

Thus, the Stafford Flint Furnace, just off the trail to the right as you cross Strafford Bridge, wasn't one of the area's original structures, even though it's been around for quite a while. It is, however, all that remains of the once thriving town of Stafford, established in 1749 and destroyed by an ice gorge in 1904. The wide gravel trail, lined with wild strawberries, parallels Deer Creek. Fishing in freshwater Deer Creek requires a nontidal fishing license. The creek serves as habitat for the federally endangered Maryland Darter and the short-nosed sturgeon. It's also popular for swimming and tubing. Several cut paths head down to this pretty waterway.

Continuing on, you'll be struck by the wealth of understory flora all about you. There are literally hundreds of species of shrubs, including honeysuckle, invasive multiflora rose, raspberry, staghorn sumac, swamp rose, winterberry, and trumpet vine. Up the hills, trillium abound, recognizable by its three-petaled flowers and three-leafed bodies. There are also Dutchman's-breeches (rare for Maryland), Virginia bluebells, dogtooth violet, windflower, and spring beauty. Rare and endangered plants include sweet-scented Indian plantain and valerian.

Cross a footbridge at 0.4 miles, going over the site of what was once the Susquehanna Tidewater Canal, built in 1835–1839 and linking Havre de Grace with Wrightsville, Pennsylvania. Make note of the little footpath to the right of the bridge, as you'll take it on the return trip. For now, continue left on the wide Heritage Greenways Trail. At 0.75 miles, you'll see the first right cut to the banks of the Susquehanna. Head down there; you'll see fishermen standing on one of the many decent-size rocks that dot the river near its banks. Many regard the Susquehanna as the best fishing grounds on the East Coast. A tidal license is required to fish here. Visiting in early spring might allow you to catch sight of the annual shad and herring runs. Among the most popular catch: smallmouth bass, largemouth bass, and channel catfish, but carp, American shad, alewife, blue backed herring, striped bass, pike, and perch are also abundant. It's a striking river, and standing on its banks—alternating as sand, mud, and rocks—is inspiring. As if the river wasn't enough, the woods behind you present one of the most biologically diverse ecosystems in North America. In addition to the flora listed above, you'll see as dominant in the overstory yellow poplar, birch, red oak, black oak, white oak, chestnut oak, American beech, black cherry, white ash, black gum, hickory, sycamore, and red maple. Among the creatures making homes here are the wood frog, eastern painted turtle, river otter, raccoon, white- tailed deer, white-footed mouse, eastern chipmunk, and red fox.

If birds are more your fancy, the river hosts many of them, mostly kingfishers, gulls, osprey, heron, and bald eagles. (For a much more comprehensive list of the bird types [well over 100] that have been spotted in and around the area of Conowingo Dam, see **www.harfordbirdclub.org/conowingo.html**.) In the woods behind, dominant species include red-headed woodpecker, wild turkey, pileated woodpecker, winter wren, house wren, wood thrush, sapsucker, downy woodpecker, and screech owl.

There's a very long boardwalk at 1 mile, which helps to protect especially sensitive wetlands; river floods often reach this area, as it's barely above sea level. The hills to the left rise very steeply and abruptly; these are gneiss columns, many of them 90 degrees. The trail soon runs alongside railroad tracks, part of the defunct Philadelphia Electric Railroad Company, and ends near 3 miles at a gate. The Conowingo Dam is just ahead. The dam, constructed in 1926, is almost 4,500 feet long and 100 feet high. Full capacity flows approach 40 million gallons per minute. If you're lucky enough to catch a release, it's an extraordinary sight.

Turn around and head back, taking advantage of one of the cuts to the river if you haven't already headed there. When you get back to the trail split you passed earlier (this time at 4.2 miles), take the packed dirt foot trail as it heads into the thick woods. This is a stunning and beautiful trail, crowded with vegetation and close to the banks of the river. As for that close vegetation, be aware of not only poison ivy, but also nettles, which can give you what feels like an intense jellyfish or bee sting and can last up to half an hour. If you get stung, don't rub the area, as that makes it worse. If water levels aren't too high, there's a great little beach that you'll pass, near a large jumble of rocks.

At 5.5 miles, cross the Deer Creek Tressel Bridge and head right, passing the Stafford Road Parking Area. Walk along Stafford for a quarter-mile until you see a hiker icon and MASON-DIXON TRAIL post to the left. This is Spur Trail #6, blazed in silver (as are all the spur trails in the park system). It will link you to the red-blazed Susquehanna Ridge Trail. The spur is a bit tough, but worth it as it winds uphill through mixed hardwood and a chorus of birdsong. After a tenth of a mile, you'll reach the Ridge Trail. Take it right. It crosses a stream at 6 miles and passes a grove of pines. Hit a cleared area and cross over a footbridge. Pass the Deer Creek Picnic Area through the woods to the right and soon the trail ends at the green-blazed Deer Creek Trail. Follow it until you reach a trail split at 7 miles—you will hear Deer Creek just preceding the split. Head downhill to Craigs Corner Road, a gravel park road. Emerge from the woods across from the private road you passed earlier in your car. Follow Craigs Corner for 0.3 miles to the parking area.

NEARBY ACTIVITIES

The Steppingstone Museum is located within the park. It demonstrates the rural arts and crafts of the 1880–1920 period. Call (410) 939-2299 or (888) 419-1762 or visit **www.steppingstonemuseum.org** for info. Also close by is the historic town of Havre de Grace (MD 155 east) with museums, lighthouses, and its famous promenade, extending 2400 feet along the Chesapeake Bay from the City Marina to the Concord Point Lighthouse, rebuilt after being destroyed in 2004 by Hurricane Isabel. In Aberdeen, check out minor league baseball at Ripken Stadium, home of the Ironbirds (**www.ironbirdsbaseball.com**). There's also the nearby Army Ordnance Museum, on the grounds of Aberdeen Proving Ground ([410] 278-3602 or **www.ordmusfound.org**).

52   SUSQUEHANNA STATE PARK: WOODLAND-FARM TRAILS

KEY AT-A-GLANCE INFORMATION

LENGTH: 8.3 miles

CONFIGURATION: Jagged loop

DIFFICULTY: Moderate–strenuous

SCENERY: Susquehanna River, Rock Run, historical sites

EXPOSURE: More shade than sun

TRAFFIC: Moderate–heavy at historical area, picnic area, campgrounds, and river; light on trails

TRAIL SURFACE: Dirt, gravel, asphalt

HIKING TIME: 3–3.5 hours

ACCESS: Sunrise–sunset

MAPS: USGS Conowingo Dam, Aberdeen. You can purchase the *Trail Guide to Susquehanna State Park* at www.easycart.net/ MarylandDepartmentofNatural Resources/Central_Maryland_Trail _Guides.html.

WHEELCHAIR ACCESS: No

FACILITIES: Restrooms, water, campground, Steppingstone Museum, picnic area, boat launch, phone

SPECIAL COMMENTS: This hike stitches together major portions of each of the trails in Susquehanna State Park except the Lower Heritage Greenways Trail, which is described in the previous hike. Length can be varied by taking spur trails, noted in the Description.

IN BRIEF

The wilder side of Susquehanna State Park: not much walking along the river, but full of old growth and blissful solitude.

DESCRIPTION

Before you begin the hike, you might want to first walk down to the river, just behind the mill. In addition to being physically beautiful, the river is awfully impressive: for the numbers, see the previous hike in this book. From behind the mill, you can see narrow Wood Island in front of you. The larger Roberts Island sits behind it, and Spencer Island is to the right. Beyond is Cecil County.

The mill was built in 1794 and operated well into the 20th century. It's open May to September on weekends 10 a.m. to 6 p.m., with grinding demonstrations from 1 p.m. to 4 p.m. A bridge once spanned the river near the mill, but it was destroyed by ice floes in 1856. The toll keeper's house, however, still remains in its position to the left of the mill. It now houses an information center for the park. The building across the road was once the Rock Run miller's house.

The red-blazed Susquehanna Ridge Trail (initially blazed in both red and blue) is a narrow foot trail. The trail runs along a western

GPS Trailhead Coordinates

UTM Zone (WGS84) 18S

Easting 401939

Northing 4384858

Latitude N 39' 36.471484"

Longitude W 76' 8.536541"

Directions ⟶

Take I-95 to Exit 89, MD Route 155 west. Go 2.5 miles to a right on MD Route 161. Go 0.3 miles to a right on Rock Run Road and follow Rock Run into the park. Follow the signs to the historic area until the road ends at the parking area to the left of the Rock Run Mill. Walk up Stafford, keeping Rock Run Mill on your left. The trailhead is 600 feet ahead, leading into the woods to the right.

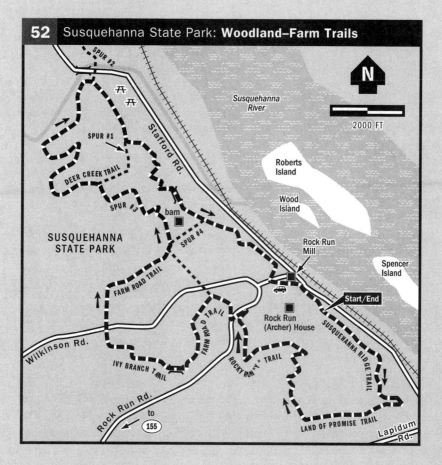

52 Susquehanna State Park: **Woodland–Farm Trails**

SPUR #2

Susquehanna River

N

2000 FT

Stafford Rd.

SPUR #1

DEER CREEK TRAIL

SPUR #3

barn

SUSQUEHANNA STATE PARK

SPUR #4

Roberts Island

Wood Island

Rock Run Mill

Spencer Island

Start/End

FARM ROAD TRAIL

FARM ROAD TRAIL

Rock Run (Archer) House

SUSQUEHANNA RIDGE TRAIL

Wilkinson Rd.

IVY BRANCH TRAIL

ROCKY RUN "Y" TRAIL

LAND OF PROMISE TRAIL

Rock Run Rd.

to
155

Lapidum Rd.

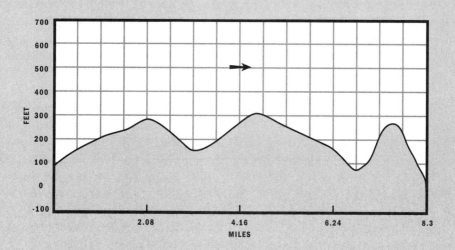

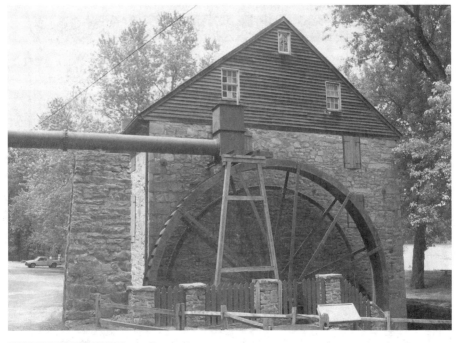

Rock Run Mill (ca. 1794)

ridge facing the Susquehanna, a few hundred feet above the river. This trail is noted for birding and wildflower viewing. Quickly, you'll cross a tiny stream and see a little cairn next to it with a hiker icon. The area is loaded with raspberry bushes. If you're seeing the berries, that means it's summer. If so, the river will be difficult to see. Still, it's a fine price to pay for the thickness of the woods.

At 0.6 miles, you'll cross an intact stone wall. This is evidence of once cleared land, not surprising in that the community of Lapidum is close by. This settlement traces its history to 1683. When you see the white-blazed Land of Promise Trail at 0.9 miles, you'll notice the Susquehanna Ridge Trail continuing straight ahead. It ends soon at Lapidum Road, entrance point for the Lapidum Boat Launch. Instead of hitting the dead end, take a right on the Land of Promise, an isolated trail that more or less follows that same stone wall.

At 1.1 miles, skirt around the edge of a cleared field, still walking astride the wall. Emerge into a field, a favorite of songbirds, as the trail moves through chest-high grass. More raspberry bushes await when you reenter the woods at 1.4 miles before quickly coming back out into the field. At 1.5 miles, cross a tree-lined road; to the right is the Steppingstone Museum. It demonstrates the rural arts and crafts of the 1880–1920 period. (**steppingstonemuseum.org**, [410] 939-2299). Across the road, you'll soon notice a little stream down the hill to the left. At about 2 miles, there's a fascinating area full of grapevine, trumpet vine, honeysuckle, and some invasive *Ailanthus altissima* trees. The admixture of these Chinese trees and all the vines creates a little scene that appears down-right semitropical.

At 2.1 miles, take a left on the yellow-blazed Rock Run "Y" Trail, noted for its grapevines, raspberry bushes, and brier patches. Make sure to take the right-ward split in the pine plantation when you see the 1A sign—otherwise, you'll end up at Quaker Bottom Road. The trail serves as the access point to where the Rock Run meets the Susquehanna at the historical area. To avoid going back to where you began, take the left at Rock Run, crossing over at 2.7 miles (take care on the loose rocks), and link up with the blue-blazed Farm Road Trail. The area around Rock Run is full of mountain laurel and mature beech trees.

Once across the run, take a right. You're likely to see many brown wood frogs, characterized by black "raccoon masks" around the eyes. Cross over the stone wall and immediately take a left. At 2.8 miles, emerge onto Rock Run Road and go left for about 50 feet and then back up into the woods to the right. The trail is recog-nizable by a series of log steps and a log handrail. Pass an orange-blazed trail to the right; in another ten feet, you'll see the same orange-blazed trail to the left. Take that; this is the Ivy Branch Trail. (Taking the first Ivy Branch rightward will bring you directly to the road leading to the historical area, where you've parked.)

There's a multitude of enormous trees along the Ivy Branch; it's stunningly beautiful and very peaceful, especially at around 3.5 miles. Pass a bog—again, many frogs—full of skunk cabbage. Cross a rocky stream shaded with hay-scented and Christmas fern; their combined aromas are reminiscent of cedar. Up the hill, you'll see a trail split: Spur #5 heads left and dead ends at Rock Run Road. Go right to stay on the Ivy Branch. Cross a little footbridge. Skirt around a pine plantation to the right and reach Wilkinson Road at 3.8. Straight ahead is the maintenance complex. Keep it to your right and walk along the tree line at the edge of the farm field. Continue in the same direction as the little gravel road at 3.9. Pass the entrance to the maintenance complex. Be on the lookout for when the groove in the grass, which is the trail, cuts leftward, away from the tree line. The top of the gradual hill affords a wonderful view: undeveloped land for miles.

There's a trail split at 4.5 miles. Take a left; this is the blue-blazed Farm Road Trail once again. You'll also see a rightward cut here. This is Trail Spur #4, which you can take if you're short on time, tired, or want to see an abandoned barn, silo, and stable—all looking very spooky in their dark, overrun state. The other end of the trail spur links to the red Susquehanna Ridge Trail, which you can follow right, back to the parking area. But to continue hiking, skip the spur and continue on the blue trail (you can see the barn later when you're on the red trail).

The Farm Road Trail cuts straight across an open field in waist-high grass full of grasshoppers, dragonflies, and green beetles in summer. Reenter the woods for good at 4.8 miles and take note of the little stream to the left. Take Spur #3 at 5.2 miles, crossing over the stream, to link to the green-blazed Deer Creek Trail. This trail winds through mature forest, noted mostly for what the

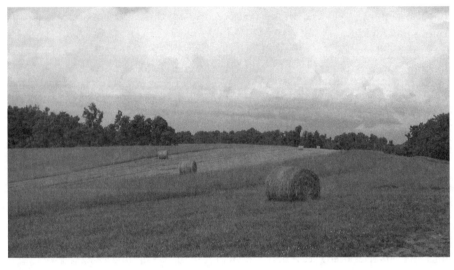

Bucolic farm trails

trail guide calls "two giant specimens of native trees, the white oak and American beech." Indeed, the girth of some of them is very impressive.

At the trail split at 6 miles, keep heading right, up the hill. Going left will take you to Craigs Corner Road. Deer Creek runs on the other side of Craigs Corner and you'll hear it for a while until you turn away and pass Trail Spur #2. Continue past Spur #1 afterward, across from the Deer Creek Picnic Area through the woods to the left, and soon the trail links up with the red Susquehanna Ridge Trail again, this time at 6.9 miles.

Cross a footbridge and a forest buffer, where a clear-cut area has been allowed to grow back naturally. Along the Ridge Trail, there's a profusion of wild mint and honeysuckle, offering a very nice aroma in summer. If you're hiking in winter and miss it, the tradeoff is that you've got great river views around the wide-girthed trees. If you didn't check it out earlier, look for the rightward Trail Spur #4 to see the abandoned barn.

Reach Rock Run at 8 miles. Cross it and take a left when you reach the park road. You're now reentering the Rock Run Historic Area, passing to the right the Rock Run House, the 1804 home of Brigadier General James Archer, who resigned from the U.S. Army to join the Confederacy. He was wounded and captured at Gettysburg in 1863. Several rooms in the mansion have been restored and stocked with period antiques; call the park for information on tours. Take a right, and the parking area is straight ahead.

NEARBY ACTIVITIES

See Susquehanna State Park: River Trails on page 257 for many nearby activities.

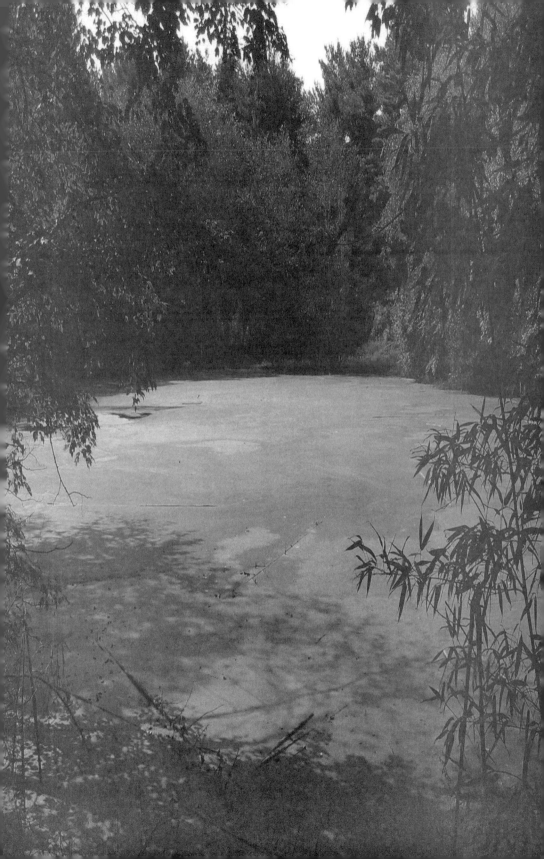

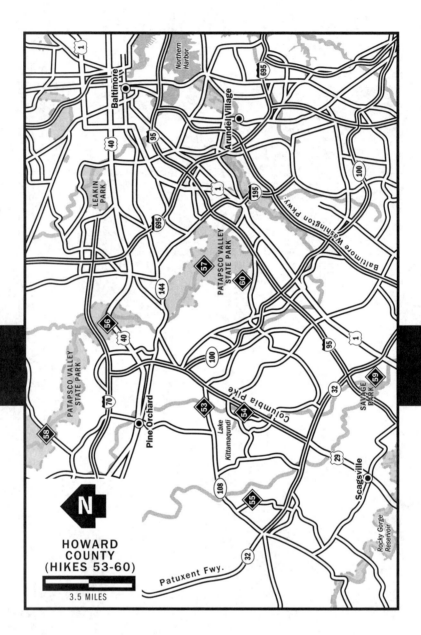

HOWARD COUNTY

53 CENTENNIAL PARK

KEY AT-A-GLANCE INFORMATION

LENGTH: 3.3 miles

CONFIGURATION: Loop

DIFFICULTY: Easy

SCENERY: Centennial Lake, Wildlife Management Area, Centennial Arboretum

EXPOSURE: Mostly sunny

TRAFFIC: Moderate–heavy

TRAIL SURFACE: Asphalt, short section of packed dirt

HIKING TIME: 1 hour

ACCESS: 7 a.m.–dusk

MAPS: USGS Savage; printable map at: www.co.ho.md.us/RAP/RAP HoCoParksCentennial.htm #anch6461

WHEELCHAIR ACCESS: Yes

FACILITIES: Bathrooms at pavilion at parking area; water fountain in front of the tennis courts. Other bathrooms and water are spread out at various parking areas around the lake. Ball fields, playgrounds, pavilions.

SPECIAL COMMENTS: For park information, call the Howard County Recreation and Parks Headquarters at (410) 313-4700.

- -

GPS Trailhead Coordinates

UTM Zone (WGS84) 18S

Easting 340273

Northing 4345039

Latitude N 39° 14.398155"

Longitude W 76° 51.048088"

IN BRIEF

Stroll around manmade 325-acre Centennial Lake, an oasis in the middle of Columbia, and enjoy the diversity of foliage in Centennial Arboretum.

DESCRIPTION

Pass a volleyball court and playgrounds at 150 feet on the right. A thick stand of trees to the left buffers the trail from Route 108. On the right is a large patch of wildflowers, a mélange of purple, yellow, and white; beyond it is a rising hill. The lake is on the other side of the hill.

Heading around to the right, the lake comes into view fairly quickly. You're likely to see in-line skaters, walkers, bicyclists, and people pushing strollers. It's obvious that Centennial is a recreational haven. Pass a parking area and pavilion, both to the left, and you'll reach the boat ramp at just under 0.6 miles. Just to the left of the boat ramp is a little wooden post with a hiker icon, denoting the trail heading into the woods. Take this packed dirt and cedar chip path as it winds through a stand of tall oaks. At 0.6 miles, still in the woods, take a left—here are lots of flowering dogwood, white oak, beech, and tulip poplar. The trail ends at a parking area. Link back up with the asphalt trail to the right toward the lake.

- -

Directions ⟶

Take I-695 to I-70 west to MD 29 south to MD 108 west toward Clarksville. Go 0.8 miles to a right into the park on Woodland Road. Take an immediate left at the sign for the pavilion. Follow to the parking area in front of the pavilion. The trailhead is between the pavilion and the tennis courts, denoted by two brown posts.

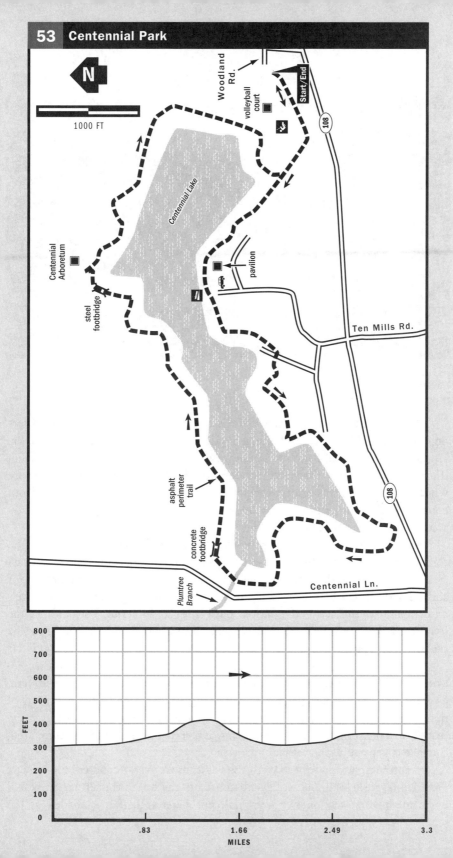

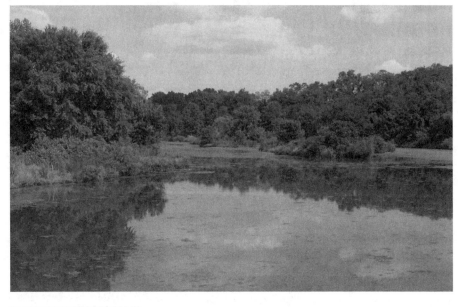

Wildlife Management Area

At just under 0.8 miles, take a left up the hill. You'll pass more wildflowers on either side. When you reach the next parking area, go right and then quickly left at the playground, heading around pavilions A and B. Go right, away from the parking area over the little wooden boardwalk at just over 1 mile. More wildflowers and cattails sit on either side of the boardwalk. The crowds thin out considerably in this section. The woods are thick on either side, but this section of the trail is entirely exposed.

At 1.2 miles, at a stand of pines to the left, the trail splits. Head to the right over another wooden boardwalk. Interestingly, the ecology changes drastically. It's now marshy wetlands—willows and cattails sway in the breeze for a few hundred feet before yielding once again to mixed hardwoods. Squirrels and chipmunks run across the path as butterflies flitter about. To the right, the Plumtree Branch of the Patuxent River leads into Centennial Lake, but it can be seen only in winter.

The trail splits again at just under 0.5 miles. Head left. The lake in this section is a maintained wildlife management area (there's no fishing allowed here, as there is elsewhere in the lake). It's full of algae and blooming lily pads; lots of ducks and the occasional gray heron make homes in this spot. You can see the rest of the lake from here and the contrast is striking—beyond this natural area, the lake is kept quite free of plant growth.

Continuing around the lake to the right, cross over a concrete footbridge. Pass tennis, basketball, and volleyball courts up the hill to the left. Soon, you'll come to the first section of the asphalt perimeter trail that is shaded as the mature trees form a canopy. At 2.3 miles, you'll come to a burgundy steel foot-bridge. On the other side is the Centennial Arboretum. Some of the trees you'll see here include black walnut, eastern red cedar, persimmon, redbud, scarlet oak, red maple, sassafras, bitternut hickory, black gum, beech, sweet cherry, black cherry, tuliptree, hornbeam (blue beech), staghorn sumac, post oak, dog-wood, and black oak. Each is labeled and immaculately maintained.

When the trail splits at 2.6 miles, head right. You'll have a nice view of the entire lake on your right. When the trail splits again at 3.1 miles, go left. You've now made a circuit of the lake. (When the trail splits again at 3.2 miles, head left for the car—if you go straight, you'll parallel Route 108 for another half mile where the trail abruptly ends.)

NEARBY ACTIVITIES

For good restaurants and shopping, head to the Columbia Town Center and Lake Kittamaqundi (see page 274). To get there, go west on Route 108 to Route 29 south and follow the signs to Town Center. For more hiking opportunities, head to The Middle Patuxent Environmental Area (see page 279), a 928-acre natu-ral area, home to 150 species of birds, more than 40 species of mammals, and numerous amphibians, reptiles, fishes, butterflies, plants, and other wildlife. To reach the MPEA, continue west on Route 108, past Centennial Park to a left on Trotter Road between Route 108 on the north and Route 32 on the south, just east of Clarksville.

54 LAKE KITTAMAQUNDI

KEY AT-A-GLANCE INFORMATION

LENGTH: 3 miles

CONFIGURATION: Loop with an out-and-back spur

DIFFICULTY: Easy

SCENERY: Lake Kittamaqundi, Patuxent River, mixed hardwoods

EXPOSURE: Half sun and half shade

TRAFFIC: Moderate–heavy

TRAIL SURFACE: Asphalt, dirt, brick

HIKING TIME: 1 hour

ACCESS: Open 24 hours a day, 7 days a week; dirt path not recommended after dark; Maryland Transit Administration (MTA) runs buses to downtown Columbia, including Columbia Mall across from Lake Kittamaqundi; for a complete MTA schedule, call (866) RIDE-MTA or visit www.mtamaryland.com.

MAPS: USGS Savage

WHEELCHAIR ACCESS: Lake loop only

FACILITIES: Food, drink, restrooms in restaurants along west side of lake

SPECIAL COMMENTS: The mileage markers included in the Description start at the entrance to the trail loop behind the Sushi Sono restaurant, but the abundance of parking in a variety of areas surrounding the lake make it possible for you to start your hike elsewhere.

GPS Trailhead Coordinates

UTM Zone (WGS84) 18S

Easting 339835

Northing 4342402

Latitude N 39' 12.968345"

Longitude W 76' 51.314914"

IN BRIEF

Take an easy stroll around Lake Kittamaqundi and, for contrast, finish with a hike through the woods between the lake and Little Patuxent River.

DESCRIPTION

Sandwiched between Little Patuxent Parkway and MD 29, the 27-acre man-made Lake Kittamaqundi bears the name of the first recorded Indian settlement in Howard County. Kittamaqundi means "meeting place," appropriate for the lake's position adjacent to the Columbia Town Center.

From the back of the Sushi Sono restaurant, head left onto the asphalt path down the hill, keeping the lake on your right. You'll see a small buffer of trees between you and the lake and some apple trees on the left. At a quarter-mile, you'll have a good view of Nomanizan Island, reachable only by boat; during the summer months you can rent a canoe, rowboat, or paddleboat at the pier.

Cross a footbridge and enter the woods at 0.3 miles; the little creek below connects Lake Kittamaqundi with Wilde Lake, a few miles to the northwest. On the left, you'll see the beginning of the Parcourse fitness circuit. Cross the creek on a wooden footbridge and

Directions

Take I-695 to I-70 west and continue to MD 29 south (toward Columbia and Washington, D.C.). Take Exit 20B, MD 175, toward Columbia Town Center. Go 1 mile and turn left onto Wincopin Circle; park anywhere in the nearby lots or garages and walk east toward the lake. The trail described in this hike starts roughly behind the Sheraton Hotel, in front of the Sushi Sono restaurant.

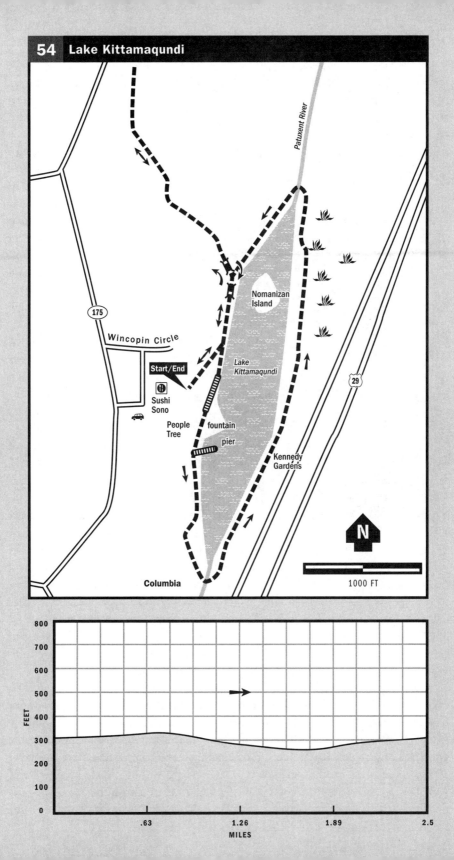

Patuxent River

175

Wincopin Circle

Nomanizan Island

Lake Kittamaqundi

Start/End

Sushi Sono

People Tree

fountain

pier

Kennedy Gardens

29

N

1000 FT

Columbia

FEET

800
700
600
500
400
300
200
100
0

.63   1.26   1.89   2.5

MILES

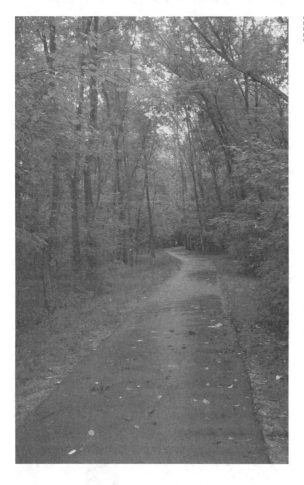

head left. The woods here are thick and mature, full of sassafras, maple, beech, sycamore, oak, gum, tulip poplar, and sumac; these fantastic foliage trees turn the path into a rainbow of color in fall.

Unfortunately, you can hear Little Patuxent Parkway as it comes into view at 0.6 miles. This section of the trail has a nice mix of fairly short, immature trees alongside centuries-old walnuts, which soar hundreds of feet above. At just under 0.75 miles, the trail connects to a sidewalk and ends unceremoniously at a bus stop on a busy intersection; turn around here.

When you see the back of the Sushi Sono restaurant again (where you began your hike), head left; you will be closer to the lake, and at 1.2 miles you'll be on a wooden boardwalk. You'll see Clyde's Restaurant (a local institution) and the Tomato Palace on the hill above the lake. Down the hill a bit, to the right of the lake, you'll see a pagoda and the People Tree, a sculpture that has come to symbolize Columbia. The boathouse here has a ramp for launching boats and canoes. The adjacent wooden pier offers nice views of the lake, which provides good habitat for hundreds of duck and geese. Facing the lake to the right is a fountain inspired by the one in Tivoli Gardens in Rome, Italy.

Walk back toward the fountain and take a left up the concrete steps; then take another left onto a brick walkway, which turns to asphalt after about ten feet. This section of the lake looks more aquatic, with a few cattails and willow trees. At 1.6 miles, the trail splits at a popular fishing spot. A short distance later, the trail splits again; continue heading left, keeping close to the lake. When you cross a creek, you'll be on the opposite end of the lake from where you started. A decent-size wooded buffer separates you from MD 29, which is not far to the right; between runs the Patuxent River. You won't be able to see the river here, but you will a little farther down the trail.

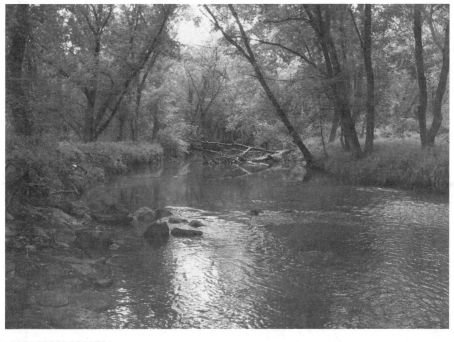

Little Patuxent River

As you walk, you'll pass through the Kennedy Gardens, dominated by black-eyed Susans, maple trees, and ornamental bushes and grasses; you'll find plenty of benches here to sit and soak in the peaceful beauty. The trail splits into a loop at 2 miles; you can head either way, but be on the lookout at the far end of the loop for a small dirt path that heads into the woods and affords a really nice hike. Note that the dirt path is not lighted so it can't be taken at night; also, it can get quite muddy after rains. Although the dirt path is easily discernible, it is a bit tight and not many people travel it; expect tall grasses on both sides of the path to sweep your legs. The Little Patuxent River runs on the right, and you'll see the remains of—or perhaps intact—beaver dams. You will be amazed at the contrast between this section of the hike and the beginning. Here, white-tailed deer run in the woods; fish, turtles, frogs, and snakes make homes in the river; and you'll probably have the trail all to yourself. The only downside is that it's brief.

At 2.3 miles, townhouses come into view on the right, but just beyond you'll see a path to the left that circles the lake. When the trail ends at a field behind the houses, zigzag through the oak trees, staying close to the lake on your left. Look for a barely discernible path that cuts abruptly to the right away from the lake; follow this path and head left over a feeder creek into the woods. The path will dump you out onto the asphalt trail in front of the wooden footbridge and Parcourse fitness circuit close to where you began; head left and continue to the start of the trail just ahead.

NEARBY ACTIVITIES

Check out what's happening at nearby Merriweather Post Pavilion, the "Mid-Atlantic Fillmore East," which has hosted virtually every big name in rock and pop music. Designed by famed architect Frank Gehry, it's been rocking for more than 40 years. You'll find it just southwest of Lake Kittamaqundi across Little Patuxent Parkway; for more information, call (410) 715-5550 or visit **www.merriweathermusic .com**. Also nearby is the African Art Museum of Maryland, which has a collection of more than 200 works of art covering a variety of cultures and styles; take MD 175 north and turn onto Vantage Point Road; continue approximately 0.2 miles to the OAKLAND sign on the right. Turn right and continue to the parking area. The large building with the white columns on the left is Oakland; the museum is on the second level. Info: (410) 730-7105; **www.africanartmuseum.org**.

MIDDLE PATUXENT ENVIRONMENTAL AREA 55

IN BRIEF

Search for varied wildlife among a swath of buffer woods around the Middle Branch of the Patuxent River.

DESCRIPTION

The varied topography and ecosystems of the 1,021-acre Middle Patuxent Environmental Area (MPEA) host an impressive diversity of wildlife, including roughly 150 birds species, more than 40 mammal species, and many amphibians, reptiles, and fishes.

Pick up an informative trail brochure at the bulletin board before you head out. At 900 feet, you'll come to a clearing with a picnic table, and you'll see wooden post #1; many species of butterflies congregate here, including monarchs, banded hairstreaks, pearl crescents, great spangled fritillaries, American ladies, and a variety of skippers. The wooden post marks the beginning of the interpretive Wildlife Loop Trail; to follow the numbers sequentially—and add a nice out-and-back with a loop in the other section of the MPEA—go straight.

You'll soon come to wooden post #2 in an area of field habitat being managed for indigo buntings, prairie warblers, American goldfinches, yellow-breasted chats, blue-winged warblers, American woodcocks, and

KEY AT-A-GLANCE INFORMATION

LENGTH: 4.7 miles

CONFIGURATION: Combination

DIFFICULTY: Easy–moderate

SCENERY: Varied flora and fauna, the Middle Branch of the Patuxent River

EXPOSURE: Slightly more shade than sun

TRAFFIC: Light–moderate

TRAIL SURFACE: Initially crushed rock and then mostly packed dirt

HIKING TIME: 1.5 hours

ACCESS: Dawn–dusk except during restricted deer hunts (see Special Comments)

MAPS: USGS Clarksville; trail maps and informational brochures available at the trailhead bulletin board and online (see Description)

WHEELCHAIR ACCESS: No

FACILITIES: None

SPECIAL COMMENTS: Middle Patuxent Environmental Area holds restricted deer hunts; call (410) 313-4726 for more information; note that the area is closed during hunts—these times are minimal, scheduled usually for very early morning hours and only on a few weekend mornings.

Directions

Take I-695 to I-70 west; continue to MD 29 south and then MD 108 west toward Clarksville. Go 5 miles and turn left onto Trotter Road; go half a mile to the gravel parking area on the left. The trail starts behind the wooden posts at the edge of the parking area next to the informational bulletin board.

GPS Trailhead Coordinates

UTM Zone (WGS84) 18S

Easting 334381

Northing 4342133

Latitude N 39' 12.761600"

Longitude W 76' 55.099547"

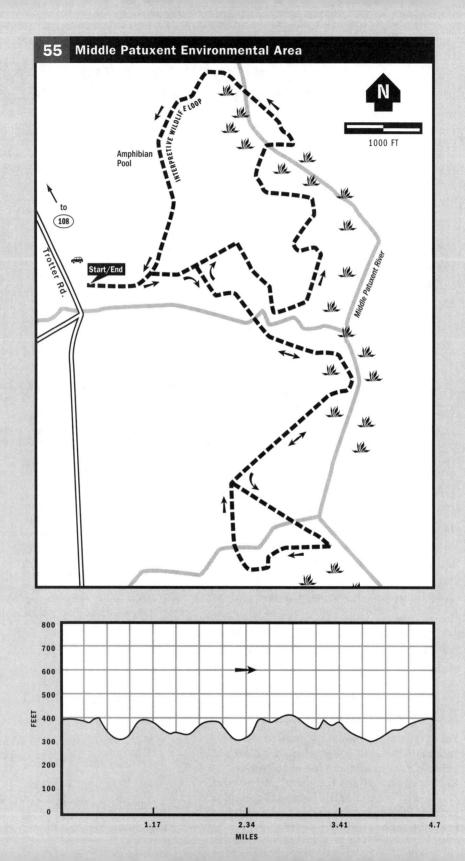

N

1000 FT

Amphibian
Pool

INTERPRETIVE WILDLIFE LOOP

to
108

Trotter Rd.

Start/End

Middle Patuxent River

FEET

800
700
600
500
400
300
200
100
0

1.17   2.34   3.41   4.7
MILES

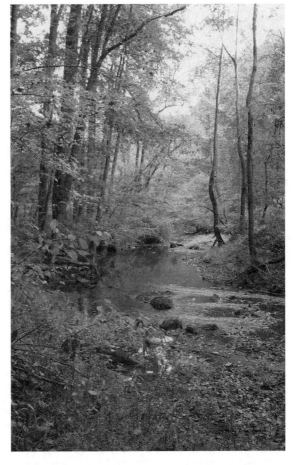

Middle Patuxent feeder stream

other birds. Head right on a path; you'll pass a bench made from the slab of what was once a very wide tree. You're now leaving the Wildlife Loop Trail, using a connector path to the Southwind Trail. No worries—you'll finish the wildlife loop on your return. Walk through a field of midlevel growth (blueberry, sweet cicely, azalea, and mountain laurel) with a few pines beyond as you head toward the Middle Branch of the Patuxent River.

The trail in this section is easy to spot but fairly wild, with much encroaching grass; it's wild enough to feel very isolated but not so much to require a bushwhack. This very lovely spot in thick woods shows no sign at all of humanity. When the trail opens at 0.5 miles, it takes on a very Appalachian feel, with ferns, big hunks of rock, moss, and the river winding its way through the big trees. You'll cross a feeder stream of the Middle Branch at 0.7 miles; on the other side, look for a hiker icon indicating the blue-blazed Southwind Trail, and follow it. The icon will help you locate the trail, which gets lost here in tall grass.

At 0.75 miles, head right into the mowed section of an open field. Known as edge habitat, this area provides important hunting and nesting grounds for a variety of animals. Many of the trees in the approaching field are persimmons. A grassland-restoration project is under way in this open area, called Clegg's Meadow, with plantings of bluestem, Indian, switch, and Eastern gamma grasses. There's also purple-martin housing here. You'll gradually head uphill following the tree line as you walk along the mowed path. When I hiked here, I was lucky to see a beautiful red fox prancing up the path ahead of me. As usual in open spaces, hawks wheel above as they look for prey.

When the trail splits at 1 mile, go straight to extend the hike; a few private homes will shatter the isolation for a while, but as you continue on the trail you'll soon regain a feeling of seclusion. Go past a cutoff path to the left, and keep going straight; turn left at the mowed path at 1.2 miles, then left again 200 feet later. In autumn, you'll smell a fantastic sweet, earthy aroma from decaying leaves, tree trunks, and mosses that haven't been disturbed for years.

The trail splits again at 1.3 miles; go left. Suddenly, the wide, open trail becomes very narrow and crowded with woods. Spicebush is dominant here, providing food for numerous songbirds, including wood thrushes and veeries. As you parallel a stream on the right, you'll begin to see numbered wooden posts again. If you still have the wildlife-loop trail brochure you picked up at the hike's beginning, you may find the numbers a bit misleading because they don't correspond to the map; that's because you left the Wildlife Loop Trail. Instead, this is the Southwind Trail. This, too, is an interpretive trail, but brochures haven't been placed at the bulletin board (at least not as of winter 2008). You can, however, retrieve the corresponding information online by clicking on "MPEA Virtual Tour" at **www.co.ho.md.us/RAP/RAP_MPEA.htm**.

As you hike a big curve up the hill and wind through mature upland forest, you'll begin to climb above the trail you were on earlier, now in the opposite direction. The trail peaks on a narrow ridge with water below on both sides. One of these waterways is Cricket Creek. Elusive minks live near the water here, but don't expect to see one during the day. At 1.8 miles, you'll be back on the trail you hiked coming in earlier. This time head right; the trail will take you past the private houses and the field before it begins running parallel to the river, this time on your right. At 2.25 miles, go left—be on the lookout for this turn because it's very easy to miss. (If you do miss it, you'll parallel the river for another quarter-mile before the trail ends, and then you'll have to turn around and come back.) Once you've turned left, you'll backtrack before you rejoin the Wildlife Loop at 2.7 miles.

Once you're back on the Wildlife Loop, the numbered wooden posts that correspond to the trail brochure come in quick succession. Wooden post #3 sits in a cluster of Virginia pines. Soon after you'll come to a deer enclosure marked with wooden post #4. At just under 3 miles, post #5 points out the varieties of grapevines in the area: fox, summer, and riverbank. Wooden post #6 sits on one of the highest points in the MPEA, more than 400 feet; the floodplain below sits at about 275 feet. When you come to the T-intersection, head right to continue onto the main section of the wildlife loop.

You'll see wooden post #7 in a mature upland forest dominated by oaks, hickories, and tulip poplars. Next you'll come to a cluster of spicebush, at 3.3 miles. Immediately after, you will see several cuts along the hills—these are drainage areas that indirectly carry runoff water to the Chesapeake Bay. The topography changes by the time you reach wooden post #10 in the floodplain. Correspondingly, the flora changes as well, and you'll see skunk cabbages, cardinal flowers, monkeyflowers, mad-dog skullcaps, green dragons, button-bushes, and American sycamores.

At 3.5 miles, you'll see a small tributary that forms an oxbow (probably once part of the Middle Branch of the Patuxent River); after you cross it, you'll come to wooden post #15, which marks dogwood trees that are dead or dying due to fungal diseases. At just under 4 miles, you'll come to a concrete wading pool that has been converted into amphibian habitat. Look to the right to see a bizarre sight: an old car of indistinguishable make. Only the hulk of the body, impaled by the trees growing through it, and clearly discernible tail fins remain.

As you continue on the trail, you'll pass a clearing on the left, the home of the MPEA's outdoor classroom for Howard County students in kindergarten through grade 12. Just beyond, at 4.2 miles, you'll rejoin the first part of trail, with wooden post #1; go right and follow the trail back to the parking area.

NEARBY ACTIVITIES

You might enjoy seeing Centennial Lake just 4 miles to the east on MD 108; take time to walk through the park's Centennial Arboretum, an immaculately maintained treasure trove of diverse tree species (see page 270). For good restaurants and shopping, head to the Columbia Town Center and Lake Kittamaqundi (see page 274); go east on MD 108 to MD 29 south and follow the TOWN CENTER signs.

56 PATAPSCO VALLEY STATE PARK: HOLLOFIELD AREA

KEY AT-A-GLANCE INFORMATION

LENGTH: 3.9 miles

CONFIGURATION: Combination

DIFFICULTY: Easy

SCENERY: Piedmont forest, Patapsco Valley overlook, pond, dam ruins

EXPOSURE: Mostly shaded

TRAFFIC: Moderate, heavy at overlook and playgrounds

TRAIL SURFACE: Packed dirt, crushed rock, asphalt

HIKING TIME: 1.5 hours

ACCESS: 10 a.m.–sunset. There is a $2 day-use fee if you enter the park at the overlook area.

MAPS: USGS Ellicott City; maps of the entire PVSP trail system can be purchased at the park headquarters or online at www.easycart.net/MarylandDepart mentofNaturalResources/Central_Maryland_Trail_Guides.html.

WHEELCHAIR ACCESS: In small sections

FACILITIES: Bathrooms, playgrounds, water, vending machines, campgrounds

- -

GPS Trailhead
Coordinates

UTM Zone (WGS84) 18S

Easting 345580

Northing 4351167

Latitude N39' 17.767324"

Longitude W76' 47.444451"

IN BRIEF

Take in one of Patapsco Valley State Park's most popular areas.

DESCRIPTION

The Peaceful Pond Trail begins as a narrow dirt path, winding among pines, hollies, tall grasses, and short stubby trees. At 500 feet, head left at the split; you'll see a sign pointing you to the pond. After another 100 feet, split to the left again, where you'll find a bench and observation deck. Unfortunately, "Peaceful Pond" is something of a misnomer with MD 40 nearby, but it's pleasant nonetheless, home to many frogs, snakes, turtles, and herons.

Moving away from the pond, head left and then back up the hill the way you came. But this time at the split, take it going the opposite direction you used to come in, past an area full of vines—looking like something out of Flash Gordon. At 0.3 miles, at the top of a steep hill, you'll see an oddly shaped oak tree with a jutting appendage at the bottom of the trunk, running horizontal for about six feet before sprouting another mature tree. Each connected tree has a different blaze—orange for Peaceful Pond and light blue for Ole Ranger Trail. Follow the the light-blue blazes.

The Ole Ranger Trail winds through tulip poplars, white pines, and multiflora

- -

Directions ─────────────────▶

Take I-695 to Exit 14, MD Route 40 west toward Ellicott City. Go 2 miles, crossing the Patapsco River, and take a right into the park. Take the first left toward the park headquarters. With the headquarters to your back, walk down the hill and to the left until you see the brown Peaceful Pond Trail sign—the blazes are orange.

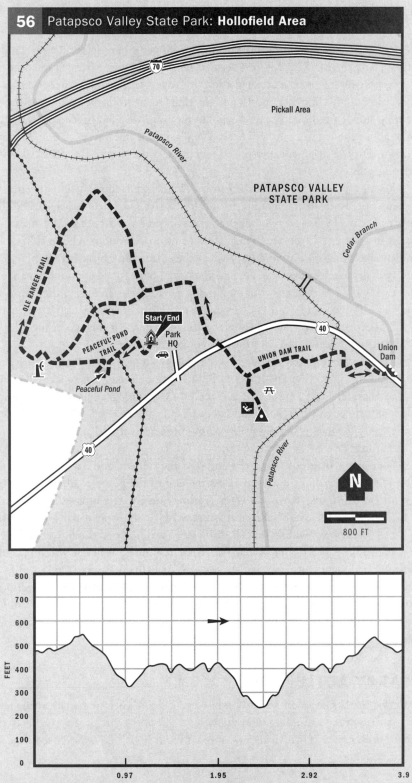

56 Patapsco Valley State Park: **Hollofield Area**

rose. It soon visits an old radio-transmission tower where in the 1940s women employed by the Maryland Forest Service kept a lookout for fires. Soon after the tower, the trail becomes a crushed-rock fire road. At 0.4 miles, there's a split—leftward runs to Church Lane Road. Go right to head deeper into the woods, the road now rutted and decayed asphalt. Sloping, wooded hills mark the trail, rising above the Patapsco River gorge. The dominant trees here are oak, hickory, and ash. On eye level, spicebush and witch hazel dominate, the perfect habitat for songbirds.

Reach a power-line cut at 0.75 miles. While a paved road runs toward the transmission lines, the Ole Ranger continues straight ahead as a packed-dirt foot trail. Cross a little stream at 0.9 miles—notice the zigzag of the stream as it runs in a series of S-curves. The trail becomes rocky and reaches a split at 1.1 miles; make note of it, as you'll take the other direction on the return hike. For now, cross the footbridge and come to the paved park road beyond it. Head left, under MD 40, and then go straight, passing the tollgate, and on to the overlook, described by park literature as "arguably the most breathtaking [vista] in the park." There are more-isolated spots that I like better, but this is a beautiful spot nonetheless, with each season offering its own splendor.

If you want to extend your hike beyond what's described here, the paved road heading right down the hill before the overlook area leads to a small campground. Though on a paved road, the walk to the campground is very pleasant, as it winds through thick woods and goes for more than a mile. Also, on the way to the campground, you'd pass the yellow-blazed River Ridge Trail, a 0.2-mile trail that leads to the Patapsco River.

Back at the overlook, head left and pass the tollgate and playgrounds to the left and picnic pavilions to the right. At the end of the paved road, you'll see the sign for the white-blazed Union Dam Trail. It immediately crosses a picnic area and goes downhill toward the river on a twisty, rock-strewn path. Notice the CSX rail line below heading into the hill you're walking on. You'll reach the dam (or what's left of it after numerous floods) at 2.3 miles. When it was intact, the dam supplied water for the J. W. Dickey Textile Mills in nearby Oella.

On the way back, return on the Ole Ranger Trail you took to the overlook. This time, at the split head left at the sign reading TOWER .5 MILE at 3.3 miles. Go left at the orange arrow pointing to the pond, and backtrack to the headquarters, reaching it at 3.9 miles.

NEARBY ACTIVITIES

Just a bit farther west on MD 40 is historic Ellicott City (**www.ellicottcity.net**), full of restaurants, antiques, museums, and shopping. In nearby Oella is the Benjamin Banneker Historical Park and Museum ([410] 887-1081; see page 78 for a hike here).

PATAPSCO VALLEY STATE PARK: ORANGE GROVE–AVALON AREAS

 57

IN BRIEF

See waterfalls, rivers, streams, upland forest, historical structures, and entire herds of deer in one of the more diverse hikes in Patapsco Valley State Park. This hike begins in the Orange Grove Area and takes in the Avalon Area before returning to Orange Grove.

DESCRIPTION

The 300-foot suspension Swinging Bridge provides one of the few places for easy access across the Patapsco River. You can cross it to go to the paved Grist Mill Trail and the Hilton Area of the state park, but to hike in the Orange Grove Area, turn around and head up the hill on the stone steps to the blue-blazed Cascade Falls Trail. It winds uphill, taking in a little switchback, before quickly coming to Cascade Falls, at 0.3 miles. Ferns, mossy rocks, and oaks surround a narrow ridge where the falls spill over; the trail becomes a series of rocks that leads across the falls and gives you an unobstructed and fantastic view. It's a superb way to start your hike.

On the other side of the falls, you'll see the orange-blazed Ridge Trail on the left;

KEY AT-A-GLANCE INFORMATION

LENGTH: 6.4 miles

CONFIGURATION: Loop

DIFFICULTY: Moderate

SCENERY: Cascade Falls, historical ruins, abundant wildlife, mature forest

EXPOSURE: Shade

TRAFFIC: Light

TRAIL SURFACE: Packed dirt

HIKING TIME: 2.5–3 hours

ACCESS: 10 a.m.–sunset daily

MAPS: USGS Relay; you can also purchase an excellent map of the entire Patapsco Valley State Park trail system from the Maryland Department of Natural Resources online at www.easycart.net/ MarylandDepartmentofNatural Resources/Central_Maryland_Trail _Guides.html.

WHEELCHAIR ACCESS: No

FACILITIES: Restrooms and water at the trailhead

SPECIAL COMMENTS: $2 day-use fee, which is usually collected by the honor system; place the money in an envelope at the tollgate.

Directions

Take I-95 to Exit 47 (BWI Airport); and travel east on I-195 to Exit 3 heading toward Elkridge. Turn right on US 1 heading south, and then take the next right onto South Street. You will see the park entrance immediately on the left. Follow the park road past the WELCOME TO ORANGE GROVE SCENIC AREA signs and turn left onto Gun Road followed by an immediate right onto River Road. Continue to the parking area on the left across from the Swinging Bridge over the Patapsco River. The trail starts at the CASCADE FALLS TRAIL sign up the hill from the parking area.

GPS Trailhead Coordinates

UTM Zone (WGS84) 18S

Easting 348989

Northing 4344967

Latitude N 39' 14.452901"

Longitude W 76' 44.990158"

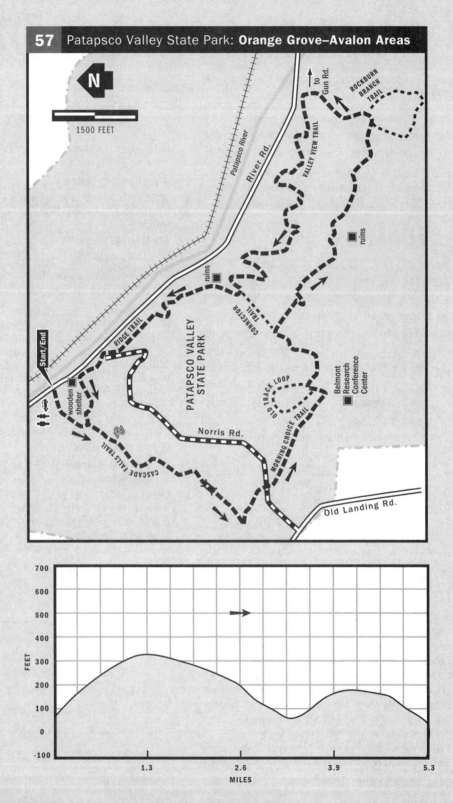

57 Patapsco Valley State Park: **Orange Grove–Avalon Areas**

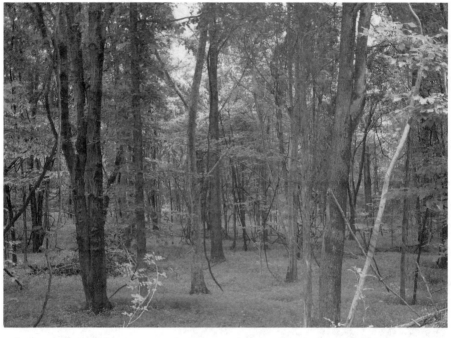

Rockburn Branch Trail

you'll take that trail on the way back, so head right instead. The trail becomes very rocky as it winds through mature beech, oak, dogwood, maple, redbud, and sassafras; you'll see and hear the stream that feeds the falls to the right. At just over 0.25 miles, cross the water again. Soon after, the trail splits; you can go either way, but I suggest heading left because the trail to the right forms a loop and after 0.8 miles will lead you to the same place you're heading now by going left. Cross the water once again and continue paralleling the stream by heading upstream. You'll come to a creek bed and small footbridge at just under 0.5 miles followed by a little gulley full of moss and ferns. There are a few eastern hemlocks visible here; look also for plant species more commonly found in mountains, including erect trillium, false hellebore, and wild sarsaparilla. Lots of rocks and fallen trees in the water create pools and small rapids that produce a pleasant babble. Cross the water again, this time on a wooden footbridge and again, on another wooden footbridge soon after (just before you come to the second footbridge, you'll see the spot where the other side of that initial loop connects to the main trail).

At 0.75 miles, the trail levels out and quiets down a bit. You're now away from water, walking among beech and oak trees in a mature forest. When the trail splits, go left up the hill heading toward the yellow-blazed Morning Choice Trail (if you go straight, you'll wind up leaving the park boundary in another 0.3 miles). In the middle of the hill, the trail splits again—stay on the Morning Choice Trail on the left; head uphill where you'll see a tangle of vines and

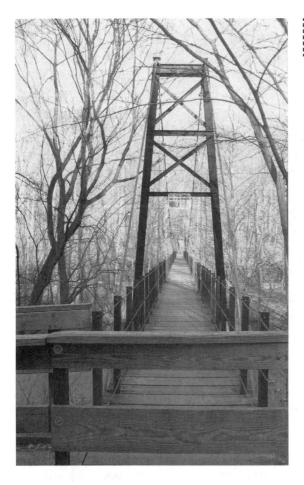

Swinging Bridge, one of the
Patapsco's few crossing points

smaller trees. Many birds flit around the tall, thin oaks and poplars; during spring and fall migrations, you might see bluebirds, scarlet tanagers, and Baltimore orioles. At 0.9 miles, cross Norris Road, a gravel park road. When you come to a T-intersection, take a left into a natural drainage area; it's usually muddy here, but boards placed at the lowest points in the trail will help keep your boots dry.

After walking through a small stand of holly, you'll come to the red-blazed Old Track Loop Trail, at 1.1 miles. For a short section, the red and yellow-blazed trails run together. On the right you'll see a huge cluster of bamboo that measures about 30 feet high and 85 feet across. When the trail splits, head left on the red-blazed path. (You can take the yellow-blazed path, which eventually leads to a nice stream crossing where wood thrushes congregate, but it's impassable in all but the lowest water levels; the trail then ends abruptly at Landing Road 1 mile later, where you'll have to turn around. The better option, I think, is to stay on the red-blazed trail; you'll soon hook back up with the yellow one so you can continue the loop.)

On the red-blazed trail, you'll soon come to an open field to the right through the woods, where you'll see the Belmont Research Conference Center up the hill. Stay within the woods for a while longer, passing evergreens and oaks covered in ivy—a nice spot of green in winter. At 1.6 miles, rejoin the yellow-blazed trail and take a left up the hill. At the top of the hill, you'll see an orange-blazed trail, which is a connector trail between the yellow Morning Choice and the orange Ridge Trail, to the east. You can take this if you're short on time, but to extend the hike and make a bigger (and very pleasant) loop, take a right and stay on the yellow-blazed trail heading toward the Avalon Area of PVSP.

The path becomes a cut groove along the tree line of the field before winding back through the woods at 1.9 miles; you'll pass the ruins of old houses on the left. Both houses have paths running to them, but it's not safe to poke around inside. Once past the house ruins, you'll come back to the field again, where you'll follow the tree line. Look across the field for deer; I've never seen fewer than two dozen in this area, and often I've spotted many more. As a bonus, you'll see loads of jays, cardinals, blackbirds, and cedar waxwings flitting about the mountain laurel and holly on the edge of the field.

At 2.4 miles, come to the purple-blazed Rockburn Branch Trail; if you take a left, you'll return to the orange-blazed Ridge Trail. Instead, take a right and do the lovely Rockburn Branch Trail. It's a 1.2-mile loop. At 2.6 miles, you'll come to Rockburn Branch, a lovely little stream that you'll parallel for another two-tenths of a mile before swinging left away from it. Now the trail winds through mature forest before heading uphill and rejoining the trail split, at 3.6 miles, where you earlier left the yellow Morning Choice Trail. This time, go right for 100 yards on the purple-blazed Rockburn Branch Trail and then go straight down the hill on the orange-blazed Ridge Trail. You'll be heading toward the Valley View Trail, which parallels the much higher Ridge Trail before the two eventually link. At the bottom of the hill, you'll come to a wide gravel path; head left and cross a stream. Then walk left toward a stone shelter where you'll see a sign pointing to the white-blazed Valley View Trail straight ahead; on the right, you'll see the orange-blazed Ridge Trail and a footbridge.

Valley View Trail begins as a narrow ridgeline in the middle of the hill following the valley amid a plenitude of evergreens. Initially, you'll parallel River Road, which doesn't provide the best scenery but does allow good views of the valley and Patapsco River beyond. The trail soon rises away from the road and very quickly climbs the hill; in winter, you can see across the entire valley from this spot. Valley View Trail provides a good sense of the topography—hills rising and falling all around, with the piedmont river valley below. You won't want for grand, sweeping views along this trail.

At 4.4 miles, take a right at the T-intersection, and you'll be back on the orange-blazed Ridge Trail, which winds along a series of drainage cuts. You've lost your valley views, but you'll gain a level area in mature upland forest, with abundant groves of mountain laurel. Head downhill and at 4.7 miles, pass the connector on the left to the yellow-blazed Morning Choice Trail you hiked earlier. You'll still see lots of mountain laurel and now also an abundance of beech trees. The ruins of a series of stone houses, some with collapsed wooden roofs still visible, mark the trail after 5 miles. At 5.2 miles, you'll cross a little stream running over beautiful pink-hued, striated rocks, and you'll see a wooden shelter ahead. At 5.6 miles, you'll see a cut that leads down to River Road; turn the other direction and head uphill to the left. You'll soon hear Cascade Falls and, at 6 miles, you'll reach the cut to the right that leads to the falls. When you reach the falls, cross the water, and head back to your car.

NEARBY ACTIVITIES

Satisfy your thirst for history by driving (or walking) on River Road through the developed section of the Avalon Area of Patapsco Valley State Park. All that remains of Avalon, a thriving mill town until wiped out by a massive flood in 1868, is one stone building that now houses the visitor center, which features exhibits on about 300 years of history in the Patapsco Valley. You'll find the 704-foot-long Thomas Viaduct about 1.5 miles south of the Swinging Bridge; completed in 1835, the viaduct is the world's largest multiple-arched stone railroad bridge. Less than a mile north of the Swinging Bridge on River Road is Bloede's Dam, which contains the world's first submerged electrical generating plant.

PATAPSCO VALLEY STATE PARK:
UNMAINTAINED AREA: GRANITE-WOODSTOCK
58

IN BRIEF

Make a loop of a section of Patapsco Valley State Park where the trails take you over tough, but rewarding, terrain.

DESCRIPTION

There are many developed areas inside PVSP that provide amenities for family outings, camping, and picnics. But there are huge tracts of the park where you're on your own. Since this area of PVSP is unmaintained, it promises solitude and a vigorous hike. There are also places where the trail seems to disappear. You'll always be able to get through, but be prepared.

From the trailhead, follow the path down a steep ridge to the river, where you'll probably scatter mallards and wood ducks, and take a left, walking upstream. The trail is initially difficult to discern, but head along the river and it will become clearer. The path is a horse trail winding along the water's edge. It's very rocky, so unless you too are wearing horseshoes, be careful. Several large trees have fallen in the path and you'll have to climb over.

Directions ⸻⸻⸻⸻➤

Take I-695 to Exit 18, Liberty Road west toward Randallstown. Go 1.9 miles to a left on Old Court Road. Go 5.7 miles, passing through Granite, past the Maryland Job Corps, and cross over the Patapsco River. As soon as you cross the river and the railroad tracks, park on the right in the gravel parking area. (Be careful not to park in front of the wooden hitching posts; these are for horses.) Alternate directions are to take I-695 to Exit 22, Greenspring Avenue south. Take the first right onto Old Court Road and go 12 miles to the parking area above. The trailhead is behind you over the tracks and to the left down the hill.

KEY AT-A-GLANCE INFORMATION

LENGTH: 7 miles

CONFIGURATION: Loop (plus out-and-back depending on water level)

DIFFICULTY: Moderate–strenuous

SCENERY: Patapsco River, wildlife, railroading accoutrements

EXPOSURE: Mostly shaded

TRAFFIC: Light

TRAIL SURFACE: Packed dirt, potential railroad track

HIKING TIME: 2.5–3 hours

ACCESS: Dawn–dusk

MAPS: USGS Ellicott City, Sykesville; a map of the McKeldin Area and/or the entire PVSP trail system is available at the park or online at www.easycart.net/MarylandDepartment ofNaturalResources/Central_Mary land_Trail_Guides.html.

WHEELCHAIR ACCESS: No

FACILITIES: No

SPECIAL COMMENTS: This is an unnamed, unmaintained section of PVSP, and I call it Granite–Woodstock because of its location between those two towns. Beware that this hike involves one river crossing (but with an alternative if crossing isn't feasible), and a potentially frightening railroad bridge crossing if water levels are high.

GPS Trailhead Coordinates

UTM Zone (WGS84) 18S

Easting 338720

Northing 4355244

Latitude N 39' 19.895360"

Longitude W 76' 52.273951"

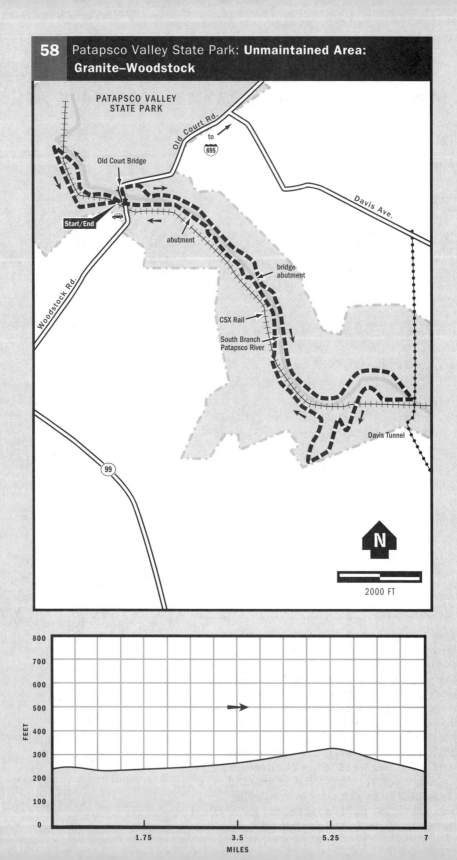

PATAPSCO VALLEY
STATE PARK

Old Court Rd.

to
695

Old Court Bridge

Davis Ave.

Start/End

abutment

Woodstock Rd.

bridge
abutment

CSX Rail

South Branch
Patapsco River

Davis Tunnel

99

N

2000 FT

Come to an oxbow at a quarter-mile. It's shallow, but it's about 20 feet across and there are no rocks for crossing. If you want to keep your boots dry, head up to the left and circle around until you find a better place to cross. After the oxbow, the trail becomes much more obvious, as a narrow groove in the grass. At half a mile is where the horses cross the Patapsco and where you can do the same if the weather is warm and you take your shoes off—the river is fairly shallow here and is only about 100 feet across, aided by a sand and rock bank that cuts into the river. I hiked here in winter and didn't want wet feet, so instead climbed the hill and walked along the railroad tracks back toward the trailhead. If you do cross the river, follow the obvious trail on the other side back toward the bridge on Old Court Road.

Whichever route you choose, you'll reach Old Court at roughly 1 mile. There's a wide shoulder on the bridge if you haven't yet crossed. The trail on the Baltimore County side is very obvious. It becomes a pleasant and easy stroll among primarily beech and oak, with briers lining the path. Generally speaking, the trail is fairly muddy in places because of horseshoes; as a result, you'll also see lots of deer prints in the mud (and probably a few deer running about as well).

At just under 2 miles, swing away from the river a bit and cross over an old abutment. If you look across the river to the Howard County side, you'll see the same abutments there where they joined before floods destroyed the bridge. The trail splits here, but keep straight instead of going left—the leftward option is a half-mile spur that ends at Davis Avenue. Cross over a little brook. This section is marked by low growth: grapevines and mountain laurel mostly. At 2.25 miles, look for a huge gash in the ground, almost like a sinkhole. A trickle of water pours from the hillside, creating a beautiful mini-waterfall, maybe eight feet in height.

Soon after, huge rock outcroppings and enormous oak and walnut dominate the left side of the trail, the river running on the right. At an island in the river, follow the trail as it heads uphill. At 2.8 miles, you'll see a grove of tulip poplars with gnaw marks at their bases, a result of beaver activity. Look in the river here and you're bound to see dams as well. More fallen trees lay in the path. As a result, the horse trails head to the left on higher ground, but there's still a path along the river, which I recommend. It makes for more difficult hiking—climbing and weaving around rocks and trees—but it's quite wild and strenuous, and invigorating.

Every now and then when you think you might have lost the trail, it reappears as an obvious alleyway among the trees. After 3 miles, there's a narrow ridge, falling off about ten feet to the right while the left is a wall of jagged rock. It's quite a spot, affording nice views of the river. Loads of grapevine, ivy, and briers dot the hillside as you make your way toward the pine forest on top of the hill. At 3.4 miles, the river curves around to the right and you'll see a bridge in the distance—keep heading toward it. If it gets too rough, you can always backtrack a bit and take one of the three or four leftward cuts—these will eventually loop back toward the bridge (if you do go with one of the leftward paths, once you come to a power-line cut, head back right toward the river—you'll be passing the bridge otherwise). Staying along the river requires some scrambling over rocks, gaining and falling in elevation as you cross over drainage areas and gullies, but it's a great way to go. During some of the upward climbs, if the sun is out and hitting at the right angle, your view gets pleasantly obstructed temporarily by the reflection of mica chips on the rocks.

Come to a grove of holly, cautious of the many briers and prickers along the way. You'll reach a few rock promontories with great views, making it well worth the strenuous climb. Come back down to level land toward the bridge. Because the bridge supports over time have blocked sediment and rock, a river crossing here isn't very difficult. In fact, it might be quite easy depending on conditions. This is recommended in all but the most difficult conditions because crossing the bridge above can be scary—it certainly isn't for children or those afraid of heights. Big gaps in the railroad ties make it a bit forbidding. Trains do run, albeit infrequently. You'll certainly hear one coming and if so, obviously don't attempt a crossing then.

Standing on the tracks, you can see the Dorsey Tunnel almost a mile in the distance behind you and the Davis Tunnel a few hundred feet ahead—you'll be heading in the direction of the Davis Tunnel. Once on the other side of the bridge, look down the hill to the right for a stream culvert that still remains from the old railroad bed used by the famous Tom Thumb, the steam-powered engine that raced a horse, coming up short due to a slipped belt. Walk toward the Davis Tunnel and head to the right. Walk up the hill on deer trails. Many layers of earth and forest sit atop the tunnel now. On top of the tunnel, you'll see a prominent path. The tracks are no longer from wildlife, but from mountain bike and hiking boot instead.

At the top of the hill, the river is a few hundred feet below to the right; every now and then when it opens up, you can see the whole valley. There are several splits around 4 miles; taking the rightward ones keeps you closest to the river— many of these are single-track made by mountain bikers. Pass through a carpet of moss, some climbing up the trunks of beech and oak, with azalea nearby as well. Go gradually downhill toward a little brook. Cross and head again toward the river. Cross over water again at 4.5 miles; this is the Davis Branch. Stay as near the river as possible—often this means simply within sight of it.

At 4.7 miles, you'll see a ridge to the right—when you see it, head toward the railroad tracks. When you reach the T, take a left at the rock escarpment. You'll be in the woods buffer alongside the tracks, but then emerge aside the tracks themselves. The trail ends here and leaves you at the tracks. Resultantly, I was a bit bummed to be out of the woods, but this was quickly tempered by the sight of a bald eagle following the river downstream, a victim of its hunting prowess hanging from its talons. Hawks and turkey vultures are also visible in

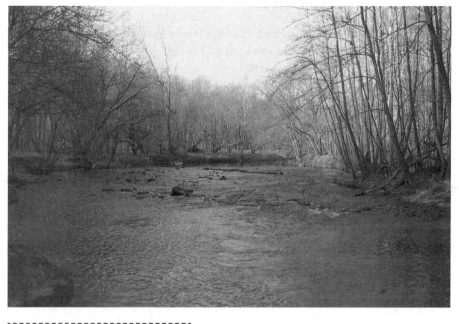

Isolated section on the Patapsco River

this open area. Additionally, Canada geese, green herons, and kingfishers populate the area year-round.

There's lots of lamb's ear and skunk cabbage along the tracks. At 4.8 miles,
it suddenly gets very narrow against the tracks, so cross over and go down the
hill. You'll soon see a groove along the river, which is the trail. It's seldom used
and easy to lose, but the woods are wide and it's easy to make your way—the
only potential snags are the occasional gullies and brooks, but these are generally crossable with one big jump or with the aid of a decent-size rock or two.

At 5.3 miles, the trail widens and becomes easy to follow. You can see the
trail on the other side where you were. Sweet gum trees give off a sweet, sharp,
and enticing aroma. The muddy banks of the river show lots of squirrel, deer,
raccoon, beaver, opossum, and fox tracks. After another quarter-mile, the trail
gets rough and passage becomes difficult as the hill drops to the river's edge—
you can always go back up and walk along the tracks until you see the trail
reemerge below and then walk back down. The best place to do this is right after
the stone abutment of an old bridge; there's also a #21 sign at the tracks. At 6.2
miles, the trail gets lost in jumble of fallen trees, but keep the river close by and
the trail reemerges. Once back down along the river, look for a section of trees
that have been felled. This is another beaver area; in fact, when I hiked here,
I scared one of the poor unsuspecting creatures. He waddled into the river,
swam to the other side, and regarded me from a safe distance.

At 6.6 miles, you can begin to see the Old Court Bridge at a leftward bend in the river. This time, don't climb the hill, but instead keep under the bridge; the trailhead will be up ahead to the left at 7 miles.

NEARBY ACTIVITIES

If you desire maintained trails, pavilions, ball fields, and picnic areas, as well as facilities, head just north to the McKeldin Area of PVSP (see page 147). Take Woodstock Road west until it ends at Old Frederick and take the first right onto Marriotsville Road. The McKeldin entrance is off Marriotsville.

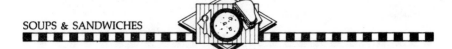

SEAFOOD IS KID FOOD

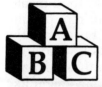

Every child loves the feel of a wiggly fish on the end of his fishin' pole, but to convince him to eat it is often another story! With a little ingenuity you can help your family (kids, too!) become avid seafood fans.

- **START CHILDREN EARLY!**
  Seafood is an ideal first protein source for toddlers. It is easy to chew and digest. Seafood is perfect as a finger food. With its mild flavor it is often more easily accepted by youngsters than red meat.

- **ONE-POT MEALS ARE GOOD!**
  A quick and easy one-pot meal to start a toddler is seafood poached in a liquid such as chicken broth or seasoned water. Start with diced potatoes and a favorite vegetable. Cover with liquid and simmer until tender. Add fish chunks and steam until fish flakes when tested with a fork.

- **CHOOSE BONELESS FISH.**
  Sometimes toddlers and younger children are afraid of bones. So choose boneless and skinless fillets or ask your seafood retailer to debone fish. Good boneless finger foods are shrimp, imitation crab, and squid.

- **START SLOWLY.**
  Serve one seafood meal per week to your family and increase gradually. For the first few meals, serve a meal of their favorite dishes and a small portion of seafood.

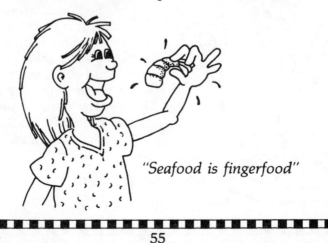

"Seafood is fingerfood"

- **GET THE KIDS INVOLVED.**

  Get the children involved in preparation of seafood meals. They are often enthusiastic helpers. Peeling shrimp, picking crab or debearding mussels are all fun chores. Encourage the kids to be part of the shopping trip. All kids love to look at the live crab and lobster tank in many seafood departments. Let them decide what type of seafood they might like to try for dinner.

  Have the kids help with the actual cooking, too. Chopping vegetables or cutting fish into chunks, with supervision, can help win them over. Let the kids help make their favorite dessert for the end of the seafood dinner. Serve recipes with familiar flavors. Try "Italian Fisherman's Spaghetti", always a favorite with its tomato base and Italian flavors.

- **IT'S A LIFETIME DIET.**

  Let seafood join your family's meal plan at least three times per week. It is important to get children off to an early start with a heart-healthy diet that may help prevent heart disease later in life. Children may surprise their parents and actually look forward to "Manhattan Shellfish Chowder" or poached salmon! Seafood is the perfect kid food!

  Suggested recipes: Lunchbox Tuna Sandwich, page 57
  Italian Fisherman's Spaghetti, page 96
  Four-Minute Flounder, page 110

Seafood eating is fun with a hint from a fisherman's wife: keep a jar of pennies by the table for your seafood dinners. Have the kids "go fishin'" for the bones. With every bone, a penny is earned. Kids will gladly clean their plates.

"Go fishin' for bones"

LUNCHBOX TUNA OR SALMON SANDWICH

It's fun to have a variety of breads on hand in the freezer. This sandwich spread is great in pita bread, on rye, whole grain breads or spread on rice cakes.

☐ 1 can (6½ oz.) water-packed tuna or salmon

☐ ½ cup low fat cottage cheese, blended

☐ 3 T. celery, finely chopped

☐ 2 T. green onion, finely chopped

☐ 8 slices of bread

☐ Suggested garnishes:
sliced tomatoes
sliced cucumbers
sliced pickle
alfalfa sprouts
lettuce

1. Drain and flake tuna or salmon with a fork.
2. Combine fish, cottage cheese and vegetables.
3. Use ¼ of mixture for each of 4 sandwiches. Garnish as desired. Serve with fresh fruit. **Makes 4 sandwiches.**

WITH TUNA:
217 calories per sandwich
6.0 grams fat per sandwich
484 mg sodium per sandwich
24 mg cholesterol per sandwich

WITH SALMON:
240 calories per sandwich
3.0 grams fat per sandwich
580 mg sodium per sandwich
48 mg cholesterol per sandwich

Substitutions:
any cooked, flaked fish

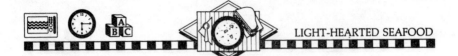

TUNA MELT SUPREME

♥ *Solid white albacore tuna is one of the best sources of omega-3 fatty acids. The canning process does not significantly reduce the omega-3 content in canned tuna or other varieties of canned seafood such as canned salmon. Chunk light tuna has only half of the amount of omega-3's as in the solid white variety. Tuna packed in water has the same omega-3 content as tuna packed in oil. But, while draining water from water-packed tuna removes only about 3% of the omega-3's, draining oil removes 15-25% (because these fatty acids are oil-soluble).*

- ☐ 1 can (6½ oz.) water-packed tuna, drained
- ☐ ¼ cup low fat cottage cheese, blended
- ☐ ¼ cup carrot, grated
- ☐ 1 T. red onion, minced
- ☐ 1 tsp. lemon juice
- ☐ ½ tsp. capers, drained
- ☐ ¼ tsp. Dijon mustard
- ☐ ⅛ tsp. pepper
- ☐ 2 English muffins, split and toasted
- ☐ 2 oz. part-skim Mozzarella cheese, grated

MICROWAVE:

1. Combine all ingredients except muffin and cheese.
2. Spoon tuna mixture onto muffin halves and top with cheese.
3. Place on paper towel on microwave-proof plate. Microwave on HIGH until cheese is melted, about 35-45 seconds. Garnish with a little grated carrot and serve hot. **Makes 4 open-faced sandwiches.**

184 calories per sandwich
4.1 grams fat per sandwich
385 mg sodium per sandwich
23 mg cholesterol per sandwich

Substitutions:
canned salmon, imitation crab

OPEN-FACED CRAB MUFFINS

Surimi seafood is a new fish product that has become available to consumers. Usually sold under a number of names, such as imitation crab meat or imitation lobster tail, surimi can be used in any recipe that calls for lobster or crab. It is currently made from Alaskan pollock, a mild white-fleshed fish, and flavored with real shellfish or shellfish extract and is fabricated into the shape, texture and color of shellfish. It can be a less expensive and still healthy alternative to the real thing!

☐ ¾ cup low fat cottage cheese, blended

☐ ¼ cup Parmesan cheese

☐ ⅓ cup green onion, finely chopped

☐ 6 drops hot pepper sauce (Tabasco)

☐ 2 tsp. Worcestershire sauce

☐ 12 oz. imitation crab, shredded

☐ 6 English muffins (split in half) or substitute rice cakes

1. Mix blended cottage cheese, Parmesan cheese, green onion, Tabasco and Worcestershire sauce together in mixing bowl. Stir in imitation crab.

2. Spread ¼ cup crab mixture on each muffin half.

3. Place on cookie sheet and bake at 400° for 10-12 minutes. Serve for lunch with a salad. As an appetizer cut into triangles. **Makes 12 open-faced sandwiches.**

112 calories per sandwich
1.4 grams fat per sandwich
303 mg sodium per sandwich
16 mg cholesterol per sandwich

Substitutions:
crab, shrimp

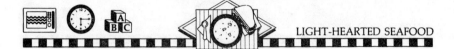
SHRIMP TOPPED RICE CAKES

These are easy to heat in the microwave, too.

- ☐ ¾ cup shrimp meat, cooked
- ☐ 3 ozs. light cream cheese, softened
- ☐ 2 T. fresh chives, chopped
- ☐ ⅛ tsp. hot pepper sauce (Tabasco)
- ☐ 8 plain rice cakes

1. Chop shrimp meat.
2. Combine cream cheese, chives and Tabasco in small bowl; beat at medium speed with electric mixer or in food processor until smooth. Stir in shrimp and blend mixture.
3. Spread the shrimp mixture evenly on rice cakes. Place rice cakes on baking sheet. Broil 5-6 inches from heat, 2 to 5 minutes or until warm. Serve immediately. **Makes 8 rice cake sandwiches.**

73 calories per sandwich
2.3 grams fat per sandwich
105 mg sodium per sandwich
27 mg cholesterol per sandwich

Substitutions:
imitation crab, lump crab meat

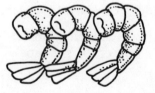

HIGHLINER'S CHOICE SALMON CHOWDER

- ☐ 1 lb. salmon fillets, boneless and skinless
- ☐ 1 cup onion, chopped
- ☐ 1 cup potato, diced
- ☐ ¼ cup celery, chopped
- ☐ 1 T. polyunsaturated margarine
- ☐ 2 T. water
- ☐ 2 T. flour
- ☐ ¼ tsp. white pepper
- ☐ ¼ tsp. dried dill weed
- ☐ 1 can (8 oz.) stewed tomatoes
- ☐ 2 cans (13 oz. each) evaporated skim milk
- ☐ 1 cup part-skim Mozarella cheese, grated
- ☐ 2 T. parsley, chopped

1. Cut salmon into 1-inch pieces; set aside.
2. In saucepan saute onion, potato and celery in margarine and water until potatoes are tender.
3. Blend in flour, add pepper, dill, tomatoes, milk and salmon. Heat until soup thickens and comes to a simmer; stir occasionally. Simmer until salmon flakes when tested with fork.
4. Stir in cheese; add parsley. Serve with whole wheat roll. **Makes 4-6 servings.**

362 calories per serving
11 grams fat per serving
452 mg sodium per serving
69 mg cholesterol per serving

Substitutions:
scallops, crab meat, shrimp meat

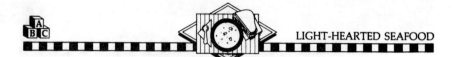

MANHATTAN SHELLFISH CHOWDER

- ☐ 1 medium onion, chopped
- ☐ 2 cloves garlic, minced
- ☐ 1 T. olive oil
- ☐ 1 can (10 oz.) low salt chicken broth
- ☐ ½ cup water
- ☐ 1 can (8 oz.) tomatoes
- ☐ 1 cup dry white wine
- ☐ 2 tsp. dried thyme
- ☐ 2 tsp. dried basil
- ☐ Pepper to taste
- ☐ 24 small or 12 medium clams, scrubbed
- ☐ ½ lb. sea scallops

1. In 8-quart saucepan over medium heat, saute onion and garlic in olive oil until tender.
2. Stir in chicken broth, water, tomatoes, wine and herbs; season with pepper. Simmer 10 minutes.
3. Increase heat to high; add clams and cook 2 minutes or until their shells open. Add scallops; cook until just done; about 2 minutes. Serve with whole wheat roll and green salad. **Makes 4 servings.**

218 calories per serving
5.0 grams fat per serving
482 mg sodium per serving
203 mg cholesterol per serving

Substitutions:
chopped clams, squid or mussels
boneless, skinless, and chunked firm white-fleshed fish

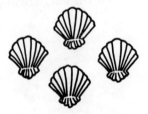

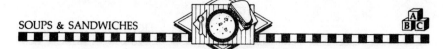

NORWEGIAN CRAB BISQUE

- ☐ 2 cups water
- ☐ 1 small onion, diced
- ☐ 2 stalks celery, chopped
- ☐ 2 medium potatoes, diced
- ☐ 2 carrots, sliced
- ☐ 1 cup frozen peas
- ☐ 6-8 whole allspice
- ☐ 1 tsp. dried dill weed
- ☐ ½ tsp. white pepper
- ☐ 2 cans (13 oz. each) evaporated skim milk
- ☐ 1 lb. imitation crab
- ☐ 1 T. parsley
- ☐ Dash of hot pepper sauce (Tabasco)

1. Place water, onions, celery, potatoes, carrots, peas, allspice, dill and white pepper in 4-quart saucepan. Bring to boil; reduce heat and simmer for 15 minutes. Remove and discard allspice.
2. Add milk and simmer (do not boil). Gently stir in imitation crab. Garnish with parsley and Tabasco. Serve with french bread. **Makes 6 servings.**

229 calories per serving
0.3 gram fat per serving
629 mg sodium per serving
38 mg cholesterol per serving

Substitutions:
scallops, shrimp, boneless, skinless, firm white-fleshed fish

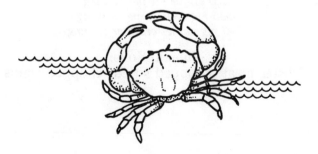

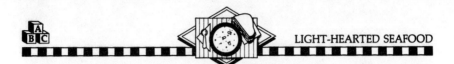

BOURBON STREET GUMBO

💜 *Okra has a sticky, "gummy" consistency and acts as a thickener in soup, stews and chowders, hence the word "gumbo"!*

- ☐ ¼ cup polyunsaturated oil
- ☐ 1 white onion, chopped
- ☐ 2 stalks celery, chopped
- ☐ 4 cloves garlic, minced
- ☐ ½ green pepper, chopped
- ☐ 1 can (8 oz.) tomato sauce
- ☐ 1 can (16 oz.) whole tomaoes, mashed

- ☐ 2 cups water
- ☐ 2 pkgs. (8 oz. each) frozen okra, cut up
- ☐ 2 bay leaves
- ☐ Pepper to taste
- ☐ 1 lb. raw shrimp, peeled and deveined
- ☐ 1 lb. crab meat
- ☐ 1 T. dried parsley

1. Heat oil in kettle. Add onion, celery, garlic and green pepper and saute over medium heat until vegetables are tender-crisp.
2. Add tomato sauce and mashed tomatoes and simmer for 5 minutes.
3. Add water, okra, bay leaves and pepper. Cover and cook until okra is tender. Discard bay leaf. At this point gumbo base can be refrigerated or frozen.
4. To complete, reheat gumbo base, add shrimp and cook until shrimp turn opaque. Add crab meat; warm through. Garnish with parsley. **Makes 6-8 servings.**

225 calories per serving
8.0 grams fat per serving
536 mg sodium per serving
140 mg cholesterol per serving

Substitutions:
lobster meat, chopped squid, chopped clams

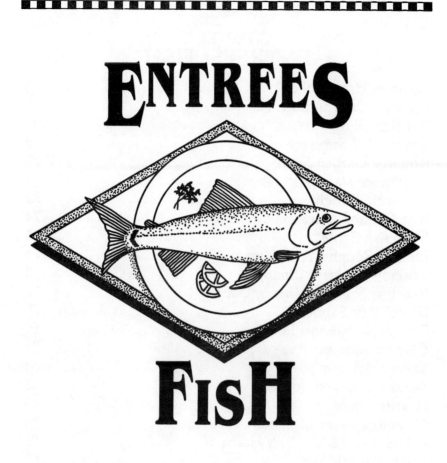

ENTREES

FISH

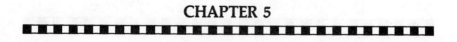

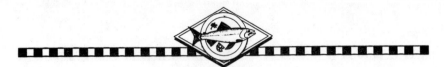

CHAPTER 5
ENTREES: FISH

WHEN IS FISH COOKED?

Perfectly cooked fish is moist and has a delicate flavor. There's no secret about cooking fish properly. Fish is done when the flesh has just begun to turn from translucent to opaque (or white) and is firm but still moist. It should flake when tested with a fork.

THE 10-MINUTE RULE FOR FISH

The 10-Minute Rule is one way to cook fish by conventional methods (but not deep-frying or microwaving). It can be used for baking (at 400° to 450°), grilling, broiling, poaching, steaming and sauteing. Here is how to use the 10-Minute Rule:

- Measure the fish at its thickest point. If the fish is stuffed or rolled, measure it after stuffing or rolling.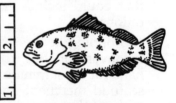

- Cook fish about 10 minutes per inch, turning it halfway through the cooking time. For example, a 1-inch fish steak should be cooked 5 minutes on each side for a total of 10 minutes. Pieces less than ½ inch thick do not have to be turned over. Test for doneness. Flake with a fork. Fish should reach an internal temperature of 145°.

- Add 5 minutes to the total cooking time for fish cooked in foil or in sauce.

- Double the cooking time for frozen fish that has not been defrosted. Use this rule as a general guideline since fillets often don't have uniform thickness.

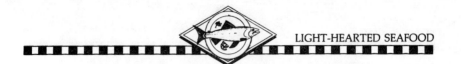

SEAFOOD ON THE RUN

 Many of us live with a hectic schedule, fix several different meals for our families and feel too often that family members are just ships passing in the night. Seafood offers an easy and quick meal choice. It is a great convenience food. Consider a last minute meal from the supermarket. Try a stir-fry, such as "Country Garden Saute," page 71, with a seafood selection from the seafood counter and vegetables from the salad bar. It's easy to purchase shrimp, scallops or halibut and pre-cut vegetables with choices that could include mushrooms, celery, carrots, broccoli or onions.

Stopping at the seafood counter 3-4 times a week can be inconvenient. But frozen seafood is excellent and always on hand for a last minute meal. Purchase frozen seafood from your seafood merchant and keep it at 0°F to -20°F. Stock up on seafood that your local supermarket or seafood store has on sale. Thaw seafood in the refrigerator, under cold running water or in the microwave. Seafood can also be cooked from the frozen state by steaming, poaching, microwaving or baking, just double the cooking time. More "frozen-at-sea" products are appearing on the market so watch for that label.

Canned seafood products are also excellent for quick and easy to fix casseroles, salads and sandwiches. Keep a can in the refrigerator, cooled and ready to serve.

Eating seafood for the health, convenience, and taste of it is fun and easy. Enjoy to your heart's content!

Suggested recipes: Country Garden Saute, page 71
Four-Minute Flounder, page 110
Garlic Shrimp, page 122
Slender Steamed Sole, page 83

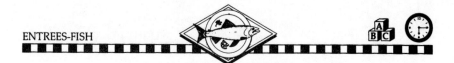

BLUEFISH DIJON

*Any type of fish is a healthier choice
than the leanest red meat or poultry.
Not only is fish low in cholesterol and saturated fat,
but it's also high in omega-3 fatty acids, which may
help lower cholesterol in the blood.*

☐ **3 T. Dijon mustard**

☐ **⅓ cup low fat yogurt**

☐ **2 lbs. bluefish**

☐ **Pepper to taste**

☐ **⅓ cup vermouth or dry white wine**

1. Combine mustard with yogurt in bowl; set aside.
2. Place fish in baking dish, season with pepper; spread fish with mustard mixture. Pour the vermouth or wine around fish.
3. Bake uncovered at 400°, until fish flakes when tested with fork. **Makes 8 servings.**

*153 calories per serving
5.2 grams fat per serving
147 mg sodium per serving
66 mg cholesterol per serving*

Substitutions:
halibut, Pacific rockfish (snapper), lingcod

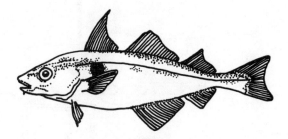

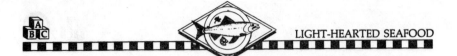

OCEAN COD SUPREME

☐ 1½ lbs. cod

☐ 1 cup dry white wine
(omit if desired)

☐ ¼ cup seasoned
bread crumbs

☐ 1 cup low fat yogurt

☐ ¼ cup green onion,
minced

☐ Paprika

1. Place fish in baking dish. Pour wine over cod and marinate in refrigerator 15-30 minutes.

2. Discard wine and pat fish dry with paper towels; dip both sides in bread crumbs. Place fish back in baking dish.

3. Combine yogurt and green onion and spread over fish. Sprinkle with paprika.

4. Bake in 400° oven about 15-20 minutes or until fish flakes when tested with fork. Serve with baked potatoes and steamed carrots. **Makes 6 servings.**

152 calories per serving
1.5 grams fat per serving
132 mg sodium per serving
47 mg cholesterol per serving

Substitutions:
Pacific rockfish (snapper), orange roughy, bluefish

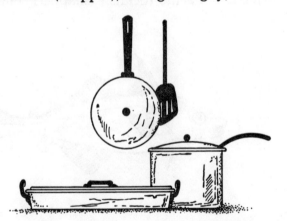

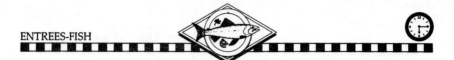

COUNTRY GARDEN SAUTE

Super salad bar dinner

♥ *A once-a-week stir-fry is a good way to use up the bits and pieces of vegetables in the produce drawer and to vary them with the season. It's a great way to stretch a pound of seafood.*

- ☐ 1 lb. firm fish, such as halibut
- ☐ Pepper
- ☐ 1 T. polyunsaturated oil or olive oil
- ☐ 1 cup carrots, sliced
- ☐ 1 cup celery, sliced
- ☐ 1 cup green onion, diagonally sliced
- ☐ 1 cup broccoli flowerets

- ☐ 1 cup mushrooms, sliced
- ☐ ¼ cup water
- ☐ ¼ cup chicken broth (low salt chicken broth may be used)
- ☐ 2 tsp. cornstarch
- ☐ ¼ tsp. fresh ginger, grated or ⅛ tsp. ground ginger
- ☐ 1 tsp. lemon peel

1. Remove bones and skin from fish; cut into 1-inch cubes. Season with pepper. Set aside.
2. In wok or frying pan, heat oil over medium-high heat. Add vegetables and water; saute until tender-crisp.
3. Add fish to pan. Combine stock, cornstarch, ginger and lemon peel; add to fish and vegetables.
4. Cook and stir until thickened and fish flakes when tested with fork. Serve with steamed rice. **Makes 4 servings.**

186 calories per serving
5.0 grams fat per serving
155 mg sodium per serving
67 mg cholesterol per serving

Substitutions:
shark, albacore tuna, salmon, prawns

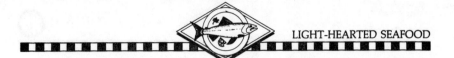

CUCUMBER HADDOCK

□ 2 cups water
□ 1 chicken-flavored bouillon cube (or eliminate water and add 2 cups low salt chicken broth)
□ ⅛ t. garlic powder
□ 2 medium cucumbers, unpeeled

□ 1 lb. haddock
□ 1 cup plain low fat yogurt
□ 1½ tsp. lemon juice
□ 2 T. cornstarch
□ ½ tsp. dried dill weed

1. In skillet, dissolve bouillon in 2 cups boiling water. Add garlic powder and reduce to medium heat.

2. With tip of vegetable peeler score cucumbers lengthwise all around and cut in half lengthwise. Remove seeds and cut crosswise in ¼-inch slices.

3. Add prepared cucumbers and fish to broth and poach 5 minutes until fish flakes when tested with fork.

4. Remove and drain cucumbers and fish with slotted spoon and place on serving dish.

5. In bowl, combine remaining ingredients and add to broth in skillet. Simmer until sauce thickens; pour over fish and cucumbers. **Makes 4 servings.**

134 calories per serving
1.5 grams fat per serving
350 mg sodium per serving
70 mg cholesterol per serving

Substitutions:
salmon, halibut, orange roughy

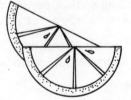

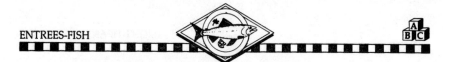

CASEROLE DELIGHT

❤️ *Water chestnuts, commonly used in Chinese cuisine, are not nuts but tubers.*
Unlike nuts, they are low in calories (about 14 calories per ounce or approximately four water chestnuts) and almost fat-free. Great for a crunch in salads, sandwiches and stir-fry.

☐ 1 cup dry vermouth
☐ 1½ lbs. cooked halibut, flaked
☐ 1 tsp. Italian Seafood Seasoning (see page 138)
☐ 1 large onion, chopped
☐ 2 cups celery, sliced
☐ 1 cup unsweetened pineapple chunks, drained

☐ 1 can (8 oz.) sliced water chestnuts
☐ 1 cup low fat cottage cheese, blended
☐ ¼ cup slivered almonds, chopped
☐ 1 cup part-skim Mozzarella cheese, grated
☐ ¼ cup chow mein noodles

1. Pour vermouth over fish in 1½-quart casserole dish. Cover and marinate for 15 minutes.
2. Drain fish. Sprinkle Italian Seafood Seasoning over fish.
3. Stir in onions, celery, pineapple chunks, chestnuts, and blended cottage cheese.
4. Sprinkle almonds, Mozzarella cheese and chow mein noodles over the top.
5. Bake at 375° for 25 minutes. Serve with rice. **Makes 6-8 servings.**

294 calories per serving
9.0 grams fat per serving
293 mg sodium per serving
61 mg cholesterol per serving

Substitutions:
canned salmon, canned tuna

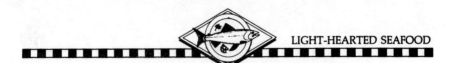

BEST DRESSED MACKEREL OR TROUT

☐ 2 lbs. dressed, whole
mackerel or trout

☐ Pepper

☐ 1 T. polyunsaturated
margarine

☐ Lemon juice

☐ 1 onion, thinly sliced

1. Pepper inside and outside of fish. Put dabs of margarine and squeeze lemon juice inside body cavity. Place onions inside of fish. Wrap in foil.

2. Bake in 400° oven or place on rack in large pot over 2-3 inches of boiling water to steam. Cooking time is 10 minutes per pound, or about 20 minutes. Cook until fish flakes when tested with fork. Serve with steamed or boiled potatoes and green salad. **Makes 8 servings.**

WITH MACKEREL:
200 calories per serving
9.6 grams fat per serving
110 mg sodium per serving
45 mg cholesterol per serving

WITH TROUT:
235 calories per serving
13.7 grams fat per serving
82 mg sodium per serving
55 mg cholesterol per serving

Substitutions:
any variety and size of whole, dressed fish,
whole, dressed salmon

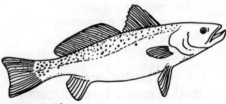

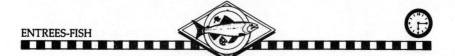

MONKFISH SAUTE

Monkfish was named in the Mediterranean Sea region. This large, ugly fish was discarded by fishermen as scrapfish, but the monks found them to be quite tasty. So came the name "monksfish". Monkfish is best prepared by cutting into thin slices. At full thickness, by steaming or baking. Poaching monkfish is also excellent.

☐ 1 pkg. (6 oz.) frozen pea pods

☐ 1½ T. olive oil

☐ 2 lbs. monkfish, cut into ½-inch slices

☐ 2 tomatoes, cut into eighths

☐ ¼ cup water

☐ 2 T. cornstarch

☐ 2 T. light soy sauce

☐ ⅛ t. pepper

1. Thaw and drain pea pods; set aside.
2. Heat olive oil in large skillet. Add monkfish and cook over medium heat for 2 minutes, stirring frequently. Add pea pods and tomatoes.
3. Combine water, cornstarch, soy sauce and pepper in small bowl.
4. Add to monkfish mixture and cook until sauce is thick and seafood is opaque, stirring frequently. Serve over steamed rice. **Makes 8 servings.**

138 calories per serving
4.0 grams fat per serving
374 mg sodium per serving
95 mg cholesterol per serving

Substitutions:
scallops, squid rings, halibut cheeks

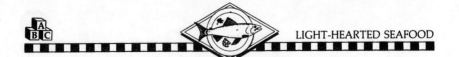

ORANGE ROUGHY WITH TOMATO-TARRAGON SAUCE

POACHED FISH:

- ☐ 1 small carrot, finely diced
- ☐ 1 small rib celery, finely diced
- ☐ 1 small onion, finely diced
- ☐ 1 can (10 oz.) low salt chicken broth
- ☐ 4 cups water
- ☐ 3 sprigs parsley
- ☐ 1 clove garlic, minced
- ☐ ½ tsp. whole black pepper
- ☐ ½ tsp. dried red pepper, crushed
- ☐ 1 lb. orange roughy

TOMATO-TARRAGON SAUCE:

- ☐ 1 T. polyunsaturated margarine
- ☐ 4 tsp. flour
- ☐ 1 cup reserved poaching liquid
- ☐ ¼ tsp. dried tarragon, crushed
- ☐ Pepper to taste
- ☐ 2 tomatoes, diced
- ☐ 2 tsp. parsley, chopped

1. To prepare poaching liquid: combine carrot, celery, onion, chicken broth, water, parsley, garlic, whole pepper and red pepper in large saucepan or poacher. Place on top of burner, bring to boil; reduce heat and simmer for 20 minutes.

2. Bring the liquid back to boil and immerse the fillets. Reduce the heat and simmer for 5-10 minutes or until fish flakes when tested with fork.

3. While fish is poaching, prepare sauce. In saucepan, heat margarine until melted, add flour and cook until bubbly, about 1 minute. Whisk in 1 cup hot poaching liquid, tarragon, pepper and tomatoes. Simmer for 5 minutes.

4. Place each serving of fish on plate and top with sauce. Garnish with parsley. **Makes 4 servings.**

137 calories per serving
3.6 grams fat per serving
145 mg sodium per serving
78 mg cholesterol per serving

Substitutions:
ocean perch, cod, sea bass

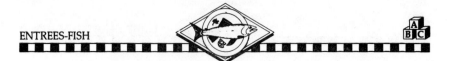

CHEESEY ROCKFISH (SNAPPER)

- ☐ 2 T. polyunsaturated margarine, melted
- ☐ ½ cup Parmesan cheese
- ☐ ¼ cup yellow cornmeal
- ☐ ¼ cup flour
- ☐ ½ tsp. pepper
- ☐ 1 tsp. Spanish paprika
- ☐ 2 lbs. Pacific rockfish (snapper), skinless and boneless

1. Pour melted margarine into baking pan.
2. Combine Parmesan cheese, cornmeal, flour, pepper and paprika together in paper bag. Place fish in bag and shake to coat each fillet.
3. Place fish in baking dish. Turn fish once to coat with margarine. Pour remaining cheese/cornmeal/flour mixture onto fish.
4. Bake at 400° until golden brown and fish flakes when tested with fork, approximately 15-20 minutes. Serve with bulgur and steamed vegetables. **Makes 8 servings.**

188 calories per serving
5.5 grams fat per serving
184 mg sodium per serving
392 mg cholesterol per serving

Substitutions:
bluefish, ocean perch, cod

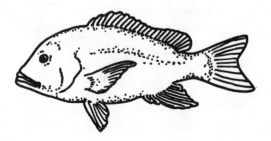

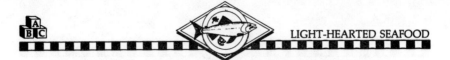
POACHED SABLEFISH (BLACK COD)

- ☐ 8 cups water
- ☐ 2 T. light soy sauce
- ☐ 2 stalks green onions, chopped
- ☐ 1 clove garlic, chopped
- ☐ Juice of ½ lemon
- ☐ 1 lb. sablefish (black cod), fillets or steaks

1. Bring water to boil in 8-quart sauce pan. Add soy sauce, green onions, garlic and lemon juice and simmer for 20 minutes.
2. Place sablefish in poaching liquid. Simmer for 8-10 minutes or until fish flakes when tested with fork. **Makes 4 servings.**

162 calories per serving
7.5 grams fat per serving
457 mg sodium per serving
73 mg cholesterol per serving

Substitutions:
bluefish, cod, salmon

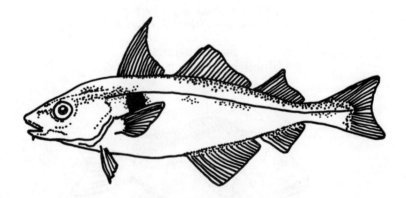

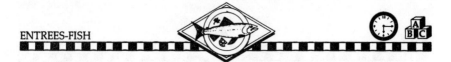

BRISTOL BAY SALMON
Elegant entertaining idea

☐ 1½ lbs. salmon fillets
    or steaks
☐ ½ cup low fat yogurt

☐ 1 T. mayonnaise
☐ 2 T. onion, minced
☐ 1 tsp. dried basil

1. Place salmon in baking pan.
2. Mix remaining ingredients together and spread over salmon.
3. Bake in 400⁰ oven for 10-15 minutes or until salmon flakes when tested with fork. Serve with boiled new potatoes and vegetables. **Makes 6 servings.**

188 calories per serving
10.0 grams fat per serving
104 mg sodium per serving
75 mg cholesterol per serving

Substitutions:
halibut, spearfish, swordfish

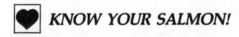 *KNOW YOUR SALMON!*

KING SALMON: also known as Chinook. Largest of all salmon with the record being 168 lbs. Color ranges from white to deep red and very high in oil content. Flavorful.

SOCKEYE SALMON: also known as red or blueback. Averages 6 lbs., deep red color and high oil content. Flavorful.

SILVER SALMON: also known as coho. Averages 4-12 lbs. Flesh is orange-red in color and oil content is fairly high.

PINK SALMON: also known as humpback or humpie because it develops a hump before spawning. Average weight is 3-8 lbs. Light colored flesh, less oil and very delicate flavor.

CHUM SALMON: also called keta, silverbrite or dog salmon. Weighs 8-10 lbs. Typically the last salmon up the river at the end of summer and into late fall. Dubbed dog salmon because it was fed to dogs when salmon was more abundant. Firm flesh which tends to be pale.

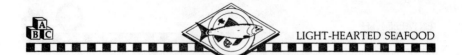

THAI-STYLE SALMON POTATO

- ☐ ½ cup onion, chopped
- ☐ 1 T. fresh ginger root, slivered
- ☐ ¼ to ½ tsp. red pepper, crushed
- ☐ 1 T. polyunsaturated oil
- ☐ 1 lb. salmon, skinned, boned and cubed
- ☐ 2 cups broccoli flowerets
- ☐ 1 cup pea pods
- ☐ 1 cup tofu cubes
- ☐ 1 cup cucumber, vertically sliced

- ☐ 2 shiitake mushrooms, rehydrated & thinly sliced
- ☐ ¾ cup water
- ☐ ¼ cup vinegar
- ☐ 4 tsp. packed brown sugar
- ☐ 1 T. cornstarch
- ☐ 1 tsp. lemon peel, grated
- ☐ Pepper to taste
- ☐ 4 large Russet potatoes, baked

1. Saute onion, ginger root and red pepper in oil until onion is tender; add salmon and cook 3 minutes.
2. Add broccoli, pea pods, tofu, cucumber and mushrooms; cook until vegetables are tender-crisp.
3. Combine water, vinegar, brown sugar, cornstarch, lemon peel and pepper; stir into vegetables. Cook until mixture thickens and boils.
4. To serve, split baked potatoes lengthwise and open by gently squeezing from the bottom. Spoon ¼ of salmon mixture over each potato. **Makes 4 servings.**

462 calories per serving
14.0 grams fat per serving
81 mg sodium per serving
72 mg cholesterol per serving

Substitutions:
canned salmon, canned, water-packed tuna

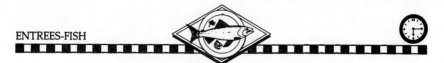

CURRIED SALMON

♥ *This recipe is especially good with milder salmon varieties such as chum, coho or pinks.*

☐ 1 cup white wine

☐ 4 green onions,
   diagonally cut

☐ 1 bay leaf

☐ 1 T. polyunsaturated
   margarine

☐ 1-2 tsp. curry powder

☐ 2 ripe pears or apples,
   cored and sliced

☐ 1 red pepper, julienne
   cut

☐ 1½ lbs. salmon fillets

1. In large, deep skillet combine wine, green onions, bay leaf, margarine and curry powder. Heat to boil.

2. Add fruit and vegetables and simmer about 5-10 minutes or until tender-crisp. Remove fruit and vegetables onto serving platter and keep warm in oven. Discard bay leaf.

3. Add salmon to liquid in skillet and cover. Steam until fish flakes when tested with fork.

4. Place fish on serving platter over vegetables and fruit. Drizzle any remaining liquid over all. **Makes 4-6 servings.**

258 calories per serving
9.7 grams fat per serving
100 mg sodium per serving
75 mg cholesterol per serving

Substitutions:
trout, black cod, scallops

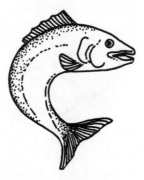

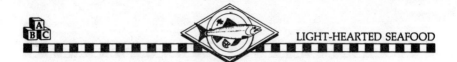

SAVORY SALMON LOAF
Fisherman's Favorite

☐ 1 can (15½ oz.) salmon
☐ 3 slices bread, torn into small pieces
☐ ⅓ cup onion, finely minced
☐ ¼ cup skim milk

☐ 2 eggs
☐ 2 T. parsley, minced
☐ 1 T. lemon juice
☐ ¼ tsp. dried dill weed
☐ Dash pepper

1. Drain salmon, reserving 2 T. liquid; flake.
2. Combine all ingredients including reserved salmon liquid. Place in lightly-oiled loaf pan.
3. Bake at 350° for 45 minutes. Serve with steamed vegetables.

ALTERNATE PREPARATION METHOD — SALMON PATTIES

1. Prepare salmon mixture as above, omitting milk.
2. Shape into 8 patties.
3. Saute in pan with 1 T. polyunsaturated oil until golden brown. Serve on hamburger buns with favorite garnishes. **Makes 6 servings.**

193 calories per serving
7.8 grams fat per serving
388 mg sodium per serving
98 mg cholesterol per serving

Substitutions:
leftover, cooked, flaked trout, salmon or halibut

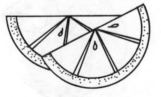

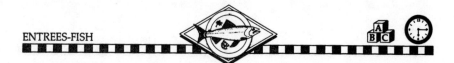

SLENDER STEAMED SOLE

SAUCE:

□ 1 T. light soy sauce

□ 2 tsp. polyunsaturated oil

□ 1 tsp. fresh ginger, finely chopped

□ 1 lb. sole fillets

1. To prepare sauce: in mixing bowl combine soy sauce, oil and chopped ginger root.
2. Arrange fish on steaming rack. Brush fish with sauce.
3. Place rack over boiling water. Cover and steam 7-10 minutes or until fish flakes when tested with fork. Serve with steamed rice and vegetables. **Makes 4 servings.**

102 calories per serving
1.8 grams fat per serving
260 mg sodium per serving
51 mg cholesterol per serving

Substitutions:
orange roughy, cod, tilefish

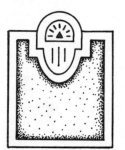

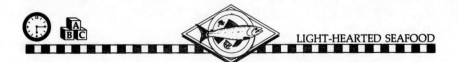

HEARTFELT SOLE

☐ 1 T. olive oil
☐ 3 shallots, minced
☐ 1 clove garlic, minced
☐ ¼ to ¾ cup white wine

☐ 1½ lbs. sole fillet
☐ ¼ tsp. dried dill weed
☐ Pepper to taste
☐ Parsley
☐ Lemon slices

1. In saute pan heat oil. Add shallots and garlic; saute for 1 minute. Add wine and heat to boiling.

2. Add sole to pan and sprinkle with dill weed. Spoon shallot and liquid over sole. Simmer 2-3 minutes or until fish flakes when tested with fork. Not necessary to turn fish. Pepper to taste.

3. Remove fish to warm serving plate. Turn pan to high heat and reduce juice. Spoon juice over sole fillets. Garnish with parsley and lemon slice. **Makes 6 servings.**

120 calories per serving
3.0 grams fat per serving
62 mg sodium per serving
50 mg cholesterol per serving

Substitutions:
pollock, orange roughy, flounder

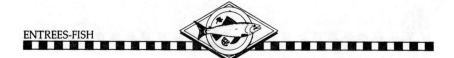

COLUMBIA RIVER STURGEON

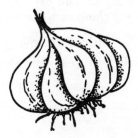 *Sturgeon is famed for its caviar, but the meat is highly prized by the locals along the Columbia River, located between the states of Oregon and Washington.*

- ☐ 1 T. fresh ginger root, sliced
- ☐ 1 tsp. pepper
- ☐ ½ cup fresh cilantro leaves
- ☐ 1 clove garlic
- ☐ 1 T. light soy sauce
- ☐ 2 T. olive oil
- ☐ Juice and rind of 2 lemons
- ☐ 1½ lbs. sturgeon steaks

1. Combine ginger root, pepper, cilantro, garlic, soy sauce, olive oil, lemon juice and lemon rind in food processor or blender and puree. Allow flavors to blend 15 minutes.
2. Place fish steaks in shallow glass dish and cover with marinade, turning fish several times to coat evenly.
3. Broil or barbecue fish, allowing ten minutes of cooking time for each inch of thickness. Baste periodically with marinade. Serve immediately. **Makes 6 servings.**

166 calories per serving
9.2 grams fat per serving
N/A mg sodium per serving
N/A mg cholesterol per serving

Substitutions:
swordfish, shark, lingcod

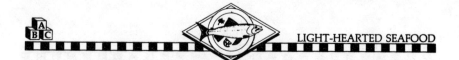
GRILLED SWORDFISH WITH HERBS

♥ *Swordfish: This firm-flesh fish with a fine grain has a distinctive flavor and can have flesh that is anywhere from white to light tan or pink. It usually is sold as steaks. The flesh tends to be dry if not basted often during cooking; use a basting sauce made with lemon juice, olive oil and herbs. Baste before broiling or baking, and use the marinade to baste the fish during cooking.*

- ☐ 1 T. olive oil
- ☐ 2 T. lime juice
- ☐ ½ cup Chardonnay wine
- ☐ 1 T. dry mustard
- ☐ 1 tsp. mustard seeds

- ☐ 1 T. chili powder
- ☐ 1 tsp. pepper
- ☐ 2 T. dried cilantro or 4 T. fresh cilantro, finely chopped
- ☐ 1 lb. swordfish steaks

1. Combine olive oil, lime juice and Chardonnay in bowl. Add spices.
2. Pour marinade over swordfish steaks and marinate for 15-20 minutes.
3. Grill swordfish over hot coals, about 5 minutes per side, or until fish turns opaque. Baste with marinade while cooking. **Makes 4 servings.**

243 calories per serving
8.5 grams fat per serving
79 mg sodium per serving
56 mg cholesterol per serving

Substitutions:
marlin, halibut, cod

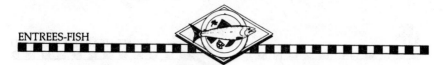

SZECHWAN STIR FRY

Tuna: Depending on the species, the flesh will range from dark pink to red but will turn white to gray-white when cooked.

SZECHWAN SAUCE:

- ☐ 2 T. rice vinegar
- ☐ 1½ T. light soy sauce
- ☐ 1 tsp. sesame oil
- ☐ ½ tsp. dried red pepper flakes

STIR FRY:

- ☐ 1 lb. albacore tuna, cut in 1-inch chunks
- ☐ 1 T. polyunsaturated oil
- ☐ 2 tsp. fresh ginger, peeled and minced
- ☐ 1 clove garlic, peeled and minced
- ☐ ¼ cup water
- ☐ 1 cup broccoli flowerets
- ☐ 1 cup carrots, thinly sliced
- ☐ ½ small red pepper, coarsely chopped
- ☐ ½ cup bamboo shoots, sliced
- ☐ ½ cup water chestnuts, sliced
- ☐ 1 cup snow peas
- ☐ 3 T. green onion, thinly sliced

1. To make Szechwan sauce: combine sauce ingredients in bowl. Add tuna to bowl to marinate.
2. Heat oil in wok over medium heat. Add ginger, garlic and water and saute for 30 seconds. Add broccoli and carrots to pan and stir fry for 3 minutes. Add red pepper, bamboo shoots, water chestnuts and snow peas; cover and simmer for 4 minutes.
3. Add marinated tuna, Szechwan sauce and green onion to wok and stir.
4. Saute 3-6 minutes or until tuna flakes when tested with fork. Serve immediately with steamed rice. **Makes 6 servings.**

158 calories per serving
5.5 grams fat per serving
244 mg sodium per serving
14 mg cholesterol per serving

Substitutions:
mahi mahi, squid rings, shrimp or prawns

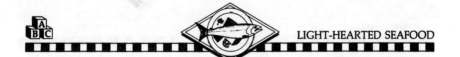

SAUCY TUNA FOR FOUR

WHITE SAUCE:

☐ 1 T. polyunsaturated margarine

☐ 1 T. flour

☐ 1 can (13 oz.) evaporated skim milk

CASSEROLE:

☐ 1 can (4 oz.) sliced mushrooms, drained

☐ 2 T. onion, minced

☐ 1 T. pimiento, chopped

☐ ¼ tsp. dried dill weed

☐ 1 T. lemon juice

☐ 1 cup frozen peas

☐ 1 can (6½ oz.) water-packed tuna, drained

☐ 1 pkg. (10 oz.) frozen broccoli spears, cooked & drained

☐ 2 T. Parmesan cheese

1. Prepare white sauce: melt margarine and blend in flour over medium heat in 4-quart saucepan. Add milk slowly while stirring.
2. Boil one minute, stirring until smooth.
3. Add remaining ingredients except broccoli spears and Parmesan cheese.
4. Lay broccoli spears in au grautin dishes and pour tuna sauce over broccoli and sprinkle with Parmesan cheese.
5. Bake uncovered at 350° for 20 minutes. Serve with green salad and whole wheat roll. **Makes 4 servings.**

243 calories per serving
4.3 grams fat per serving
539 mg sodium per serving
17 mg cholesterol per serving

Substitutions:
canned salmon, shrimp, peeled and deveined

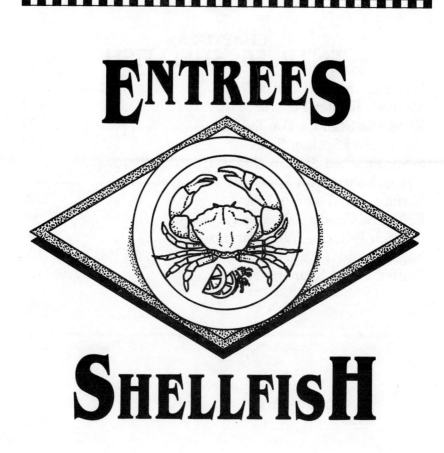

ENTREES

SHELLFISH

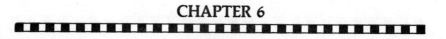

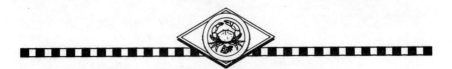

ENTREES: SHELLFISH

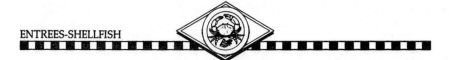

WHEN IS SHELLFISH COOKED?

Shellfish, like fish, should not be overcooked. If it's cooked too long, it becomes tough and dry and loses much of its fine flavor.

Some shellfish and all surimi seafood are already cooked when purchased. Merely heat them for a few minutes until they are uniformly heated.

Cook raw shellfish, shucked or in the shell, very lightly. You can actually see when shellfish is cooked:

- Raw shrimp turn pink and firm. Cooking time depends on the size. It takes from 3 to 5 minutes to boil or steam 1 pound of medium-size shrimp in the shell.

- Shucked shellfish (oysters, clams and mussels) become plump and opaque. The edges of oysters start to curl. Overcooking causes them to shrink and toughen.

- Oysters, clams and mussels, in the shell, open. Remove them one-by-one as they open and continue cooking until all are done.

- Scallops turn milky-white or opaque and firm. Sea scallops take 3 to 4 minutes to cook through; the smaller bay scallops take 30 to 60 seconds.

- Boiled lobster turns bright red. Allow 18 to 20 minutes per pound, starting from the time the water comes back to the boil. Broiled split lobster takes about 15 minutes.

- Cooking time for crabs depends on the type and preparation method. Sauteed or deep-fried soft-shell crabs take about 3 minutes each. Steamed hard-shell blue crabs or rock crabs take about 25 to 30 minutes for a large pot of them.

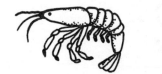

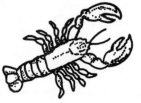

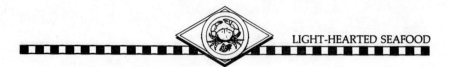

MOTHER'S OYSTER PIE

- ☐ ¾ cup seasoned bread crumbs
- ☐ 1 can (17 oz.) creamed corn
- ☐ Pepper to taste

- ☐ 2 jars (8 oz. each) small, whole oysters with liquid
- ☐ 1 jar (2 oz.) pimiento, chopped
- ☐ 4 tsp. polyunsaturated margarine

1. Divide equally into the bottom of 4 au grautin baking dishes the following: 6 tablespoons bread crumbs, ½ can corn, pepper, and 1 jar of oysters.
2. Repeat layers. Top with remaining bread crumbs and pimiento. Dot with margarine.
3. Bake at 400⁰ for 20 minutes. **Makes 4 servings.**

210 calories per serving
6.5 grams fat per serving
550 mg sodium per serving
56 mg cholesterol per serving

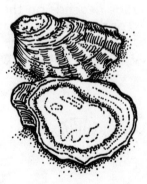

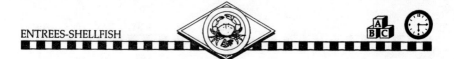

ROMANTIC SCALLOPS FOR TWO

 *Olive oils range in smell and taste from light and subtly fruity to unpleasantly strong. So try different brands. Many health professionals now recommend it for all-purpose use, spawning a new product, "extra light" olive oil, which has little taste.*

- ☐ ½ lb. sea scallops
- ☐ Skim milk
- ☐ 2 T. flour
- ☐ 1 T. olive oil
- ☐ ¼ cup wine
- ☐ ¼ cup shallots, chopped
- ☐ 2 T. green onion, chopped
- ☐ 2 tsp. dried parsley
- ☐ 1 lemon
- ☐ Lemon pepper to taste

1. Flatten scallops with a cleaver and dip in milk and flour.
2. Saute scallops in a saucepan with olive oil.
3. Remove scallops from pan and deglaze pan with white wine. Add shallots, green onion and chopped parsley. Simmer and pour over scallops. Squeeze lemon over scallops and season with lemon pepper. **Makes 2 servings.**

200 calories per serving
5.7 grams fat per serving
245 mg sodium per serving
55 mg cholesterol per serving

Substitutions:
oysters, monkfish medallions

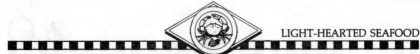
PRAWN AND SCALLOP SAUTE

♥ *Peanut oil: The taste of peanuts adds intrigue to stir-fries and sweetness to salad dressings.*

- ☐ 2 T. peanut oil
- ☐ 1 T. sesame seeds
- ☐ 1 clove garlic, minced
- ☐ Juice of half lemon
- ☐ ¼ lb. sugar peas
- ☐ ½ cup green onion, finely chopped

- ☐ ½ red pepper, seeded and chopped
- ☐ 1 cup mushrooms, sliced
- ☐ ½ tsp. dried basil
- ☐ 1 lb. small prawns, peeled and deveined
- ☐ ½ lb. sea scallops
- ☐ Pepper to taste

1. In large skillet, melt margarine; saute sesame seeds and garlic until lightly browned. Add lemon juice.
2. Add sugar peas, green onion, red pepper, mushrooms and basil; saute until tender-crisp.
3. Push vegetables aside and saute prawns and scallops until opaque. Pepper to taste. Serve with pasta and french bread. **Makes 6 servings.**

175 calories per serving
5.2 grams fat per serving
209 mg sodium per serving
135 mg cholesterol per serving

Substitutions:
albacore tuna, halibut, salmon

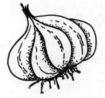

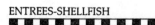
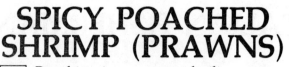

SPICY POACHED SHRIMP (PRAWNS)

♥ *Poaching is as easy as boiling water.
It is also among the healthiest ways
to prepare fish, since no fat is used when you cook;
instead, you simmer the fish in a flavorful liquid for a
moist and tasty meal every time.*

☐ 2 T. mustard seed
☐ 1 T. whole black pepper
☐ 1 tsp. Spanish paprika
☐ 1 tsp. garlic, minced

☐ ½ tsp. onion powder
☐ 4 cups water
☐ 1 lb. raw shrimp or prawns

1. Place mustard seed and whole black pepper in cheesecloth bag.
2. Place all spices, including spice bag, in water and bring to boil; reduce heat and simmer for 10 minutes.
3. Add shrimp or prawns and cook for 3 minutes or until shrimp/prawns turn opaque. Remove shrimp/prawns from water and rinse in cold water to stop cooking process. Chill. Serve with cocktail sauce as an appetizer or in salad. **Makes 4 servings.**

*90 calories per serving
0.8 gram fat per serving
140 mg sodium per serving
158 mg cholesterol per serving*

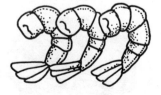

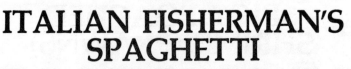

ITALIAN FISHERMAN'S SPAGHETTI

 About 99% of all shrimp you buy has been frozen. This does no harm to the nutritional value of the shrimp and it tastes as delicious as fresh.

- ☐ 1 cup onion, chopped
- ☐ 2 cloves garlic, minced
- ☐ 1 T. olive oil
- ☐ 1 can (8 oz.) tomato sauce
- ☐ 1 can (28 oz.) whole tomatoes, undrained and mashed
- ☐ 1 tsp. each dried basil, thyme, marjoram and oregano

- ☐ 1 bay leaf
- ☐ ¼ tsp. pepper
- ☐ 1 T. parsley, minced
- ☐ 1 lb. raw medium shrimp, peeled and deveined

1. In large kettle, saute onion and garlic in oil until tender.
2. Add tomato sauce, tomatoes and spices. Let simmer 20-30 minutes, stirring occasionally. Remove and discard bay leaf.
3. Add shrimp; cover and simmer 3-5 minutes or until shrimp turns opaque. Stir occasionally. Serve over hot spaghetti. **Makes 6-8 servings.**

106 calories per serving
2.2 grams fat per serving
375 mg sodium per serving
89 mg cholesterol per serving

Substitutions:
clams, mussels, squid rings

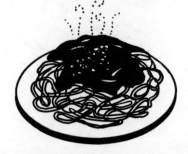

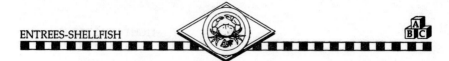

SHRIMP AND TOMATO TOSTADA

SALSA:

- ☐ 2½ cups fresh tomatoes, chopped
- ☐ ½ cup green pepper, chopped
- ☐ ½ cup onion, minced
- ☐ 1 can (4 oz.) green chiles, diced
- ☐ 1 T. sugar

- ☐ ¾ tsp. cilantro (chopped) or coriander
- ☐ ½ tsp. dried whole oregano
- ☐ 2½ T. lemon or lime juice
- ☐ 1 can (8 oz.) tomato sauce

TOSTADA:

- ☐ 3 cups water
- ☐ 1 lb. raw shrimp, unpeeled, medium size
- ☐ 8 tortillas (flour or corn)

- ☐ Suggested garnishes: shredded lettuce part-skim Mozzarella cheese, grated

1. Combine salsa ingredients in medium bowl; stir well. Cover mixture and let stand at room temperature for 1 hour.
2. Bring water to boil in saucepan; add shrimp, and cook 3 minutes or until shrimp turns opaque. Drain shrimp well, and rinse with cold water. Peel and devein shrimp.
3. Layer shredded lettuce and Mozzarella cheese on tortillas. Top with shrimp and salsa. Also excellent as a salad. **Makes 8 servings.**

196 calories per tostada
2.5 grams fat per tostada
314 mg sodium per tostada
89 mg cholesterol per tostada

Substitutions:
imitation crab, crayfish

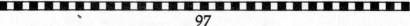

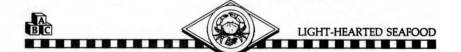

PHILIPPINE PANSIT

☐ 1 pkg. (6½ oz.) Maifun (rice sticks)

☐ 1 T. polyunsaturated oil

☐ 2 cups frozen peas

☐ 1 medium onion, sliced

☐ 1 cup mushrooms, sliced

☐ ½ cup carrots, grated

☐ 1 cup cabbage, shredded

☐ ¼ cup light soy sauce

☐ 1 cup chicken broth or low salt chicken broth

☐ ½ lb. cooked shrimp, peeled and deveined

1. Soak Maifun in hot water (enough to cover) until soft (about 10 minutes). Drain and cut into shorter lengths; set aside.
2. Heat oil in frying pan. Add peas, onion, mushrooms, carrots, cabbage, soy sauce and chicken broth. Mix and bring to full boil.
3. Lower heat, add shrimp and Maifun. Cook until Maifun is tender or until liquid is gone. **Makes 6-8 servings.**

Made with low salt broth:
165 calories per serving
2.6 grams fat per serving
404 mg sodium per serving
33 mg cholesterol per serving

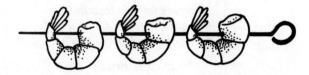

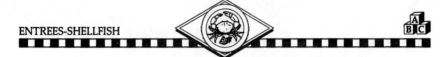

SPINACH FETTUCINE WITH SHRIMP

- ☐ 2 ozs. dry spinach fettucine
- ☐ 1 tsp. cornstarch
- ☐ ½ cup orange juice
- ☐ 2 tsp. polyunsaturated margarine
- ☐ 4 large shrimp, peeled, deveined and sliced lengthwise in half

- ☐ ½ cup snow peas
- ☐ ¼ cup mushrooms, sliced
- ☐ ½ cup tomato, chopped
- ☐ 1 carrot, cut into curls
- ☐ Fresh chives for garnish

1. Cook fettucine according to package directions.
2. Meanwhile, blend cornstarch and orange juice together in small bowl until smooth; set aside.
3. In skillet, over high heat, melt margarine and add shrimp, snow peas, mushrooms and tomatoes and saute just until shrimp curl and become opaque, about 2 minutes.
4. Stir in orange sauce; cook until sauce thickens, about 1 minute. Remove from heat.
5. When pasta is almost done, toss in carrot curls, cook 1 minute longer and drain.
6. Toss with sauce and mushrooms and season with fresh black pepper; garnish with fresh chives. Serve with french bread. **Makes 2 servings.**

268 calories per serving
7.0 grams fat per serving
124 mg sodium per serving
79 mg cholesterol per serving

SAUCY SQUID

☐ 12 large squid

STUFFING:

☐ ⅓ cup uncooked brown rice

☐ ½ cup celery, chopped

☐ ½ cup onion, chopped

☐ ½ tsp. garlic powder

☐ ½ tsp. cumin

☐ 2 cups water

SAUCE:

☐ 1 can (28 oz.) tomatoes, undrained

☐ 2 T. lemon juice

☐ 1 green pepper, seeded and chopped

☐ 1 cup mushrooms, sliced

☐ 1 T. fresh dill weed, finely chopped or 1 tsp. dried dill weed

☐ ¼ tsp. saffron

☐ Reserved chopped squid, if desired

1. Clean squid, leaving mantles (bodies) whole for stuffing. The tentacles may be chopped and reserved for adding to sauce.

2. To make stuffing: place all stuffing ingredients in 2-quart sauce pan. Stir. Bring to boil, reduce heat and simmer for 40 minutes. If any liquid remains, drain off. Let the rice mixture cool for ease of handling in stuffing the squid.

3. To make sauce: combine all ingredients for sauce, stir and set aside.

4. Lightly stuff each squid mantle. The amount to use depends on the size of each squid. Do not overstuff as the squid tends to shrink as it cooks, while the rice may continue to swell. Reserve any extra stuffing. Close openings and secure with toothpicks.

5. Lay the stuffed squid in a single layer in a 8″ x 11″ x 2″ casserole dish. Pour the sauce over squid. Place in 350⁰ oven and bake 45 minutes. If there is extra stuffing, it may be reheated in the oven the last 15 minutes of baking time and served as a side dish with squid and sauce. **Makes 4-6 servings.**

135 calories per serving
1.5 grams fat per serving
380 mg sodium per serving
230 mg cholesterol per serving

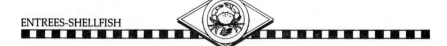

STUFFED SQUID SUPREME

☐ 12 large squid

SAUCE:

☐ ½ cup onion, chopped

☐ 1 clove garlic, minced

☐ 2 T. olive oil

☐ 1 can (6 oz.) tomato paste

☐ ¾ cup water

☐ ¼ cup celery, chopped

☐ 1 T. oyster sauce

☐ ⅛ tsp. lemon pepper

☐ 3 bay leaves

STUFFING:

☐ 16 oz. part-skim
   Ricotta cheese

☐ ¼ cup fresh parsley, chopped

☐ 3-4 cooked artichoke
   hearts, chopped

1. Clean squid, leaving mantles (bodies whole for stuffing. Remove tentacles from squid. Chop and reserve for stuffing.

2. Saute onion and garlic in oil until lightly browned. Add tomato paste and water. Add celery, oyster sauce, lemon pepper and bay leaves. Cover and simmer for 20 minutes, or until sauce is thick.

3. To make stuffing: combine Ricotta cheese, chopped tentacles, parsley and artichokes. Fill the squid with cheese stuffing (a pastry gun works well). Close openings and secure with toothpicks.

4. Place filled squid in large, 2-inch deep baking dish and pour sauce on top; remove bay leaves. Bake at 325⁰ for 20-25 minutes. **Makes 4-6 servings.**

296 calories per serving
12.0 grams fat per serving
270 mg sodium per serving
240 mg cholesterol per serving

MICROWAVE

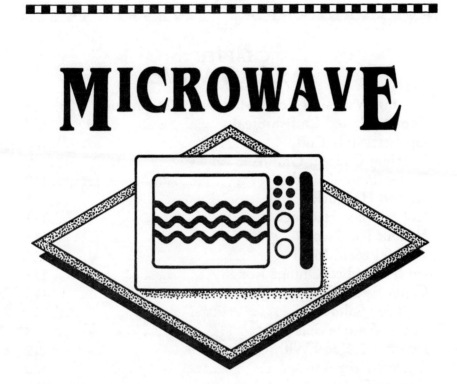

CHAPTER 7

MICROWAVE

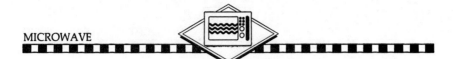

MAKING WAVES

SEAFOOD MICROWAVE TECHNIQUES

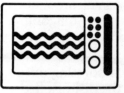

Seafood cooks perfectly in the microwave oven. It remains tender, moist and flavorful. Almost all kinds of seafood can be prepared in the microwave oven. However, there are many microwave ovens on the market and they vary in power. You may need to experiment to find the right cooking time for a particular recipe.

Watch closely when you try a new recipe for the first time. If a range of times is given, start with the shortest one. You can always put the dish back in the oven and cook it a little longer, but you cannot turn the clock back if it has cooked too long. Write the correct time down on the recipe for future reference.

Split-second timing is the secret to cooking seafood in the microwave. Seafood cooked by microwave is done when the flesh has just begun to change from translucent to opaque or white and when it is firm but still moist. Seafood will continue to cook after it has been removed from the microwave, so take the dish out before it looks done — when the outer edges are opaque with the center still slightly translucent. Allow the fish to stand, covered, for a few minutes before serving.

Getting everyone to sit down to dinner at the same time is a rare feat. The solution: a meal of microwaved foods that will "hold" and remain at the ideal serving temperature. Holding time is the length of time a properly wrapped or covered food will stay hot after cooking is complete. It should not be confused with standing time, during which microwaved food is still cooking. Fish can be tented with foil or wrapped in plastic to retain heat. Whole fish (2-3 lbs.) will hold its serving temperature for 7 minutes; fish fillets (4 1-lb. fillets) will hold its temperature also for 7 minutes!

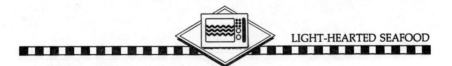

COOKING FISH IN THE MICROWAVE OVEN

- Use a shallow microwave-proof dish to hold the fish.
- Shield the head and tail of a whole fish with aluminum foil to guard against excess drying. (It is safe to use small amounts of foil in newer microwave ovens.) Make several diagonal slashes through the skin of the fish to prevent it from bursting.
- Arrange fillets in a dish with the thicker parts pointing outward and the thinner parts toward center of the dish. Rolled fillets cook more evenly by microwave than flat fillets.
- Cover the dish with plastic wrap and vent by turning back a corner.
- Allow 3 to 6 minutes per pound of boneless fish cooked on high (100% power) as a guide. Rotate the dish halfway through the cooking time.
- Fish may also be poached in a liquid in the microwave. Bring the liquid (fish stock or water and wine) to a boil, then add fish. Cover with plastic wrap and cook as described above.
- Cook side-dishes first and keep them covered while cooking the fish. They will retain heat longer than fish.

COOKING SHELLFISH IN THE MICROWAVE

- Arrange a single layer of shellfish in a shallow dish and cover with plastic wrap turned back at one corner for venting.
- Allow 2 to 3 minutes per pound of thawed, shucked shellfish cooked on high (100% power). Stir and rotate halfway through the cooking time. Allow to stand for one-third of the cooking time after removing from the oven. (For example, if you cook ½ pound of shucked shellfish for 1 minute and 30 seconds, allow it to stand for 30 seconds before serving.) Be careful not to overcook.
- Place clams, mussels or oysters in the shell in a single layer in a shallow dish. Cover with plastic wrap, venting at one corner. Cook for 2 to 3 minutes on high (100% power). Check and remove pieces as they open. Continue until all have opened. 1 pound will take 12 to 15 minutes.

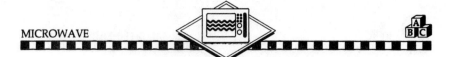

TOMATO-BASTED CATFISH STEAKS

- ☐ ¼ cup tomato sauce
- ☐ ¼ cup vinegar
- ☐ ½ tsp. dried dill weed
- ☐ ⅛ tsp. paprika
- ☐ ¼ tsp. pepper
- ☐ ½ tsp. Worcestershire sauce
- ☐ ½ tsp. polyunsaturated vegetable oil
- ☐ 1 lb. catfish fillets or steaks
- ☐ Vegetable cooking spray

MICROWAVE:
1. Combine tomato sauce with vinegar, spices, Worcestershire sauce and oil in small bowl; stir well.
2. Place catfish in microwave-proof pan. Spread tomato mixture over both sides of fish.
3. Cover and microwave on HIGH 3-6 minutes or until fish just begins to flake. Take out of microwave and let stand a few minutes until fish flakes easily when tested with fork.

CONVENTIONAL OVEN:
1. Prepare as in 1 above. Then, brush half of mixture over one side of fish. Coat rack of broiler pan with cooking spray. Place steaks on rack; broil 4-5 inches from heat source. Cook 5 minutes.
2. Turn fish over; brush with remaining tomato mixture. Broil an additional 5 minutes or until fish flakes easily when tested with fork. Serve with pasta and fruit plate. **Makes 4 servings.**

130 calories per serving
4.0 grams fat per serving
156 mg sodium per serving
62 mg cholesterol per serving

Substitutions:
orange roughy, sea bass, flounder

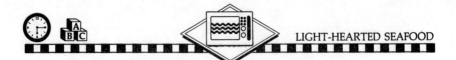

JAPANESE STYLE COD

*Seafood cooks to moist perfection
in the microwave — fast!*

☐ 1 lb. cod fillets
☐ 1 T. mayonnaise
☐ 1 T. light soy sauce

☐ ½ cup Panko
(Japanese-style
bread crumbs)
☐ ⅛ tsp. paprika
☐ ⅛ tsp. pepper

MICROWAVE:

1. Place fish in microwave-proof baking dish.
2. Combine mayonnaise, soy sauce, Panko, paprika and pepper in small bowl. Spread mixture over fish.
3. Cover and cook on HIGH for 3-5 minutes, turning dish halfway through cooking time. Remove fish from oven and let sit 3-5 minutes until fish flakes when tested with fork. Serve with steamed rice and vegetables.

CONVENTIONAL OVEN:

1. Follow directions for microwave method, except place fish in baking pan.
2. Bake in 400° oven until fish flakes when tested with fork. **Makes 4 servings.**

150 calories per serving
4.0 grams fat per serving
348 mg sodium per serving
46 mg cholesterol per serving

Substitutions:
flounder, Pacific rockfish (snapper), ocean perch

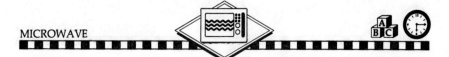

ZUCCHINI COD AU GRATIN

- ☐ 1 lb. cod fillets
- ☐ Pepper
- ☐ ¼ cup dry white wine
- ☐ 4 cups zucchini, shredded
- ☐ 3 T. Parmesan cheese
- ☐ 6 T. seasoned bread crumbs
- ☐ 2 T. parsley, chopped
- ☐ 2 T. green onion, finely chopped
- ☐ ½ tsp. dried basil

MICROWAVE:

1. Cut cod into serving-sized pieces; season with pepper. Sprinkle with wine; let stand 10 minutes. Discard wine after marinating.
2. Combine zucchini, Parmesan cheese, bread crumbs, parsley, green onion and basil in bowl; mix well.
3. Spread half zucchini mixture evenly over bottom of microwave-proof individual serving dishes.
4. Arrange cod on zucchini mixture. Spread remaining zucchini mixture over fish.
5. Microwave covered with waxed paper on HIGH for 3-5 minutes or until fish just flakes when tested with fork. Turn dish halfway through cooking. Remove from oven and let stand for several minutes to complete cooking. **Makes 4 servings.**

196 calories per serving
2.0 grams fat per serving
230 mg sodium per serving
50 mg cholesterol per serving

Substitutions:
bluefish, haddock, flounder

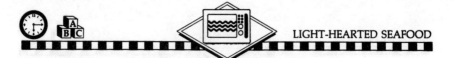

FOUR-MINUTE FLOUNDER

A microwave is a dieter's best friend;
it doesn't need added fat and it often intensifies flavors!

- ☐ 1 cup water
- ☐ ½ cup dry white wine
- ☐ 1 small onion, sliced
- ☐ 2 sprigs parsley
- ☐ 5 peppercorns
- ☐ 1 lb. flounder

MICROWAVE:

1. In 1-quart microwave-proof bowl combine water, wine, onion, parsley and peppercorns; mix well.
2. Microwave on HIGH 2-3 minutes or until mixture boils.
3. Place flounder in microwave-proof dish; pour wine mixture over flounder.
4. Microwave on HIGH for 3-5 minutes or until fish just begins to flake when tested with fork. Turn dish halfway through cooking time. Remove from oven and let stand to complete cooking. **Makes 4 servings.**

139 calories per serving
1.6 grams fat per serving
67 mg sodium per serving
56 mg cholesterol per serving

Substitutions:
salmon, cod, black cod

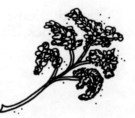

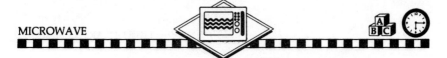

HERBED HADDOCK

☐ 1 lb. haddock

☐ 2 T. polyunsaturated
   margarine

☐ 2 T. dry white wine

☐ 1 T. green onion, chopped

☐ 1 T. parsley, chopped

☐ ⅛ tsp. thyme

☐ ⅛ tsp. marjoram

☐ Lemon slices

MICROWAVE:

1. Cut fish into serving-sized pieces.
2. Melt margarine in microwave-proof bowl; add remaining ingredients except lemon.
3. Place fish in microwave-proof dish; baste with margarine mixture. Arrange lemon slices on fish.
4. Microwave on HIGH, covered, for 3-5 minutes or until fish just flakes when tested with fork. Turn dish halfway through cooking time, basting fish with margarine mixture. Let stand several minutes to complete cooking. **Makes 4 servings.**

145 calories per serving
6.0 grams fat per serving
160 mg sodium per serving
68 mg cholesterol per serving

Substitutions:
catfish, pollock, grouper

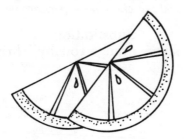

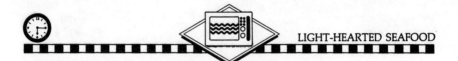

HOT & SPICY HADDOCK

☐ 1 tsp. onion powder
☐ 2 tsp. curry powder
☐ 1 tsp. cumin
☐ 1 tsp. fresh ginger, grated
   or ½ tsp. ground ginger

☐ ½ tsp. tumeric
☐ ½ clove garlic, minced
☐ 1 lb. haddock

MICROWAVE:
1. Mix spices together in paper bag. Put fish in bag and shake to coat.
2. Arrange fish in shallow microwave-proof baking dish, placing thickest portions toward outside of dish. Sprinkle with remaining coating. Cover with paper towel.
3. Microwave on HIGH 3-6 minutes, turning dish halfway through cooking time. Microwave just until fish begins to flake when tested with fork. Let stand covered for 2-3 additional minutes.

CONVENTIONAL OVEN:
1. Mix spices together as in number 1 above.
2. Place fish in baking pan. Sprinkle with remaining coating.
3. Bake, grill or broil fish until it flakes when tested with fork.
Makes 4 servings.

80 calories per serving
15.0 grams fat per serving
60 mg sodium per serving
50 mg cholesterol per serving

Substitutions:
croaker, orange roughy, shrimp

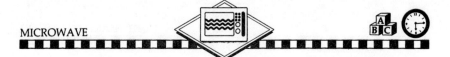

HALIBUT FOR TWO

- ☐ 1 lb. halibut steaks or fillets
- ☐ 1 T. olive oil
- ☐ Dash garlic powder
- ☐ Dash pepper

MICROWAVE:
1. Brush fillets or steaks with olive oil. Sprinkle with garlic powder and pepper.
2. Place fish in microwave-proof dish. Cover with paper towel.
3. Microwave on HIGH 3-6 minutes, turning dish halfway through cooking time. Microwave just until fish begins to flake when tested with fork. Let stand covered for 2-3 minutes to continue cooking until fish flakes easily when tested with fork.

CONVENTIONAL OVEN:
1. Same as number 1 above.
2. Grill or broil for 8-10 minutes or until fish flakes when tested with fork. Serve with boiled new potatoes and steamed carrots. **Makes 4 servings.**

150 calories per serving
4.9 grams fat per serving
68 mg sodium per serving
68 mg cholesterol per serving

Substitutions:
Northern pike, lingcod, haddock

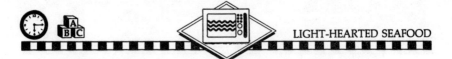

WAIKIKI MAHI MAHI

☐ 1 lb. mahi mahi
☐ Pepper
☐ 1 medium tomato, diced
☐ ¼ cup fresh
  mushrooms, sliced
☐ ¼ cup onion, sliced

☐ ¼ cup celery, diced
☐ 1 T. lemon juice
☐ 1 T. polyunsaturated oil
☐ ¼ tsp. thyme
☐ Dash pepper
☐ Chopped parsley

MICROWAVE:
1. Sprinkle mahi mahi with pepper and place in microwave-proof dish. Spoon tomato over fish.
2. In microwave-proof bowl combine mushrooms, onion, celery, lemon juice, oil, thyme, and dash of pepper; mix well. Microwave on HIGH, covered with plastic wrap for 2-3 minutes or until tender-crisp.
3. Spoon vegetable mixture over fish. Microwave on HIGH, covered, for 3-5 minutes or until fish just flakes when tested with fork. Let stand several minutes to complete cooking. Garnish with parlsey. **Makes 4 servings.**

162 calories per serving
4.7 grams fat per serving
160 mg sodium per serving
96 mg cholesterol per serving

Substitutions:
grouper, tilefish, trout

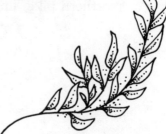

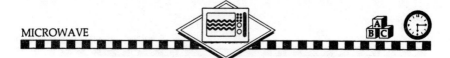

HERB-CRUMBED ORANGE ROUGHY

- ☐ 1 lb. orange roughy
- ☐ 1 T. olive oil
- ☐ ¼ cup seasoned bread crumbs
- ☐ 1 T. parsley, finely chopped
- ☐ Pepper to taste
- ☐ ⅛ tsp. dried thyme, crushed

MICROWAVE:
1. Place fish in microwave-proof dish. Brush with olive oil. Combine bread crumbs, parsley, pepper and thyme. Sprinkle the seasoned crumb mixture onto the fish. Cover with paper towel.
2. Microwave for 3-6 minutes per pound, turning dish halfway through cooking time. Microwave until fish just begins to flake when tested with fork.
3. Let stand covered for additional 2-3 minutes or until fish flakes when tested with fork.

CONVENTIONAL OVEN:
1. Place fish in baking pan. Brush with olive oil. Combine bread crumbs, parlsey, pepper and thyme. Sprinkle the seasoned crumb mixture onto the fish.
2. Bake in 450⁰ oven for about 10 minutes or until fish flakes when tested with fork. Serve immediately with wedges of lemon or lime. **Makes 4 servings.**

125 calories per serving
4.0 grams fat per serving
110 mg sodium per serving
22 mg cholesterol per serving

Substitutions:
Pacific rockfish (snapper), cod

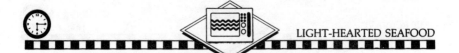

CAJUN BAKED ROCKFISH (SNAPPER)

☐ ⅓ cup light mayonnaise
☐ ½ tsp. ground cumin
☐ ½ tsp. onion powder
☐ ¼ tsp. ground red pepper

☐ ¼ tsp. garlic powder
☐ 1 lb. Pacific rockfish (snapper) fillets
☐ 8 sesame crackers, crushed

MICROWAVE:
1. Combine mayonnaise and seasonings in bowl. Brush red snapper with mayonnaise mixture; coat with sesame cracker crumbs.
2. Arrange fish in shallow microwave-proof baking dish, placing thickest portions toward outside of dish. Cover with paper towel. Microwave on HIGH 3-6 minutes; turning dish halfway through cooking time until fish just begins to flake when tested with fork. Let stand, covered, 2-3 minutes to complete cooking.

CONVENTIONAL OVEN:
1. Combine mayonnaise and seasoning in bowl.
2. Brush red snapper with mayonnaise mixture; coat with sesame cracker crumbs.
3. Place in baking dish. Bake in 400° oven for 15-20 minutes or until fish flakes when tested with fork. Serve with corn meal muffins and steamed vegetables. **Makes 4 servings.**

168 calories per serving
6.8 grams fat per serving
177 mg sodium per serving
45 mg cholesterol per serving

Substitutions:
catfish, tilefish

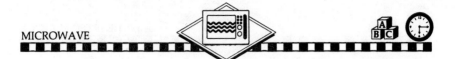

POPEYE'S SALMON

- ☐ 1 lb. salmon fillets, skinless and boneless
- ☐ Pepper to taste
- ☐ 1 medium onion, thinly sliced and halved
- ☐ 1 T. polyunsaturated margarine

- ☐ 4 cups packed spinach leaves (about 8 oz.) or 8 oz. frozen whole spinach, thawed and drained
- ☐ 1 tsp. lemon juice
- ☐ 1 tsp. olive oil
- ☐ ½ tsp. light soy sauce
- ☐ ¼ tsp. sugar

MICROWAVE:

1. Season salmon with pepper; place in microwave-proof dish. Microwave covered with plastic wrap at HIGH power 3-5 minutes or until fish just flakes when tested with fork. Turn dish halfway through cooking time. Keep warm.

2. Place onion and margarine on large microwave-proof serving platter. Microwave covered with plastic wrap at HIGH 3 minutes or until onion is tender: turn dish halfway through cooking.

3. Place spinach leaves over onion mixture. Microwave, covered, on HIGH 2 minutes or until spinach is wilted.

4. Combine lemon juice, olive oil, soy sauce and sugar; mix well. Drizzle over spinach. Place salmon on spinach mixture. **Makes 4 servings.**

221 calories per serving
11.0 grams fat per serving
192 mg sodium per serving
73 mg cholesterol per serving

Substitutions:
ocean perch, orange roughy, bluefish

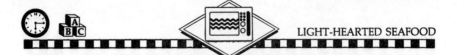

GINGER-SESAME SOLE FILLETS

- ☐ ½ T. sesame seeds
- ☐ 2 tsp. fresh ginger, minced
- ☐ 1 clove garlic, minced
- ☐ 1 T. sesame oil
- ☐ 1 tsp. light soy sauce
- ☐ 1 lb. sole fillets
- ☐ Pepper to taste
- ☐ 1 T. fresh ginger, thinly slivered

MICROWAVE:

1. Toast sesame seeds in small dry skillet over low heat.
2. Combine minced ginger and garlic, sesame oil and soy sauce in small bowl; set aside.
3. Season fillets lightly with pepper and arrange in single layer in microwave-proof baking dish.
4. Spread ginger mixture over fillets, then sprinkle with slivered ginger.
5. Cover dish with plastic wrap. Microwave on HIGH for 3-5 minutes, turning dish halfway through cooking time. Remove from oven and let stand until fish flakes when tested with fork.
6. Sprinkle with sesame seeds and serve. **Makes 4 servings.**

140 calories per serving
4.7 grams fat per serving
260 mg sodium per serving
50 mg cholesterol per serving

Substitutions:
grouper, flounder, tilefish, trout

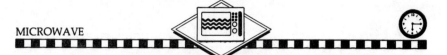

HOLIDAY SEAFOOD WITH CHAMPAGNE

Microwave in minutes

☐ 2 lbs. firm fish fillets, boneless and skinless

☐ 1 cup champagne

☐ 1 cup mushrooms, sliced

☐ 1 cup onions, sliced thin in rings

☐ 1 T. polyunsaturated margarine

☐ 1 cup plain low fat yogurt

☐ 1 T. cornstarch

☐ 1 cup part-skim Mozzarella cheese, grated

☐ 1 tsp. dried tarragon

☐ ½ tsp. white pepper

☐ Paprika

MICROWAVE:

1. Place fish fillets in microwave-proof pan. Cover with champagne and marinate for 10 minutes.

2. Microwave mushrooms and onions in margarine for 4 minutes in separate microwave-proof container.

3. Drain champagne from fish. Discard.

4. Mix yogurt, cornstarch, Mozzarella cheese, tarragon and white pepper together. Spread over fish. Spread vegetables over fish and top with paprika.

5. Cover and microwave on HIGH for 5-10 minutes or until fish just begins to flake when tested with fork. Turn dish halfway through cooking time. Let stand for several minutes to complete cooking. **Makes 8 servings.**

223 calories per serving
7.3 grams fat per serving
225 mg sodium per serving
87 mg cholesterol per serving

Substitutions:
halibut, Pacific rockfish (snapper), cod

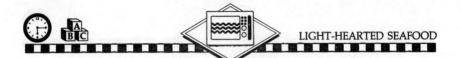

OYSTERS PARMESAN

 Oysters are an excellent source of iron and are low in cholesterol and calories.

- ☐ ¼ cup green onion, chopped
- ☐ ¼ cup fresh parsley, chopped
- ☐ 3 cloves garlic, minced
- ☐ 2 tsp. polyunsaturated margarine
- ☐ 1 T. lime juice
- ☐ 4 drops hot pepper sauce (Tabasco)
- ☐ 1 jar (10 oz.) small oysters
- ☐ ¼ tsp. cracked black pepper
- ☐ ¼ cup Parmesan cheese
- ☐ ¼ cup bread crumbs

MICROWAVE:

1. Place green onion, parsley, garlic, margarine, lime juice and Tabasco in microwave-proof dish. Stir; microwave on HIGH for 1 minute.

2. Add oysters to dish and stir to coat with mixture. Sprinkle pepper, Parmesan cheese and bread crumbs over top of oysters.

3. Microwave on HIGH for 3-5 minutes or until oysters are done. Can be served in individual seafood shells as an appetizer or as an entree. **Makes 2-4 servings.**

130 calories per serving
4.5 grams fat per serving
23 mg sodium per serving
39 mg cholesterol per serving

Substitutions:
mussels

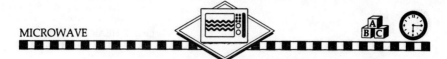

CANCUN SHRIMP

☐ 2 T. olive oil
☐ 2 cloves garlic, minced
☐ 2 lbs. shrimp or prawns,
   peeled and deveined

☐ Cumin
☐ Lemon juice
☐ Pepper to taste

MICROWAVE:
1. Microwave olive oil with garlic on HIGH for 30 seconds in microwave-proof dish.
2. Stir in shrimp with cumin, lemon juice and pepper. Arrange shrimp/prawns in single layer.
3. Cover casserole tightly and cook on HIGH for 2-3 minutes, stirring every minute until shrimp just begin to turn opaque. Remove from oven and let stand additional 2-3 minutes to complete cooking. Serve hot or cold with bowl of cocktail sauce on side. Can also be prepared and served with shells. **Makes 8 servings or several appetizers.**

132 calories per serving
4.4 grams fat per serving
158 mg sodium per serving
178 mg cholesterol per serving

Substitutions:
oysters, crayfish, lobster

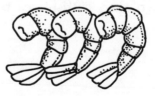

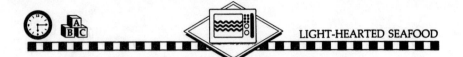

GARLIC SHRIMP

☐ 6 cloves garlic,
  coarsely chopped

☐ 2 T. olive oil

☐ 1 tsp. red chile pepper,
  seeded and minced or
  ½ tsp. dried red pepper flakes

☐ 2 lbs. large shrimp or
  prawns, peeled
  and deveined

☐ 1 T. lime juice

MICROWAVE:
1. Microwave garlic in oil on HIGH for 1 minute.
2. Add chile pepper and shrimp and cover; microwave on HIGH for 1 minute.
3. Add lime juice and cook an additional 2 minutes or until shrimp begin to turn opaque. Let stand 2-3 additional minutes to complete cooking.

CONVENTIONAL OVEN:
1. Saute garlic in oil in large, heavy skillet over medium-high heat for 1 minute.
2. Add chile pepper and shrimp and cook 4 minutes, stirring constantly.
3. Add lime juice and cook an additional 2 minutes or until shrimp turn opaque. Serve as an appetizer or entree. **Makes 8 servings.**

133 calories per serving
4.4 grams fat per serving
158 mg sodium per serving
178 mg cholesterol per serving

Substitutions:
croaker, catfish, sea bass

SAUCES

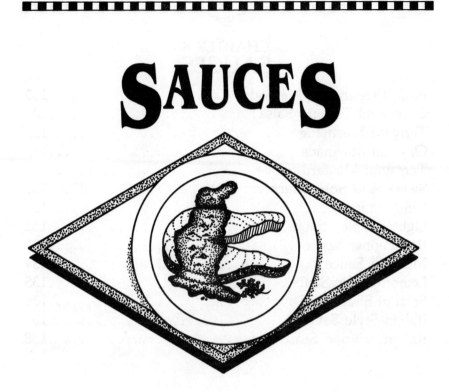

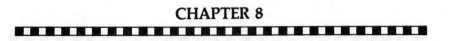

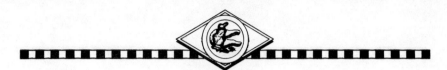

CHAPTER 8
SAUCES

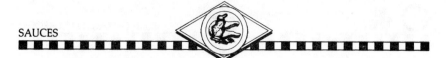

BASIC PREPARATION METHODS

The following preparation methods serve as basic guidelines to preparing seafood in a heart-healthy manner.

1. Select a sauce from this chapter.
2. Select desired seafood.
3. Prepare and serve seafood and sauce as per recipe directions.

- **BAKE**
  Place seafood in baking dish. Add sauce or topping to keep moist. Cover and bake at 400-450°F. until done.

- **BROIL**
  Place seafood in broiler pan. Brush with marinade, sauce, a small amount of polyunsaturate margarine or other topping. Flavor as desired. Broil 4-5 inches from heat source without turning. Cook until done.

- **POACH**
  Estimate amount of liquid needed to cover seafood in poaching pan or saucepan. Liquids could include skim milk, water, low-salt chicken broth or wine. Season as desired. Bring to boil; cover & simmer about 10 minutes. Add seafood and bring to boil. Reduce heat and simmer until done.

- **STEAMING**
  Place seafood on a steaming rack, set 2 inches above boiling liquid, in deep pot. Season as desired. Cover tightly. Reduce heat and steam until done.

- **GRILLING OR BARBECUING**
  Place seafood on lightly-oiled grill. Baste with sauce or marinade as desired. Turn halfway through cooking time. Continue to baste throughout cooking time. Cook until done.

- **SAUTEING**
  Heat a small amount of polyun-saturated margarine or oil with liquid, such as white wine, in frying pan or saute pan. Add vegetables as desired. Add seafood and saute over medium heat until done.

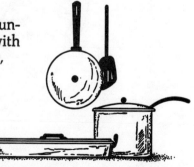

- **MICROWAVE**
  See pages 105, 106.

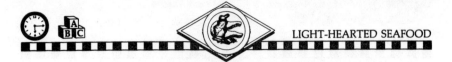

CORN AND TOMATO SALSA

One of our favorites

♥ *Excellent as a sauce on a seafood tostada.*

☐ ½ cup onion, finely chopped

☐ 1 large, ripe tomato, chopped

☐ 1 box frozen corn

☐ Juice from 1 lime

☐ 1 tsp. ground cumin

☐ 1 tsp. garlic powder

☐ 1 can (4 oz.) green chiles, chopped

1. Mix all ingredients together in medium-size bowl. Let stand until frozen corn is thawed. Serve chilled on barbecued seafood or cold poached fish. **Makes 4 servings. Sauce for 1 lb. of seafood.**

47 calories per serving
0.7 gram fat per serving
30 mg sodium per serving
0 mg cholesterol per serving

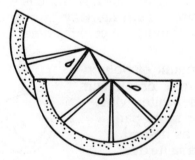

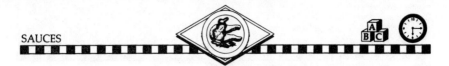

TERIYAKI MARINADE

□ 1½ T. pineapple juice
□ 1½ T. light soy sauce
□ 1 T. polyunsaturated oil
□ 1 T. sherry

□ 1 T. fresh ginger, grated
□ ¼ tsp. dry mustard
□ 1 clove garlic, minced
□ ½ tsp. brown sugar

1. Combine ingredients in bowl.
2. Pour marinade over fish and marinate about 15 minutes, turning over once.
3. Drain fish, reserving marinade.
4. Prepare fish for cooking. Baste with marinade as fish cooks. Suggested methods of cooking include grilling, broiling, steaming, or microwaving. Marinade may be reserved in the refrigerator for up to 2 weeks. **Makes 4 servings. Marinade for 1 lb. of seafood.**

40 calories per serving
3.6 grams fat per serving
246 mg sodium per serving
0 mg cholesterol per serving

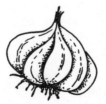

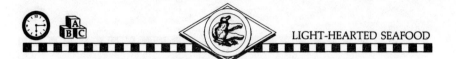

ORIENTAL MARINADE

☐ 2 T. orange juice
☐ 2 T. light soy sauce
☐ 1 T. catsup
☐ 1 T. polyunsaturated oil

☐ 1 T. parsley, chopped
☐ 1 T. lemon juice
☐ ½ clove garlic, minced
☐ Dash pepper

1. Combine all marinade ingredients in bowl. Pour marinade over fish and let stand for 15 minutes, turning once.
2. Drain fish, reserving marinade. Grill, broil or steam fish as desired, basting with sauce during cooking. **Makes 8 servings. Marinade for 2 lbs. of seafood.**

22 calories per serving
1.8 grams fat per serving
215 mg sodium per serving
0 mg cholesterol per serving

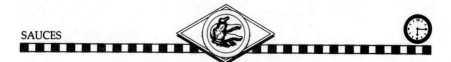

TARRAGON MUSTARD SAUCE

- [ ] 2 T. tarragon vinegar
- [ ] 2 T. Dijon mustard
- [ ] 1 tsp. dried tarragon

- [ ] ¼ cup plus 2 T. plain low fat yogurt
- [ ] ¼ cup light mayonnaise

1. Combine tarragon vinegar, mustard and dried tarragon in small bowl.
2. Add yogurt and mayonnaise; stir until well blended. Spread over fish. Bake or microwave seafood.
3. Alternative method: serve over cooked seafood such as leftover grilled or cold poached seafood. **Makes 6 servings. Sauce for 1½ lbs. seafood.**

45 calories per serving
4.0 grams fat per serving
142 mg sodium per serving
0 mg cholesterol per serving

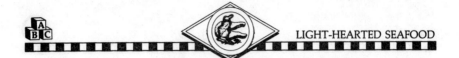

SWEET AND SOUR SAUCE
Family favorite

- ☐ 1 small onion, chopped
- ☐ ¼ cup catsup
- ☐ 1 jar (2 oz.) pimiento, sliced
- ☐ 1 T. polyunsaturated oil
- ☐ ¼ cup white wine vinegar
- ☐ 1 T. Worcestershire sauce
- ☐ ½ tsp. pepper
- ☐ 1 tsp. paprika

- ☐ 2 tsp. chili powder
- ☐ 1 tsp. fresh garlic, minced
- ☐ 1 tsp. fresh ginger, minced
- ☐ 2 T. sugar
- ☐ 1 cup water
- ☐ 1 cup mushrooms, sliced

1. Combine all ingredients in saucepan.
2. Bring to boil; lower heat and simmer at least fifteen minutes; set aside.
3. Pour sauce over seafood and bake or broil as desired; or pour heated sauce over grilled seafood. Sauce may be refrigerated for 2 weeks. **Makes 6 servings. Sauce for 1½ lbs. of seafood.**

46 calories per serving
0 grams fat per serving
130 mg sodium per serving
0 mg cholesterol per serving

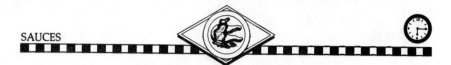

WINE SAUCE

Excellent as a saute sauce

- ☐ 1 T. olive oil
- ☐ 3 T. dry white wine
- ☐ 2 T. parsley, minced
- ☐ 2 cloves garlic, minced
- ☐ Pepper

1. Combine all ingredients in bowl. Brush on fish and broil or grill seafood as desired. **Makes 4 servings. Sauce for 1 lb. of seafood.**

44 calories per serving
3.5 grams fat per serving
0 mg sodium per serving
0 mg cholesterol per serving

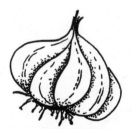

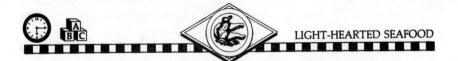

LIGHT & SPICY SAUCE

- ☐ 1 T. polyunsaturated oil
- ☐ 1 T. parsley, finely chopped
- ☐ 1 T. light soy sauce
- ☐ 1 tsp. Worcestershire sauce
- ☐ ½ tsp. garlic, minced
- ☐ ¼ tsp. pepper
- ☐ 3 T. lemon juice

1. In small mixing bowl combine all ingredients. Marinate fish briefly before cooking; brush on marinade during baking, microwaving, or broiling. **Makes 4 servings. Sauce for 1 lb. of seafood.**

41 calories per serving
3.5 grams fat per serving
210 mg sodium per serving
0 mg cholesterol per serving

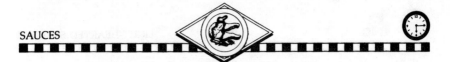

RED PEPPER SAUCE

- ☐ 1 T. olive oil
- ☐ 1 T. shallots, chopped
- ☐ 3 cloves garlic, chopped
- ☐ 1 T. parsley, chopped

- ☐ 1 medium red pepper, sliced into narrow strips
- ☐ ⅛ tsp. cayenne pepper
- ☐ ¼ tsp. pepper

1. In small saute pan, heat olive oil; add shallots and garlic. Saute until tender.
2. Add parsley, red peppers, cayenne and pepper; saute until pepper is tender-crisp. Remove from heat. Set aside. Makes excellent topping for grilled fish. **Makes 4 servings. Sauce for 1 lb. of seafood.**

37 calories per serving
3.5 grams fat per serving
6.5 mg sodium per serving
0 mg cholesterol per serving

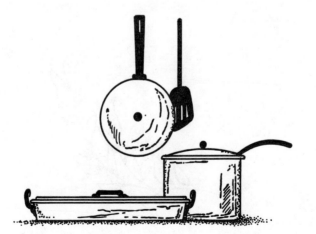

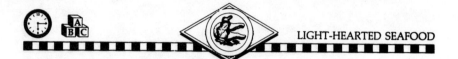

MEXICALI SAUCE

- ☐ 1¼ cups prepared chunky salsa
- ☐ 1 T. lime juice
- ☐ ½ tsp. dried oregano
- ☐ ½ clove garlic, minced
- ☐ ¼ tsp. cumin
- ☐ Fresh lime wedges

1. Combine salsa, lime juice, oregano, garlic and cumin in small bowl; set aside.
2. Spread sauce over prepared fish (baking, steaming or poaching are good methods) and serve with lime wedges. **Makes 4 servings. Sauce for 1 lb. of seafood.**

20 calories per serving
0 grams fat per serving
100 mg sodium per serving
0 mg cholesterol per serving

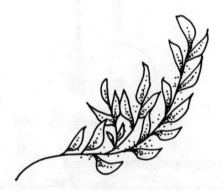

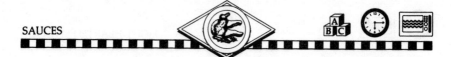

LEMON-GARLIC SAUCE

Excellent as a saute sauce.

♥ Save time by peeling garlic in advance and storing it, covered with olive oil, in a jar. It will stay fresh for at least two weeks in the refrigerator and perk up the oil, too.

☐ 1 T. polyunsaturated margarine, melted

☐ 1 clove garlic, finely chopped

☐ 2 T. lemon juice

☐ Pinch pepper

☐ Fresh parsley, chopped

1. In small saucepan, melt margarine. Add garlic and saute until tender. Remove from heat. Add lemon juice, pepper and parsley. Spread over fish and cook as desired.

MICROWAVE:

1. Microwave margarine and garlic on HIGH until tender (about 1 minute) in microwave-proof pan. Add lemon juice, pepper and parsley. Spread over fish and cook as desired. **Makes 4 servings. Sauce for 1 lb. of seafood.**

25 calories per serving
3.0 grams fat per serving
35 mg sodium per serving
0 mg cholesterol per serving

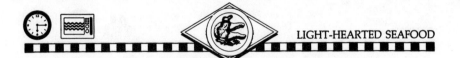

SCAMPI SAUCE

☐ 1 tsp. olive oil
☐ 4 cloves garlic, minced
☐ 2 T. dry vermouth
☐ 1 tsp. dried red pepper flakes

☐ 1 tsp. paprika
☐ 1 T. lemon juice
☐ ½ cup fresh parsley, chopped

1. Heat oil in saute pan; add garlic and cook over medium heat until tender.
2. Stir in vermouth, pepper flakes, paprika and lemon juice. Brush on fish and cook in desired manner.

MICROWAVE:
1. Combine oil and garlic in 10-inch pie plate. Cook on HIGH for 1-2 minutes or until tender.
2. Stir in vermouth, pepper flakes, paprika and lemon juice. Brush on fish and bake or grill. **Makes 4 servings. Sauce for 1 lb. of seafood.**

15 calories per serving
1.2 grams fat per serving
0 mg sodium per serving
0 mg cholesterol per serving

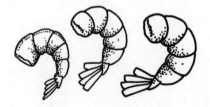

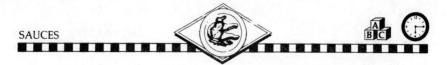

ITALIAN-STYLE SAUCE

☐ 1 T. olive oil

☐ Juice from 1 lemon
(about 2 T.)

☐ ¼ tsp. garlic powder

☐ ¼ tsp. onion powder

☐ 1 T. Italian Seafood
Seasoning
(see page 138)

1. In large bowl, mix olive oil, lemon juice, garlic, onion powder and Italian Seafood Seasoning.
2. Add seafood into seasoning bowl and coat thoroughly.
3. Saute, bake or grill seafood as desired. **Makes 4 servings. Sauce for 1 lb. of seafood.**

38 calories per serving
3.5 grams fat per serving
0 mg sodium per serving
0 mg cholesterol per serving

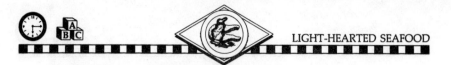

ITALIAN
SEAFOOD SEASONING

Great all around spice mixture for seafood preparation.

☐ **2 tsp. dried rosemary** ☐ **2 T. dried thyme**
☐ **2 T. dried oregano** ☐ **3 T. dried basil**
☐ **3 T. dried marjoram**

1. Mix all ingredients together. Grind in blender or food processor until finely ground.
2. Place in jar and cover tightly.
3. Shake before using. Shake on microwave, baked or grilled seafood.

0 calories per serving
0 grams fat per serving
0 mg sodium per serving
0 mg cholesterol per serving

GENERAL

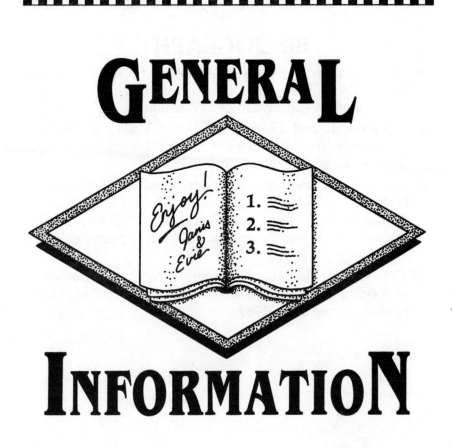

INFORMATION

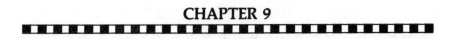

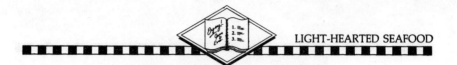

BIBLIOGRAPHY

Adams, C.: *Nutritive Value of American Foods in Common Units*, Agriculture Handbook No. 456, USDA, U.S. Government Printing Office, Washington, D.C., 1975.

Pennington, J. and Church, H.: *Food Values of Portions Commonly Used*, Bowes and Church (13th edition). Harper & Row, Publisher, New York, 1980.

Sidwell, V.: *Chemical and Nutritional Composition of Finfishes, Whales, Crustaceans, Mollusks, and Their Products*, U.S. Dept. of Commerce, NOAA, NMFS, National Technical Information Service, Springfield, VA, 1985.

USDA, Human Nutrition Information Service: *Composition of Foods: Finfish and Shellfish Products*, Agriculture Handbook Number 8-15, 1987.

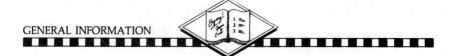

ABOUT THE AUTHORS

Practically born into the world of seafood, both Janis Harsila and Evie Hansen were reared in families who relied on the commercial fishing industry for their earnings. Later, both married commercial fishermen. They met on a fishing dock in the San Juan Islands in the state of Washington. A fast friendship grew into a solid partnership when they both realized they shared a deep love of seafood. Moreover, each had a commitment to bring their world to those who want to eat fish but know little of how to handle, prepare or serve it. National Seafood Educators was formed in 1977 to provide education, training and recipe development to retailers, health professionals and consumers and to make the culinary pleasures of healthful seafood accessible to all.

In 1983, National Seafood Educators introduced one of the first seafood and health awareness programs in the nation. Their efforts were recognized by the American Heart Association — Washington Affiliate who as co-sponsors, produced a seafood consumer awareness campaign called, "Seafood Is Heart Food", which was used throughout the nation. In 1986, National Seafood Educators published a highly-regarded, seafood cookbook called *Seafood: A Collection of Heart-Healthy Recipes*. The book, now in its fifth printing, is recommended by the American Dietetic Association, the Tufts University Diet and Nutrition Letter and the Center for Science in the Public Interest. Additionally, it has been endorsed by the *Los Angeles Times, Washington Post, Seattle Times, Dallas Morning News*, the *Oregonian*, the *Boston Globe, Parade, Cosmopolitan, Cooking Light* and a host of other consumer publications.

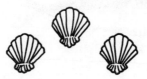

Janis Harsila, Director of Nutrition Education, is a registered dietitian. She keeps up-to-date on the latest research linking seafood diets with health benefits. She also educates health care professionals and consumers in the links between seafood and health. Harsila knows how to prepare flavorful meals which can keep people both happy and healthy. She is a member of the American Dietetic Association and Omicron Nu Honor Society.

Evie Hansen, Director of Seafood Marketing, has a lifetime of experience in consulting. Formerly a special education teacher, Hansen utilizes her training with retailers, offering them needed skills in seafood marketing and merchandising. Hansen completed a seafood merchandising program at Oregon State University and was the recipient of a Seafood Quality Control Certificate from the University of Washington. In addition, she is the co-author of a merchandising manual, *Selling Seafood,* published by the Alaska Seafood Marketing Institute, which has been sold in over twelve countries. She has been selected to appear in *Who's Who in Business and Finance* and *Who's Who in the West in 1989.*

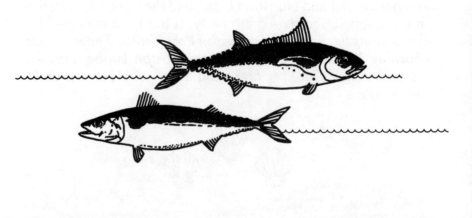

ORDERING INFORMATION

*For more copies of **Light-Hearted Seafood:***

		Quantity Purchases	
Price per book	$10.95	3 books	$29.95
Tax for WA state residents	$ .89	Tax for WA state residents	$ 2.43
Postage and Handling	$2.00	Postage and Handling	$ 4.00

*For copies of our first cookbook, **Seafood: A Collection of Heart-Healthy Recipes:***

		Quantity Purchases	
Price per book	$11.95	3 books	$32.95
Tax for WA state residents	$ .97	Tax for WA state residents	$ 2.67
Postage and Handling	$ 2.00	Postage and Handling	$ 4.00

Send personal check, VISA or MASTERCARD number (with expiration date) to:

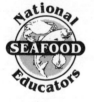

National Seafood Educators
P.O. Box 60006
Richmond Beach, WA 98160
(206) 546-6410

DIABETIC EXCHANGES

RECIPE	Pg. No.	Bread	MEAT lean	MEAT med.	MEAT high	Veg.	Fruit	MILK skim	MILK low	MILK whole	Fat	COMMENTS
Salmon Cheesecake	29	1							½		½	
Lomi Lomi Salmon	30	1				1						
Creamy Clam Dip	31	½										
Flintstone Seafood Dip	32	¼				¼						
Light & Versatile Dill Dressing	33										½	
Aleck Bay Steamer Clams	34	2	2				1					Fruit for alcohol calories
Mussels on the Half Shell	35	½	1½									
Herb Stuffed Oysters	36		1			½						
Bay Scallops & Shrimp in Pasta Shells	37	2	2			1						
Shrimp & Cucumber Salad	38		1			1						
Marinated Halibut Salad	41		3½			1	1					Allow 1 fat ex. extra
Tarragon Salmon Salad	42		1½			1						
Sweet & Sour Tuna Salad	43		2			1½	1½					
Greek Style Salad	44		2½			2						
Seashell Salad	45	2	1½			2						
Chinese Seafood Salad	46	1	1			3					½	
Pasta & Crab Salad	47	1	½			1						
Sensational Seafood Salad	48		1			2						
Cilantro Potato Salad	49	2	½			1						
Marinated Spanish Seafood Salad	50		2½			2						Allow 1 fat ex. extra

RECIPE	Pg. No.	Bread	MEAT lean	MEAT med.	MEAT high	Veg.	Fruit	MILK skim	MILK low	MILK whole	Fat	COMMENTS
Curry Shrimp & Rice Salad	51	1	1			1						
Shrimp Coleslaw	52		1			1						Allow ½ fat ex. extra
Lunchbox Tuna or Salmon Sandwich	57	2	2			3						Allow ½ fat ex. extra salmon sandwich
Tuna Melt Supreme	58	1	2			½						Allow ½ fat ex. extra
Open-faced Crab Muffin	59	1	½					½				
Shrimp Topped Rice Cakes	60	½		½								
Highliner's Choice Salmon Chowder	61	1	2	1		½						
Manhattan Shellfish Chowder	62		2			2	1					Fruit for alcohol calories
Norwegian Crab Bisque	63	1	2			4		1				Allow 1 fat ex. extra
Bourbon Street Gumbo	64	½	3			1						
Corn & Tomato Salsa	126	½				1						
Teriyaki Marinade	127					½					¾	
Oriental Marinade	128					½					⅓	
Tarragon Mustard Sauce	129					½					¾	
Sweet & Sour Sauce	130					1	½					
Wine Sauce	131					¼					¾	
Light & Spicy Sauce	132					½					¾	
Red Pepper Sauce	133					½					¾	
Mexicali Sauce	134					1						
Lemon-Garlic Sauce	135						⅓				¾	
Scampi Sauce	136					1						
Italian-Style Sauce	137					½					¾	

RECIPE	Pg. No.	Bread	MEAT lean	MEAT med.	MEAT high	Veg.	Fruit	MILK skim	MILK low	MILK whole	Fat	COMMENTS
Italian Seafood Seasoning	138											Free Food
Bluefish Dijon	69	3				¼						Allow ½ fat ex. extra
Ocean Cod Supreme	70	2½						½	⅓			Allow 1 fat ex. extra. Fruit for alcohol.
Country Garden Saute	71	3				3						Allow 1 fat ex. extra
Cucumber Haddock	72	3				2						Allow 1½ fat ex. extra
Casserole Delight	73	4				1	1					Fruit for alcohol calories
Best Dressed Mackerel	74	2									1	
Best Dressed Trout	74			2							1	
Monkfish Saute	75	2				1½						
Orange Roughy with Tomato-Tarragon Sauce	76	2				2						Allow ½ fat ex. extra
Cheesey Rockfish	77	½	3									Allow ½ fat ex. extra
Poached Sablefish	78	3				½						Allow ½ fat ex. extra
Bristol Bay Salmon	79	3										
Thai-style Salmon Potato	80	1	3	1		3						
Curried Salmon	81	3				1	1					½ fruit ex. for fruit, ½ fruit ex. for alcohol.
Savory Salmon Loaf	82	½	2½									
Slender Steamed Sole	83	2½										Allow 1 fat ex. extra
Heartfelt Sole	84	2½					½					Allow ½ fat ex. extra. Fruit for alcohol.
Columbia River Sturgeon	85	2									½	
Swordfish & Herbs	86	3				1	1					Fruit for wine calories
Szechwan Stirfry	87	2				2						
Savory Tuna for Four	88	2½				4		½				Allow ½ fat ex. extra

RECIPE	Pg. No.	Bread	MEAT			Veg.	Fruit	MILK			Fat	COMMENTS
			lean	med.	high			skim	low	whole		
Mother's Oyster Pie	92	2	1								½	
Romantic Scallops For Two	93		1½			1						
Prawn and Scallop Saute	94		3			1						
Spicy Poached Shrimp	95		3									Allow 2 fat ex. extra
Italian Fisherman's Spaghetti	96		1			1½						
Shrimp & Tomato Tostada	97	1	1			3						
Phillipine Pansit	98	1	1			2						
Spinach Fettucine With Shrimp	99	1	1½			3	½				½	
Saucy Squid	100	½	2			2						
Stuffed Squid Supreme	101		1	1		2	1					
Tomato-Basted Catfish Steaks	107		3			½						Allow 1 fat ex. extra
Japanese-Style Cod	108	½	2½									Allow ½ fat ex. extra
Zucchini Cod Au Gratin	109	1	2½			3						Allow 1 fat ex. extra
Four-Minute Flounder	110		3			½	½					Allow 1½ fat ex. extra. Fruit for alcohol.
Herbed Haddock	111		3			½						Allow ½ fat ex. extra
Hot & Spicy Haddock	112		3									Allow 1½ fat ex. extra
Halibut For Two	113		3½									Allow 1 fat ex. extra
Waikiki Mahi Mahi	114		3			1						Allow 1 fat ex. extra
Herb-Crumbed Orange Roughy	115		2½									Allow ½ fat ex. extra
Cajun Baked Rockfish	116	⅓	3									Allow ½ fat ex. extra
Popeye's Salmon	117		3½			1						
Ginger-Sesame Sole Fillets	118		2½									Allow ½ fat ex. extra

RECIPE	Pg. No.	Bread	MEAT			Veg.	Fruit	MILK			Fat	COMMENTS
			lean	med.	high			skim	low	whole		
Holiday Seafood With Champagne	119		4			1						Allow 1 fat ex. extra
Oysters Parmesan	120	½	1½			1						
Cancun Shrimp	121		3									Allow 1 fat ex. extra
Garlic Shrimp	122		3									Allow 1 fat ex. extra

ex. - exchange

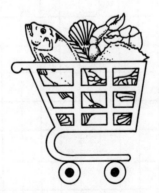

INDEX BY TITLE

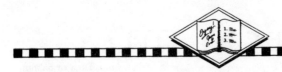

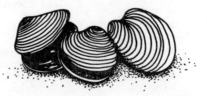

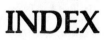

INDEX

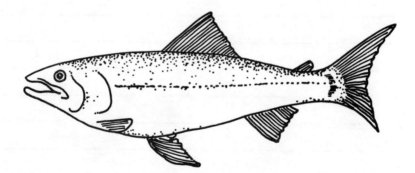

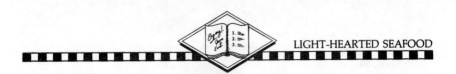

We would love to hear from you...send us your favorite recipes and ideas!

_____

_____

_____

_____

_____

_____

_____

_____

_____

_____

_____

_____

_____

_____

_____

_____

_____

_____

_____

_____

_____

_____

NOTES:

NOTES:

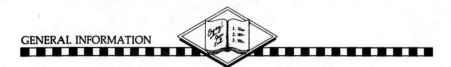

Crestwood Public
Library District
4955 W. 135th Street
Crestwood, IL 60445

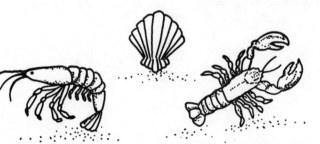